Optical Coherence Tomography in Neurological Diseases

Optical Coherence Tomography in Neurological Diseases

Edited by

Peter A. Calabresi, MD, FAAN, FANA

Professor of Neurology, Director of the Richard T. Johnson Division of Neuroimmunology and Neuroinfectious Diseases, and Director of the Johns Hopkins Multiple Sclerosis Center, Johns Hopkins University School of Medicine, Baltimore, MD, USA

Laura J. Balcer, MD, MSCE, FANA

Professor of Neurology, Population Health and Opthalmology; Vice Chair, Department of Neurology, NYU School of Medicine, NY, USA

Elliot M. Frohman, MD, PhD, FAAN

Professor of Neurology and Ophthalmology
Distinguished Teaching Professor
Kenney-Marie Dixon Pickens Distinguished Professor of MS Research
Irene Wadel & Robert Atha Distinguished Chair in Neurology
Director, Multiple Sclerosis and Neuroimmunology Program and Clinical Center for Multiple Sclerosis
University of Texas Southwestern School of Medicine

CAMBRIDGE
UNIVERSITY PRESS

CAMBRIDGE
UNIVERSITY PRESS

University Printing House, Cambridge CB2 8BS, United Kingdom

Cambridge University Press is part of the University of Cambridge.

It furthers the University's mission by disseminating knowledge in the pursuit of education, learning and research at the highest international levels of excellence.

www.cambridge.org
Information on this title: www.cambridge.org/9781107041301

Printed in the United Kingdom by Bell and Bain Ltd

A catalogue record for this publication is available from the British Library

Library of Congress Cataloging in Publication Data
Optical coherence tomography in neurological diseases / edited by Peter A. Calabresi, Laura J. Balcer, Elliot M. Frohman.
p. ; cm.
ISBN 978-1-107-04130-1 (hardback)
I. Calabresi, Peter A., editor. II. Balcer, Laura J., editor. III. Frohman, Elliot M., editor.
[DNLM: 1. Nervous System Diseases – diagnosis. 2. Tomography, Optical Coherence. WN 206]
RC349.T65
616.8′04757–dc23

2014048628

ISBN 978-1-107-04130-1 Hardback

Contents

Contributors

Laura J. Balcer
Professor of Neurology, Population Health and Ophthalmology; Vice Chair, Department of Neurology, NYU School of Medicine, NY, USA

Shin C. Beh
Assistant Professor of Neurology & Neurotherapeutics Director Vestibular Neurology & Neurovisual Disorders Multiple Sclerosis & Neuroimmunology Program UT Southwestern School of Medicine at Dallas, TX, USA

Robert A. Bermel
Mellen Center for MS Treatment and Research, Neurological Institute, Cleveland Clinic, Cleveland, OH, USA

Alexander Ulrich Brandt
NeuroCure Clinical Research Center, Charité – Universitätsmedizin Berlin, Germany

Peter A. Calabresi
Professor of Neurology, Director of the Richard T. Johnson Division of Neuroimmunology and Neuroinfectious Diseases, and Director of the Johns Hopkins Multiple Sclerosis Center, Johns Hopkins University School of Medicine, Baltimore, MD, USA

Amy Conger
Senior Neuro-Ophthalmic Imaging Specialist Clinical Center for Multiple Sclerosis UT Southwestern Medical Center Dallas, Tx, USA

Darrel Conger
Co-Director, Neuro-Ophthalmology Testing Lab Department of Neurology & Neurotherapeutics UT Southwestern School of Medicine at Dallas, TX, USA

Fiona Costello
Associate Professor of Neurology Department of Clinical Neurosciences, University of Calgary, Calgary, Alberta, Canada

C. L. Fraser
Sydney Eye Hospital, Save Sight Institute, Sydney, Australia

Elliot M. Frohman
Professor of Neurology and Ophthalmology Distinguished Teaching Professor Kenney-Marie Dixon Pickens Distinguished Professor of MS Research Irene Wadel & Robert Atha Distinguished Chair in Neurology Director, Multiple Sclerosis and Neuroimmunology Program and Clinical Center for Multiple Sclerosis University of Texas Southwestern School of Medicine at Dallas, TX, USA

Teresa C. Frohman
Director Multiple Sclerosis Neuro-Ophthalmology Research Laboratory Executive Director Multiple Sclerosis and Neuroimmunology Program Executive Director UT Southwestern & National Multiple Sclerosis Society Comprehensive Treatment Training Program Multiple Sclerosis Advanced Clinical Practitioner Department of Neurology & Neurotherapeutics UT Southwestern School of Medicine at Dallas, TX, USA

Steven L. Galetta, MD
Professor and Chair, Department of Neurology, New York University Langone Medical Center, New York, NY, USA

S. L. Graham
Macquarie University, Sydney, Australia

Ari J. Green
Associate Professor of Neurology and Ophthalmology Clinic Medical Director Neurodiagnostics Center Director UCSF MS Center, Department of Neurology, University of Californa, San Francisco, CA, USA

Benjamin M Greenberg
Associate Professor of Neurology Director, Transverse Myelitis, Neuromyelitis Optical and Pediatric Demyelinating Disease Programs Director, Neurosciences Clinical Research Center at Dallas, TX, USA UT Southwestern School of Medicine

Andrew P. D. Henderson
NMR Research Unit, UCL Institute of Neurology, London, UK

Hiroshi Ishikawa
Ocular Imaging Center, University of Pittsburgh School of Medicine, Pittsburgh, PA, USA

Peter K. Kaiser
Cole Eye Institute, Cleveland Clinic, Cleveland, OH, USA

A. Klistorner
The University of Sydney, and Macquarie University, Sydney, Australia

Devin D. Mackay
Clinical Fellow in Neurology, Department of Neurology, Brigham and Women's Hospital, Harvard Medical School, Boston, MA, USA

Elena H. Martinez-Lapiscina
Center of Neuroimmunology, Institut d'Investigacions Biomèdiques August Pi i Sunyer (IDIBAPS), Hospital Clinic of Barcelona, Barcelona, Spain

David H. Miller
Professor of Clinical Neurology, University Department of Clinical Neurology, National Hospital for Neurology and Neurosurgery, London, UK

Robert T. Naismith
Assistant Professor of Neurology, Washington University, Saint Louis, MO, USA

Scott Newsome
Assistant Professor of Neurology, Department of Neurology, The Johns Hopkins University School of Medicine, Baltimore, MD, USA

Friedemann Paul
Professor of Clinical Neuroimmunology, NeuroCure Clinical Research Center, Charité – Universitätsmedizin Berlin, Germany

Axel Petzold
Consultant Neurologist, VUMC, MS Center Amsterdam, NL and UCL Institute of Neurology, Department of Neuroinflammation, London, UK

Sashank Prasad
Department of Neurology, Brigham and Women's Hospital, Harvard Medical School, Boston, MA, USA

John N. Ratchford
Department of Neurology, The Johns Hopkins University School of Medicine, Baltimore, MD, USA

Anand Trip
Professor of Clinical Neurology, University Department of Clinical Neurology, National Hospital for Neurology and Neurosurgery, London, UK

Shiv Saidha
Assistant Professor of Neurology, Department of Neurology, Johns Hopkins University School of Medicine, Baltimore, MD, USA

Bernardo Sanchez-Dalmau
Center of Neuroimmunology and Department of Ophthalmology, Institut d'Investigacions Biomèdiques August Pi i Sunyer (IDIBAPS), Hospital Clinic of Barcelona, Barcelona, Spain

Sven Schippling
Department of Neurology, University Hospital, Zurich, Switzerland

Zane Schnurman
Departments of Neurology, University of Texas Southwestern School of Medicine at Dallas, TX, USA

Joel S. Schuman
Eye & Ear Foundation Professor and Chairman, Department of Ophthalmology
Director of UPMC Eye Center
Director, Louis J. Fox Center for Vision Restoration
Professor of Bioengineering
Professor of Clinical and Translational Science
Glaucoma and Cataract Service
University of Pittsburgh School of Medicine
Eye and Ear Institute, Pittsburgh, PA, USA

Elias S. Sotirchos
Resident Physician, The Johns Hopkins Hospital, Baltimore, MD, USA

Pablo Villoslada
Center of Neuroimmunology, Institut d'Investigacions Biomèdiques August Pi i Sunyer (IDIBAPS), Hospital Clinic of Barcelona, Barcelona, Spain

C. Yiannikas
Concord Hospital, Sydney, Australia

Preface

Shortly after the invention of the first two-dimensional optical coherence tomography (OCT) scans by James Fujimoto and colleagues at the Massachusetts Institute of Technology in 1991, ophthalmologists recognized the extraordinary potential for OCT to facilitate quantitative assessment of the neuroretina. OCT rapidly became a commonplace tool in ophthalmologic practice to identify both inflammatory and degenerative conditions affecting the optic nerve and retina. The utility of OCT to detect and quantify sequelae of optic neuropathies, including glaucoma and those associated with primary neurological diseases, was soon brought to the forefront. Rapid advances in the technology have followed and have included faster acquisition rates enabling higher-resolution images, eye tracking to minimize motion artifacts, and post-processing algorithms that permit segmentation of the nine layers of the retina. Such improvements have led to exponential growth in the application of OCT in neurological disease, both clinically and scientifically.

We now believe that OCT should become a mainstay of the neurological evaluation, as it is quite simply a quantitative ophthalmoscope. This technology is already commonplace in neuro-ophthalmology offices, and facilitates rapid and accurate assessment of the neuroretina for unexplained causes of visual loss for many neurologists. This compendium is designed to provide a useful overview for clinicians and scientists new to the field, and to serve as a resource for the more seasoned expert. Herein, we emphasize the emerging concept that the eye can indeed be considered a window into the brain, with the visual networks constituting perhaps the most elegant of the eloquent neuroscience systems from which to dissect pathophysiologic mechanisms of disease, and to detect and monitor the preventative, protective, and even restorative properties of novel neurotherapeutic agents, an exciting dividend of scientific discovery in the eye.

Perhaps one of the most gratifying aspects of editing this book has been the collaborative nature of the interactions among the authors, as well as the gracious contributions of those who did not have opportunities for their writing to be incorporated into this book. Remarkably, such unprecedented camaraderie reflects the scientific and clinical community's dedication to the exploration of vision in multiple sclerosis (MS) and other neurological diseases. Indeed, we attribute the exponential expansion of OCT in neurological diseases to these exemplary scientific interactions. Extensive documentation of reproducibility and validity for OCT measurements from independent sites around the world has rendered this technology a meaningful and cost-effective contribution to neurologic care and scientific investigation. Thanks to the many scientific and technological advancements, OCT measures now provide structural markers for aspects of neurological disease that are potentially amenable to novel therapies for protection and repair. This body of work, made reality by countless experts, epitomizes how, in just two decades, we can revolutionize our ability to practice medicine and underscores the power and productivity of collaborative works, with the ultimate shared goal of improving the quality of life for our deserving patients.

Chapter 1

Introduction to optical coherence tomography in neurological diseases

Peter A. Calabresi, Laura J. Balcer, and Elliot M. Frohman

While the neurological examination represents a time-honored gold standard for diagnosing and tracking the clinical course of disease, the sensitive and accurate assessment of central nervous system integrity remains a challenge. Optical coherence tomography (OCT) is an effective tool that has emerged over the past decade for measuring structure–function correlations and quantifying pathological changes invisible to the human eye. OCT can complement the clinical neurological examination in ways that are similar to magnetic resonance imaging (MRI), a tool that has given us tremendous structural insights into the nervous system. As we begin to understand the remarkable capacity of the brain to compensate for neurological injury, the links between structure, function, and electrophysiology that are provided uniquely by the afferent visual pathway will be critical. The relative timing of injury to the retinal ganglion cells (neurons), retinal nerve fiber layer (axons), and other ocular structures may be unique to each neurologic disorder. Such similarities outweigh differences, and the visual pathway represents an attractive global model for understanding and monitoring disease.

Neurologists acknowledge the capacity for noninvasive imaging technologies to accelerate and optimize neurologic diagnosis and follow-up. This is perhaps best illustrated by the pivotal role of MRI in the diagnosis and management of multiple sclerosis (MS). The field of neurology has witnessed a monumental transformation from near complete reliance on clinical history and examination to the addition of MRI and other noninvasive imaging techniques. An extension of the clinical examination, MRI has revolutionized care not only in MS but in the case of other neurologic disorders. For example, the relative specificity of MRI findings in some cases is helpful diagnostically. In this regard, OCT continues to evolve in its capacity to identify findings unique to any single neurologic or ocular disorder. While the architecture of the neural retina has been nearly totally inaccessible even with the application of the most sophisticated and high-precision MRI methods, the advent of high-resolution spectral-domain (SD) OCT has fundamentally changed our ability to qualitatively and quantitatively assess the eye – the most visible part of the human brain.

Neurological disorders frequently present with, or ultimately involve, visual impairment. Greater than 50% of the brain's pathways are dedicated to functional networks related to the visual system. While ocular motility is germane to foveation and subsequent image processing, the determination of the location and underlying mechanisms that compromise vision and visual perception can represent one of the most formidably challenging aspects of neurologic consultation. This is especially true given the intimate and yet highly distributed expanse of both the anterior and posterior, as well as afferent and efferent, visual processing networks, all of which require careful and systematic examination. Even the most expert clinical assessment of the visual pathway can be augmented by technological tools such as OCT. When considering all of the highly salient limitations associated with the bedside clinical neurologic and neuro-ophthalmologic examinations, we can begin to appreciate the impact on medical practice and clinical investigation that OCT has provided.

Rapid advances in OCT imaging technology have provided unprecedented, noninvasive, in vivo imaging of the retina. Spectral-domain OCT has

Optical Coherence Tomography in Neurological Disease, ed. Peter A. Calabresi, Laura J. Balcer, and Elliot M. Frohman. Published by Cambridge University Press.

spectacular image resolution and very low test-retest variability. Furthermore, ultrafast acquisition rates have minimized motion artifacts, facilitated intra-subject/inter-scan co-registration with high precision, and led to post-processing algorithms for automated segmentation analyses for measurement of retinal layer thicknesses.

Considerable improvements in both the technical and practical performance characteristics of OCT have led to an exponential growth in its application to a variety of neurological diseases. This has benefited clinical practice with respect to the rapid and accurate assessment of the neuroretina, while also catalyzing a literal scientific revolution in terms of viewing the eye as a noninvasive "window" into the brain.

The neuroretina is part of the brain, comprised of first-order neurons that relay visual information to the lateral geniculate nucleus in the thalamus. While these ganglion cell layer (GCL) neurons are susceptible to primary pathologies affecting the retinal nerve fiber layer (RNFL) axons, secondary pathology that arises in other areas of the brain such as the hypothalamus and superior colliculus can also be detected in the retina.

All forms of optic neuropathy have a characteristic signature of RNFL thinning and retinal GCL atrophy that can be quantified by OCT. More remarkably, several neurodegenerative diseases with well-known brain pathology, such as Alzheimer's disease, frontotemporal dementia, and Parkinson's disease, are now recognized to have concomitant retinal neuronal layer degeneration that can be demonstrated by OCT. Neurological diseases traditionally linked with the peripheral nervous system are increasingly reported to have central nervous system manifestations; these include type 2a Charcot-Marie-Tooth disease, in which abnormalities in mitofusin can manifest as optic nerve disease. Deeper retinal neuronal layers, including the inner and outer nuclear layers, have been shown to be abnormal in several diseases classically associated only with primary axonal demyelination, such as MS. This supports theories that neurons may be a direct target of neurological disease processes not previously thought to have a primary degenerative mechanism. As the potential applications of OCT continue to grow, its role in neurological disease is of increasing interest and importance in discovery biology as well as in the context of clinical assessment.

In this new book we provide an extensive review of the application of OCT across a broad landscape of neurological diseases. A basic-level introduction to the underlying principles of the technology is provided for the reader. This is followed by a review of the neuroanatomy of the visual system, especially the retina, the target tissue for OCT imaging. No imaging device should be employed without proper examination of the critical link with clinical function and outcomes, most notably vision. Several chapters are dedicated to the clinical validation of the utility of OCT in neurological diseases. As expected, there are significant cross-sectional associations between retinal pathology detected by OCT and low-contrast letter acuity, high-contrast visual acuity, and color perception. Perhaps more importantly, retinal imaging appears to have predictive value for estimating cerebral pathology in gray matter structures of the central nervous system. Involvement of these structures is notoriously inconspicuous early on in many neurological diseases, and therefore an understanding of gray matter pathology may facilitate early detection and prognostication for those patients with neurodegenerative disorders. The underlying tissue pathological substrates captured with OCT-generated images are limited, and, therefore, several chapters are dedicated to elucidating the promising correlations between OCT images and histopathology, vascular pathology, as well as functional electrophysiology.

Because this new technology increasingly takes its place in the clinic, OCT has also found application in clinical trials of putative neuroprotective drugs. Indeed, the rapid thinning of the RNFL and the GCL following acute optic neuritis is a logical outcome measure for phase II trials of drugs that could exert neuroprotective or neurorepair properties. The reproducible and accurate quantitation of the axonal and neuronal layers that undergo thinning in the three to six months following an acute optic neuritis make OCT an appealing tool, which is easily employed across multiple centers in clinical trials. Therefore, we have dedicated several chapters to reviewing the rationale, approach, and practicality of using OCT in clinical research trials. Whether retinal neuronal imaging will find the same application in neurodegenerative diseases, which manifest with changes that take place over years to decades, remains to be fully determined, but evidence supporting such a role in this context is rapidly mounting. Finally, the book concludes with a look to the future and a discussion of how the rapid evolution of this technology and associated retinal imaging devices may facilitate even more progress in structural and functional assessments of the retinal manifestations of neurological diseases. We now believe that OCT should become a mainstay of the neurological evaluation, because it is, quite simply, a *quantitative ophthalmoscope*.

Chapter 2

Basic principles of optical coherence tomography

Sven Schippling

Introduction

Optical coherence tomography (OCT) uses low-coherent, near infrared light to generate tomographic, two-dimensional (2-D) structural in vivo images of biological tissues based on the physical concept of time-of-flight delay and intensity of backscattered light from microscopic constituents within these tissues [1, 2]. Therefore, OCT can be considered an optical analogue of ultrasound-based tomographic imaging [3]. As is the case in ultrasonography, time gating of backscattered reflexes leads to a line profile, the so-called A-scan [1–3]. The first 2-D or so-called B-scan images, repeating the A-scanning process while changing a reference mirror′s position, were provided by Huang and colleagues from the group of James Fujimoto at the Massachusetts Institute of Technology (MIT) in 1991 [3]. It took another five years until the first OCT device with an axial resolution of 15 μm became commercially available (OCT 1; System 2000 Humphrey Instruments, Inc.). Since then, the technique has undergone a remarkable technical development. Also, the traditional application of OCT in ophthalmological diseases like glaucoma and macular edema has more recently been extended and introduced into neurology [4, 5]. Here, within a reasonably short time period, OCT has inspired a remarkable body of literature demonstrating both primary and secondary (e.g., following multiple sclerosis-associated optic neuritis) retinal pathology in a number of different disease models [4–9]. Some of this work is described in detail in the following chapters within this compendium. This section will describe basic technical principles of OCT as well as the development of this exciting methodology within the last two decades.

Basic principles of OCT in retinal imaging

OCT is based on the physical principle of partial interference between light backscattered by tissues and a reference light beam reflected from a reference mirror [1–3]. In retinal OCT imaging, low-coherent, near infrared light is emitted from a superluminescent diode and directed onto the retina through the pupil of the person being scanned [2]. The scans can be acquired with or without pupillary mydriasis. The process of generating anteroposterior tomographic scans is based on the splitting of this light beam into a sample and a reference fraction by a beamsplitter (Figure 2.1). Whereas the first is entering the patient′s eye, the latter is directed towards a (mobile) reference mirror (Figure 2.1). The light directed onto the retina crosses the transparent structures of the eye and is partially absorbed, whereas a larger fraction is backscattered by the different retinal layers [1,2]. Both the reference beam and the sample beam are reflected backward and simultaneously registered by a photodetector or spectrometer in which the co-occurrence of the two wave fronts induces an interference signal [2]. The false color or gray contrast OCT image itself is based on the distribution and amplitudes of the repeatedly incoming interference signals [2, 3].

As of this date, two different OCT technologies are still available, the older time-domain (TD) and the more recent spectral-domain (SD) OCT, also called Fourier-domain (FD) OCT [10]. The latter name refers to Jean-Baptiste Joseph Fourier (1768–1830), a French Professor at the École Polytechnique, who is known for his work on the Fourier Transform [11].

Optical Coherence Tomography in Neurological Disease, ed. Peter A. Calabresi, Laura J. Balcer, and Elliot M. Frohman. Published by Cambridge University Press.

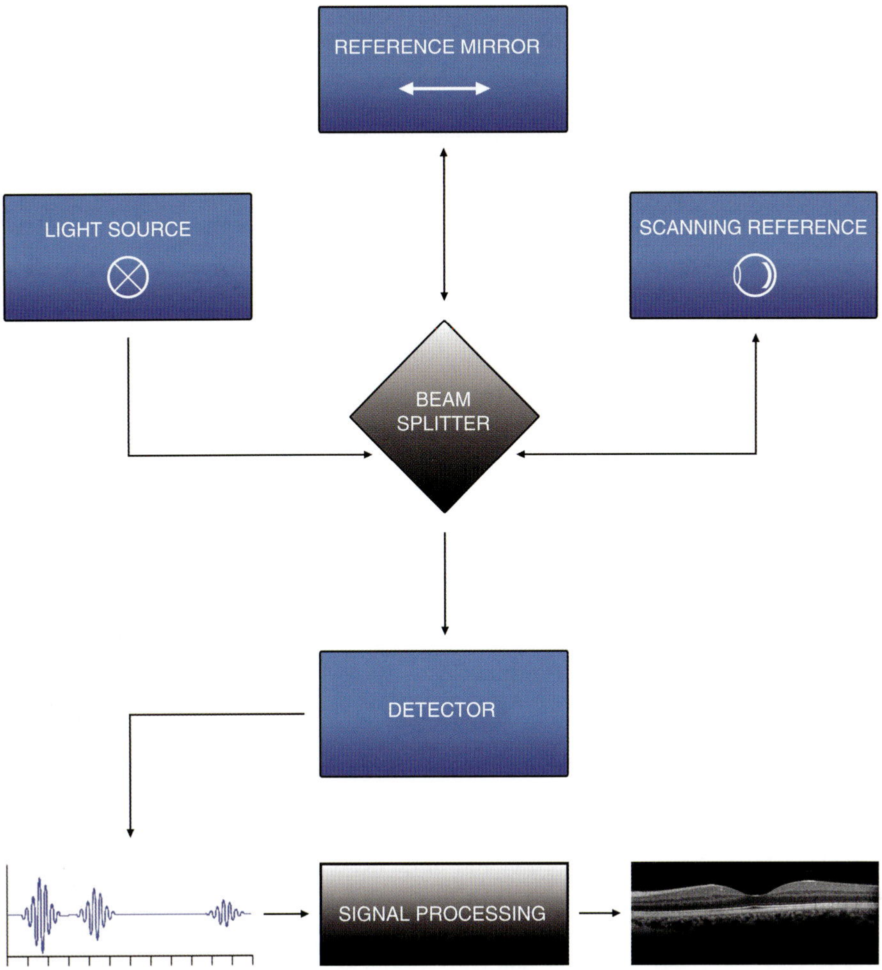

Figure 2.1 Basic principles of time-domain OCT. Interference of reference and reflected light beams from different layers within the tissue occurs as a function of axial transition of the reference mirror.

Time-domain (TD) optical coherence tomography

The basic components and setup of a TD-OCT system are detailed in Figure 2.1. As the name of this technology suggests, TD-OCT is based on the difference in the time delay of the sample light echoes reflected from the different retinal layers as a function of their depth within the tissue (here, the retina) and the reference beam echo, a single echo that is varied by changing the position of the mobile reference mirror (i.e., the reference arm-length).

Interference of light beams with low coherence only occurs in cases where the distance traveled by the light in both arms of the interferometer is equivalent to within the coherence length in order to allow interference by co-occurrence on the level of the photodetector. This phenomenon allows accurate measurement of the echo time delay. Light reflected from superficial structures of the retina or uppermost retinal layers has a shorter echo time delay than light reflected from deeper retinal structures (innermost layers) [2, 5]. The reference mirror is axially translocated in order to match echo time delays from various tissue layers. As the path length of the moving reference mirror is known, it is possible to calculate the depth of the tissue from which the fraction of reflected light arises based on the specific time delay. Based on the amplitude of the interference signals that arise from interference of the reflected light from retinal layers of different depths and the reference light from various path lengths, a single axial scan, the so-called

A-scan, is deduced. Key to longitudinal scanning is the fact that the reference mirror can be mechanically mobilized, resulting in a shift of the reference beam, extending the reference path. The reference mirror moves with a specific distance- and time-interval constant, leading to multiple adjacent A-scans, which, in sum, generate the cross-sectional 2-D or longitudinal B-scan of the retina (Figure 2.1). In TD-OCT the cross-sectional image representing the different retinal layers is generated as a function of time delay of the reflected sample light beams. In turn, the time delay depends on the composition and depth of the different layers and the position or axial translation of the reference mirror. These basic principles have led to the name of this technology: *time-domain OCT*.

TD-OCT has an axial resolution of approximately 10 μm or less (Table 2.1). Image acquisition speed is limited in TD-OCT, however, because the reference mirror needs to be moved.

Spectral-domain (SD) optical coherence tomography

The most recent, so-called fourth-generation or spectral-domain (SD) OCT technology, is based on the mathematical Fourier transform equation. This methodology is, therefore, also known as Fourier-domain technology. The Fourier transform eliminates the need for a movement of the reference beam mirror. SD-OCT replaces the photodetector from TD-OCT with a spectrometer capable of analyzing the full spectrum of interference signals at one time point generated when the sample and the reference beam meet along the same path. It allows the analysis of all frequencies simultaneously. As opposed to TD-OCT, in SD-OCT the interference signal is a function of the different wavelengths and not of the different echo time delays. The whole wavelength spectrum is converted into time delay signals by the Fourier transform. In retinal OCT imaging, this allows the analysis of all echoes from the different retinal layers simultaneously. As a consequence, SD-OCT is much more rapid than its counterpart, while at the same time providing excellent resolution. In TD-OCT, high-resolution imaging can only be achieved at the expense of an increase in acquisition times. Scanning speed is 50–100 times faster with SD-OCT than with TD-OCT [10,11].

Rapid scanning allows larger numbers of B-scans per time interval, and high-speed macular scans with an increasing B-scan density have become possible with the latest devices (see Table 2.1). SD-OCT achieves an axial resolution in the range of 5–6 μm, while digital resolution can be even higher (Table 2.1). High-resolution scans together with real-time averaging significantly increase the signal-to-noise ratio (SNR), ensuring superior image resolution and quality in SD-OCT.

Currently, a number of TD- and SD-OCT devices are commercially available. Technical characteristics of different OCT devices are detailed in Table 2.1.

Swept source (SS) optical coherence tomography

The light source in swept source (SS) OCT systems is a tunable narrow bandwidth laser. The interferences at different wavelengths are measured over time. Through rapid adjustment of the laser, scan speeds of up to 249,000 A-scans/second can be achieved [12]. SS-OCT technique was used for the first time in retinal imaging in 2006 [13].

As with TD-OCT, SS-OCT uses a photodetector instead of the combination of a CCD camera and spectrometer, as in SD-OCT. In addition, a light source with wavelengths around 1,000 nm is applied. The longer wavelengths penetrate deeper into the retina and optic nerve head. This might be useful in assessing the choroid and the lamina cribrosa, as well as the optic nerve head. A disadvantage of using longer wavelengths is a reduction of axial resolution compared to the SD-OCT (which uses light with a wavelength of around 840–880 nm) [14].

Advantages of spectral over time-domain OCT

In TD-OCT depth of the tissue is sampled point by point axially transferring the reference mirror. Compared to SD-OCT this renders TD-OCT inefficient [10,11].

Replacing the photodetector in TD-OCT with a spectrometer in SD-OCT allows spectral OCT to detect the entire wavelength spectrum corresponding to reflections from the entire depth range [11]. SD-OCT allows acquisition speeds of 27,000 to 53,000 A-scans per second in clinical application as compared to a maximum of approximately 400 A-scans per second in TD-OCT (see Table 2.1) [10–12]. In experimental settings A-scan speeds of even up to 312,500 scans per second have been

Table 2.1 Technical characteristics of commercially available OCT devices

	Fundus image			OCT image									
Device	Live image	Size	Optional modes	Technology	Light source	Scan Speed A-scans/sec	Transverse resolution**	Axial resolution**	Scan depth	Min. pupil diameter	Max. no. of A-scans/B-scan	Manufacturer	Web address
SPECTRALIS	cSLO	30°, 55°, 165°	AF, ICGA, FA, MC	SD	870 nm	40000	14 µm	7 µm	1.9 mm	2 mm	1536	Heidelberg Engineering	www.heidelberg engineering.com
Stratus	IR Cam	26° × 20.5°		TD	820 nm	400	20 µm	10 µm	2 mm	3.2 mm	768	Zeiss Meditec AG	www.meditec.zeiss.com
CIRRUS 4000	SLO	36° × 30°		SD	840 nm	27000	15 µm	5 µm	2 mm	2 mm	4096	Zeiss Meditec AG	www.meditec.zeiss.com
3D OCT 2000	IR Cam	45°	CF Camera, AF*, FA*	SD	840 nm	50000	20 µm	6 µm	2.3 mm	2.5 mm	1024	Topcon	www.topcon-medical.eu
DR 1	SLO	43°		SwS	1050 nm	100000	20 µm	8 µm		2.5 mm	1024	Topcon	www.topcon-medical.eu
iVue	IR Cam	32° × 23°		SD	840 nm	25000	15 µm	5 µm	2.3 mm	3 mm	1024	Optovue	www.optovue.com
RS-3000	SLO	40°x 30°		SD	880 nm	53000	20 µm	7 µm	2.1 mm	2.5 mm		Nidek	www.nidek-intl.com
OCT SLO	cSLO	29°		SD	830 nm	25000	20 µm	10 µm	2 mm	3 mm		Optos	www.optos.com
Copernicus HR	IR Cam	30°		SD	850 nm	52000	12 µm	3 µm	2 mm	3 mm	20000	Optopol	www.optopol.com
Canon OCT HS-100	SLO	44° × 33°		SD	855 nm	70000	20 µm	3 µm	2 mm	3 mm		Canon	www.canon-europe.com

cSLO confocal Scanning Laser Ophthalmoscope
SLO Scanning Laser Ophthalmoscope
AF Auto Fluorescence
ICGA Indocyanin Green Angiographay
FA Fluorescence Angiography
MC Multicolor
* only 3-D OCT FA Plus
** optical resolution

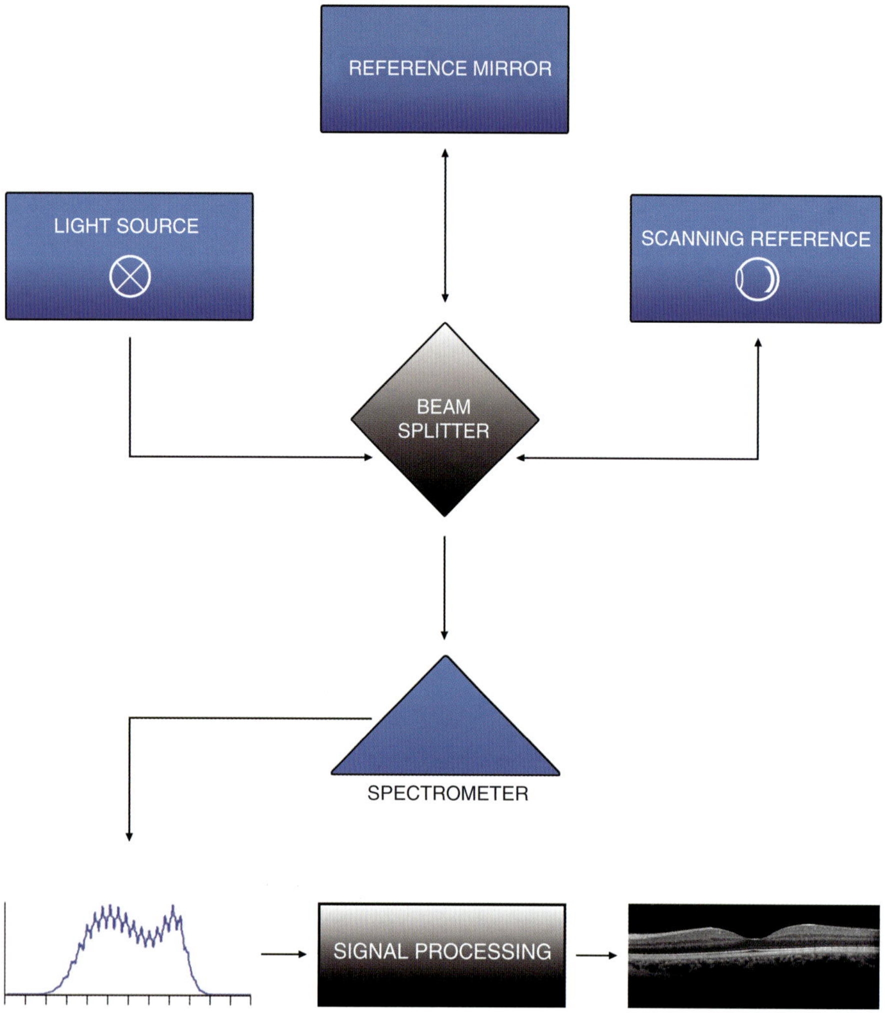

Figure 2.2 Basic principles of spectral-domain OCT. Note that in SD-OCT a complete spectrum of interference signals is processed simultaneously because of the introduction of a spectrometer, allowing faster scan acquisition, while the reference mirror is fixed.

reported with ultrahigh-speed SD-OCT devices [12]. Another advantage that comes with increasing scanning speed is that motion artifacts produced by involuntary eye movements of the person being scanned are reduced [10,11]. Averaging of multiple frames helps increasing the signal-to-noise ratio, further improving image quality [11]. In TD-OCT, scanning of the macular is based on a lower number of B-scans, and the full macula scan is extrapolated from these few B-scans. Limited retinal pathology can be missed by this extrapolation, because it may fall in a gap between two neighboring B-scans.

However, even with the increased speed of SD-OCT, physiological involuntary eye movements can be an issue during acquisition [11]. A standard volume scan (200 A-scans/B-scan; 200 B-scans at 27,000 A-scans/sec) takes about 1.48 seconds (1,480 ms). Involuntary saccades are much faster and occur at 30–50 μs (micro-saccades) or 150 ms (macro-saccades). This can result in motion artifacts of the OCT scan. In order to reduce the above mentioned motion artifacts induced by physiological saccades and to increase intra-rater and inter-rater reliability, while at the same time increasing scanning frequency, an active eye-tracking technology has been introduced in the SPECTRALIS® SD-OCT device (Heidelberg Engineering GmbH, Heidelberg, Germany). The active eye tracker (TruTrack™)

recognizes eye movements on the infrared fundus image, continuously correcting the OCT scan line and compensating according to the extent of the involuntary saccades. This feature enables the device to acquire larger data sets with higher numbers of averaged single B-scans (up to 100), while increasing the SNR and avoiding motion artifacts. A further advantage is the automatic follow-up function that comes with the active eye-tracking system. Given that each retina is unique (like an individual fingerprint), the scan is exactly repositioned for the follow-up scan with only a little variability. As a consequence, it allows monitoring of minimal changes that appear longitudinally in the context of both pathological retinal conditions and in neurodegenerative diseases such as multiple sclerosis (MS).

Optic nerve head and macular scan protocols

For the so-called peripapillary ring scan, the A-scans (Figure 2.3) are centered on a circle around the optic nerve head. A circle-diameter of 12° (approximately) 3.4 mm has been shown to provide good reproducibility [15]. As a consequence, this diameter has widely been used irrespective of the size of the optic nerve head [16]. Standard TD-OCT scanning protocols of the optic nerve head involve 256 A-scans around the optic disc. To minimize the effect of involuntary eye movements during scanning, a series of three scans is performed.

From these peripapillary ring scans the mean overall retinal nerve fiber layer (RNFL) thickness is calculated, as are the thicknesses of the four RNFL quadrants (temporal, superior, nasal, and inferior) and 12 segments around the optic nerve head (Figure 2.3). The optic nerve head or peripapillary ring scan, shows a typical morphology in which RNFL thickness is greatest at the superior and inferior poles, whereas the lowest thickness values are registered nasally and temporally. The anatomical reason behind this distribution is the fact that the majority of ganglion cell axons that – in sum – form the optic nerve enter the optic disc from the superior and inferior quadrants.

At the time that OCT was introduced into neurology only TD-OCT technology was been available. As mentioned above, TD-OCT was capable of acquiring only 400 A-scans per second. Consequently, the available scan patterns were limited. The most common scan pattern used in those devices is the peripapillary circle scan. Boundaries of the RNFL are automatically detected, and the mean overall RNFL thickness is calculated.

In TD-OCT macular assessment is performed by a set of 6 B-scans (128 A-scans each) centered in a star pattern on the fovea. For analysis the macula is divided into sectors using the ETDRS (Early Treatment of Diabetic Retinopathy Study) grid [17]. The grid layout consists of three concentric circles: one central ring with a diameter of 1 mm, an intermediate ring with a diameter of 3 mm, and an outer circle with 6 mm. The intermediate and outer rings are divided into sectors (superior, inferior, nasal, and temporal). The measures extrapolated from this macular scan are the total macular volume and mean thickness values of the respective sectors. The boundaries of the inner limiting membrane (ILM), nerve fiber layer (NFL), and Bruch's membrane (BM) are already automatically defined. Due to the low axial resolution, in the range of 10 μm, and moderate image quality an automated segmentation of deeper retinal layers was less reliable.

With the introduction of the Fourier-domain OCT technology, axial transition of the reference mirror to change path lengths was no longer needed [10, 11]. Scanning speeds increased significantly, now allowing scan patterns with a higher number of B-scans and much higher resolution. As a consequence, SD-OCT allows a much more comprehensive picture of the entire retina and a more in-depth view of retinal pathology [10,11]. However, the parameters obtained from these scans are still the same. Depending on the device the circle is calculated from a squared volumetric scan pattern (CIRRUS®, Carl Zeiss Meditec AG, Dublin CA), or consists of up to 1,536 A-scans (SPECTRALIS®, Heidelberg Engineering GmbH, Heidelberg) in the form of a circle centered on the optic nerve head. Notably, the macular volume scans differ in size, spacing between B-scans, and the number of A-scans acquired. In all devices the 3-D reconstruction of the macular cube scan is still based on extrapolation from the acquired B-scans.

It took another several years of software development until automated or semi-automated algorithms became available to perform segmentation of macular B-scans (see 2.9) that allowed the quantification of deeper retinal layers, like the ganglion cell layer, the

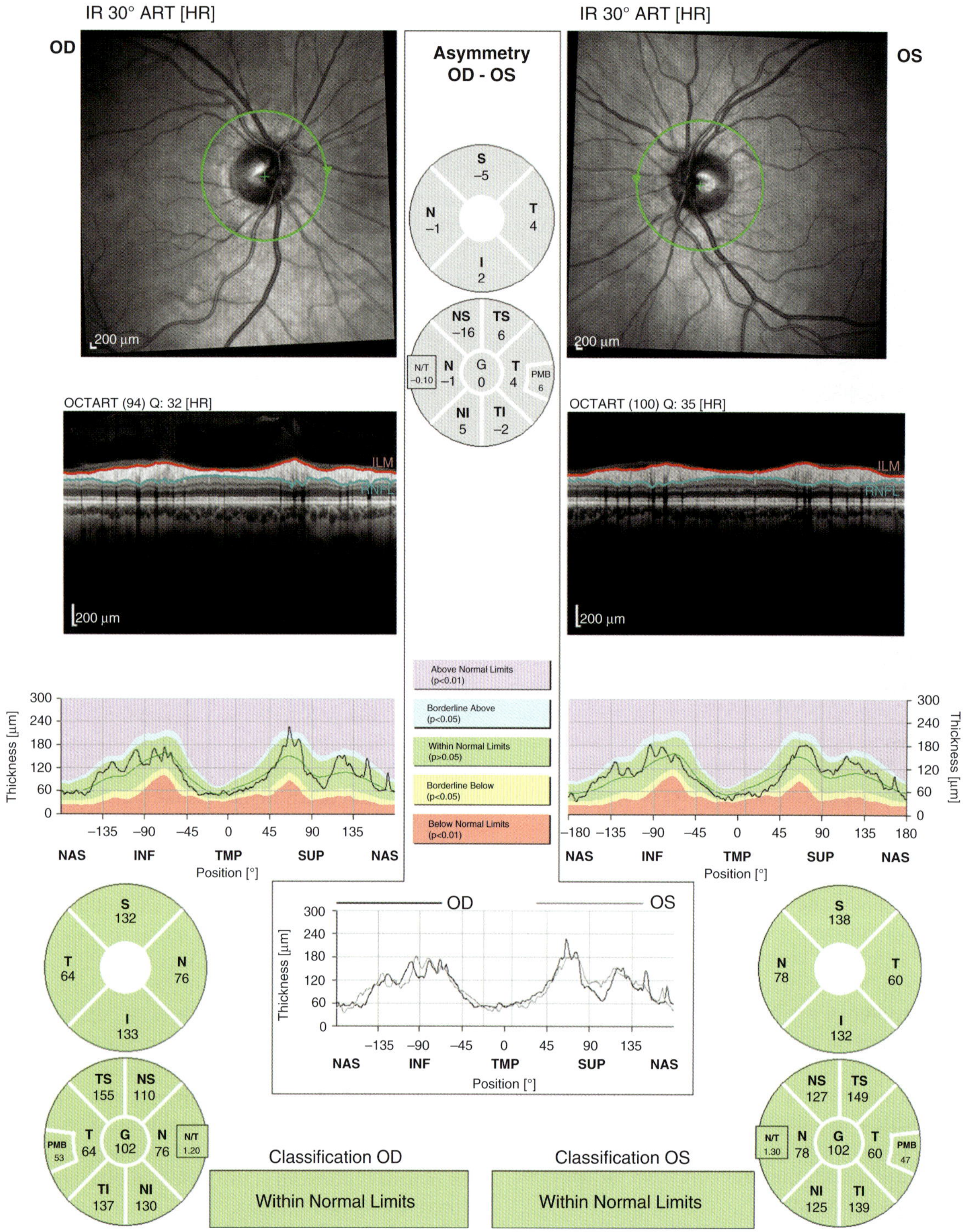

Figure 2.3 Report of a peripapillary spectral-domain OCT scan performed on a normal subject. Top left and right are the infrared fundus images of the right (OD) and left eye (OS) followed by the B-scans. Automatic segmentation of the retinal nerve fiber layer (inner limiting membrane (ILM)/red line; retinal nerve fiber layer (RNFL)/blue line).

Individual thickness shown as solid black lines for the left and right eye (within 95% confidence interval/green area). Thickness of the superior, nasal, inferior, and temporal quadrants.

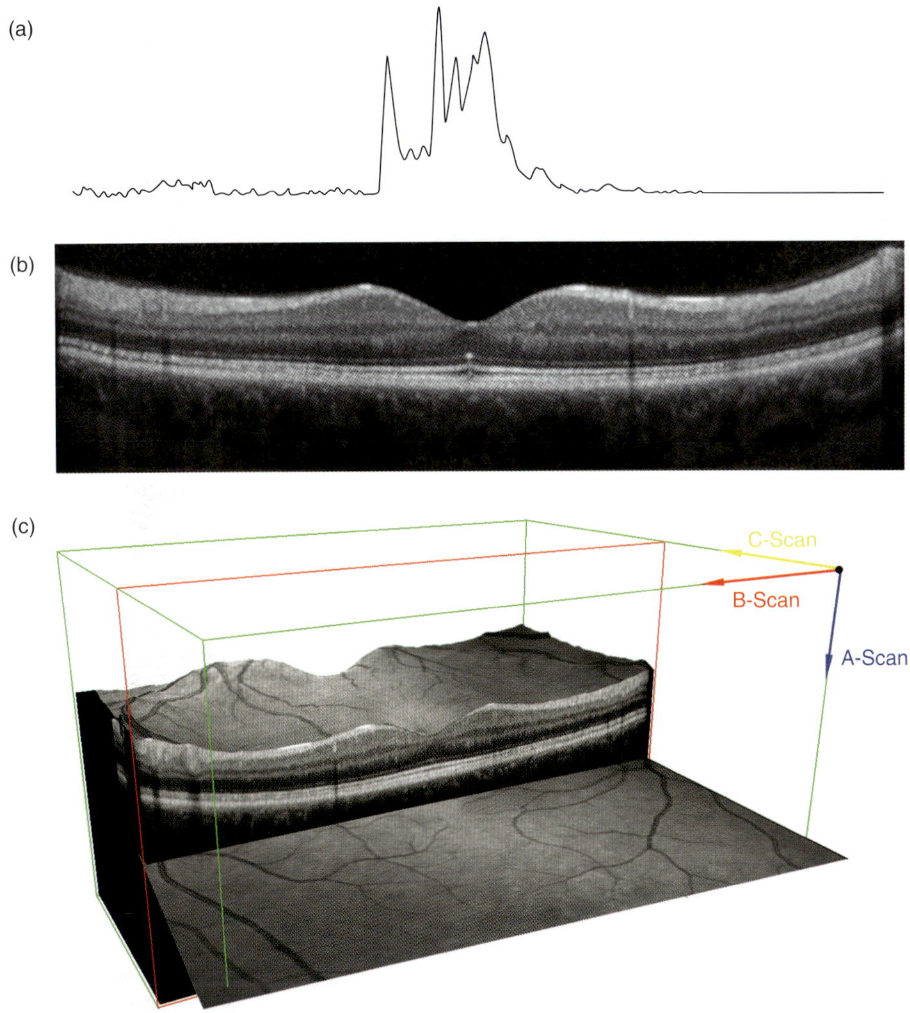

Figure 2.4 Spectral-domain OCT scan. Single A-scan profile (a). Central macular B-scan (b). 3-D macular scan generated by co-registration of fundus image and consecutive macular B-scans (c).

inner and outer nuclear, and the inner and outer plexiform layers.

3-D visualization

The scanning frequency and the number of B-scans acquired in SD-OCT allows 3-D reconstruction of macular and optic nerve head images (Figure 2.4). Usually 3-D visualization scanning laser ophthalmoscopic (SLO) or fundus images and OCT B-scans are co-registered. Current software allows reconstruction of 3-D images in a frontal or coronal plane (C-scan/en face mode) (Figure 2.5), which might help to screen and identify retinal pathologies in more detail [18].

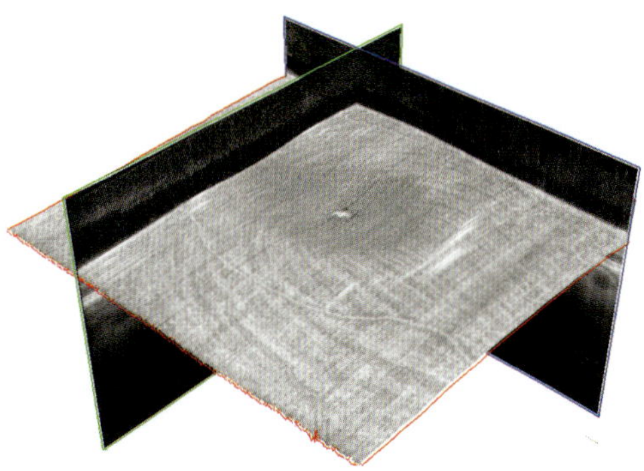

Figure 2.5 Reconstruction of macular B-scans in a frontal plane generates a C-scan perpendicular to the coronal view, as shown in Figure 2.4 (en face image).

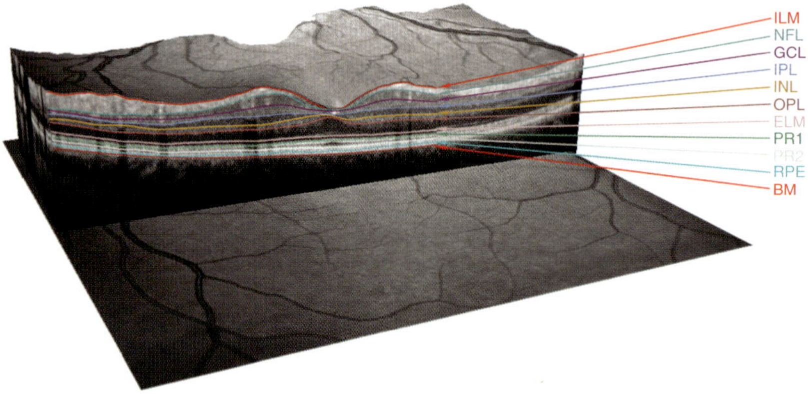

Figure 2.6 Segmented macular B-scan. Inner limiting membrane (ILM), nerve fiber layer (NFL), ganglion cell layer (GCL), inner plexiform layer (IPL), inner nuclear layer (INL), outer plexiform layer (OPL), external limiting membrane (ELM), photoreceptor layer 1 (PR1), photoreceptor layer 2 (PR2), retinal pigment epithelium (RPE), Bruch membrane (BM).

Segmentation of OCT macular B-scans

Most of today's SD-OCT devices include commercially available software capable of segmenting retinal layers beyond the RNFL. However, being able to discriminate the different layers in the retina strongly depends on the quality of the OCT scan, which is also dependent on signal strength and averaging of the single B-scan.

The quality of all SD-OCT devices is sufficient to automatically define six to seven boundaries within the retina (ILM, RNFL/GCL, IPL/INL, OPL/ONL, IS/OS, RPE/BM), but with some of the devices increased resolution allows identification of up to 11 retinal layers (Figure 2.6). Yet again, proper identification of the borders between the layers (especially in the case of GCL/IPL) is only possible in B-scans of sufficiently high quality. Most device manufacturers are coming out with automated segmentation software in addition to manual segmentation. Recent studies suggest that both automated and semi-automated as well as manual segmentation of macular B-scans show excellent intra- and inter-rater reliability when performed by experienced OCT readers [19].

References

1 Frohman EM, Fujimoto JG, Frohman TC, et al. Optical coherence tomography: a window into the mechanisms of multiple sclerosis. *Nat Clin Pract Neurol* 2008; **4**: 664–75.

2 Schuman JS, Puliafito CA, Fujimoto JG. *Optical coherence tomography of ocular diseases*. Slack, Inc., New Jersey 2004.

3 Huang D, Swanson EA, Lin CP, et al. Optical coherence tomography. *Science* 1991; **254**: 1178–81.

4 Petzold A, de Boer JF, Schippling S, et al. Optical coherence tomography in multiple sclerosis: a systematic review and meta-analysis. *Lancet Neurol* 2010; **9**: 921–32.

5 Jindahra P, Hedges TR, Mendoza-Santiesteban CE, Plant GT. Optical coherence tomography of the retina: applications in neurology. *Curr Opin Neurol* 2010; **23**: 16–23.

6 Saidha S, Syc SB, Ibrahim MA, et al. Primary retinal pathology in multiple sclerosis as detected by optical coherence tomography. *Brain* 2011; **134**: 518–33.

7 Costello F, Coupland S, Hodge W, et al. Quantifying axonal loss after optic neuritis with optical coherence tomography. *Ann Neurol* 2006; **59**: 963–9.

8 Sotirchos ES, Saidha S, Byraiah G, et al. In vivo identification of morphologic retinal abnormalities in neuromyelitis optica. *Neurology* 2013; **80**: 1406–14.

9 Brandt AU, Zimmermann H, Kaufhold F, et al. Patterns of retinal damage facilitate differential diagnosis between Susac syndrome and MS. *PLoS One* 2012; **7**: e38741.

10 Forooghian F, Cukras C, Meyerle CB, et al. Evaluation of time domain and spectral domain optical coherence tomography in the measurement of diabetic macular edema. *Invest Ophthalmol Vis Sci* 2008; **49**: 4290–6.

11 Yaqoob Z, Wu J, Yang C. Spectral domain optical coherence tomography: a better OCT imaging strategy. *Biotechniques*. 2005; **39**: S6–13.

12 Potsaid B, Gorczynska I, Srinivasan VJ, et al. Ultrahigh speed spectral / Fourier domain OCT ophthalmic

imaging at 70,000 to 312,500 axial scans per second. *Opt Express* 2008; **16**: 15149–69.

13 Lee EC, de Boer JF, Mujat M, Lim H, Yun SH. In vivo optical frequency domain imaging of human retina and choroid. *Opt Express* 2006; **14**: 4403–11.

14 Gabriele ML, Wollstein G, Ishikawa H, et al. Optical coherence tomography: history, current status, and laboratory work. *Invest Ophthalmol Vis Sci* 2011; **52**: 2425–36.

15 Schuman JS, Pedut-Kloizman T, Hertzmark E, et al. Reproducibility of nerve fiber layer thickness measurements using optical coherence tomography. *Ophthalmology* 1996; **103**: 1889–98.

16 Savini G, Zanini M, Carelli V, et al. Correlation between retinal nerve fibre layer thickness and optic nerve head size: an optical coherence tomography study. *Br J Ophthalmol* 2005; **894**: 489–92.

17 Photocoagulation for diabetic macular edema. Early Treatment Diabetic Retinopathy Study report number 1. Early Treatment Diabetic Retinopathy Study research group. *Arch Ophthalmol* 1985; **103**: 1796–806.

18 Wolff B, Matet A, Vasseur V, et al. En face OCT imaging for the diagnosis of outer retinal tubulations in age-related macular degeneration. *J Ophthalmol* 2012; 542417.

19 Seigo MA, Sotirchos ES, Newsome S, et al. In vivo assessment of retinal neuronal layers in multiple sclerosis with manual and automated optical coherence tomography segmentation techniques. *J Neurol* 2012; **259**: 2119–30.

Chapter 3

Anatomy of the anterior visual pathway

Devin D. Mackay, Steven L. Galetta, and Sashank Prasad

Introduction

Since its development in the 1990s, optical coherence tomography (OCT) has ushered in a new era of noninvasive diagnostic imaging of the eye [1]. OCT measures the optical backscattering of near-infrared light in a way that is analogous to B-scan ultrasound, which measures the acoustic backscattering properties of a tissue. OCT imaging of the visual pathways is limited to structures accessible by light, which include the conjunctiva, cornea, lens, layers of the retina, optic disc, and optic nerve head. Earlier time-domain OCT technology has been largely replaced by high-speed spectral-Fourier-domain (SD/FD) methods, which allow for much faster image acquisition and improved quality. SD-OCT images can have high axial spatial resolution (2–3 μm), although the resolution of most commercially available machines is 4–7 μm. OCT is a powerful tool for neurologists, neuro-ophthalmologists, ophthalmologists, and radiologists interested in the clinical evaluation of the anterior visual pathways. In this chapter, we illustrate the use of OCT to depict the normal anatomy of the anterior visual pathway.

Anterior eye

The anterior eye can be imaged with OCT using an adapter module or a dedicated OCT instrument specifically designed for this purpose. Structures of the anterior eye visible with OCT include the corneal epithelium, corneal stroma, corneal endothelium, sclera, trabecular meshwork, iris, canal of Schlemm, corneoscleral limbus, Schwalbe's ring, and Descemet's membrane (Figures 3.1A–D and 3.2).

Anterior chamber

Anterior chamber depth and anterior chamber angle (Figure 3.1B) can be assessed with OCT. These measures often complement findings that are observed clinically during gonioscopy. Since the overlying sclera can be highly optically backscattering, detailed features of the anterior chamber are sometimes difficult to resolve.

The anterior angle (Figure 3.1B) can also be evaluated with OCT. The corneal epithelium (Figure 3.1C) continues laterally until it meets with the sclera at the corneoscleral limbus (Figure 3.1D), just anterior to the anterior angle. Schwalbe's ring is a ring of collagenous fibers found on the posterior corneal surface at the termination of Descemet's membrane (the basal lamina of the corneal endothelium).

The canal of Schlemm is found lateral to Schwalbe's ring in the depth of the anterior angle and is the site of aqueous drainage from the anterior chamber (Figure 3.1B). Aqueous outflow proceeds through the trabecular meshwork and into the canal of Schlemm, where aqueous humor enters the aqueous veins. Aqueous veins are distinguished from blood-filled veins by the lack of optical shadows cast on deeper structures. From aqueous veins, the aqueous humor enters the scleral veins, sometimes by way of an intervening vascular plexus. Schlemm's canal and the aqueous outflow pathways that lead to the scleral veins can be visualized with commercially available SD-OCT. 3-D OCT imaging allows for more detailed visualization of the outflow channel networks [2].

Sclera

The sclera is the dense, white protective covering of the eye, composed almost entirely of collagen

Optical Coherence Tomography in Neurological Disease, ed. Peter A. Calabresi, Laura J. Balcer, and Elliot M. Frohman. Published by Cambridge University Press.

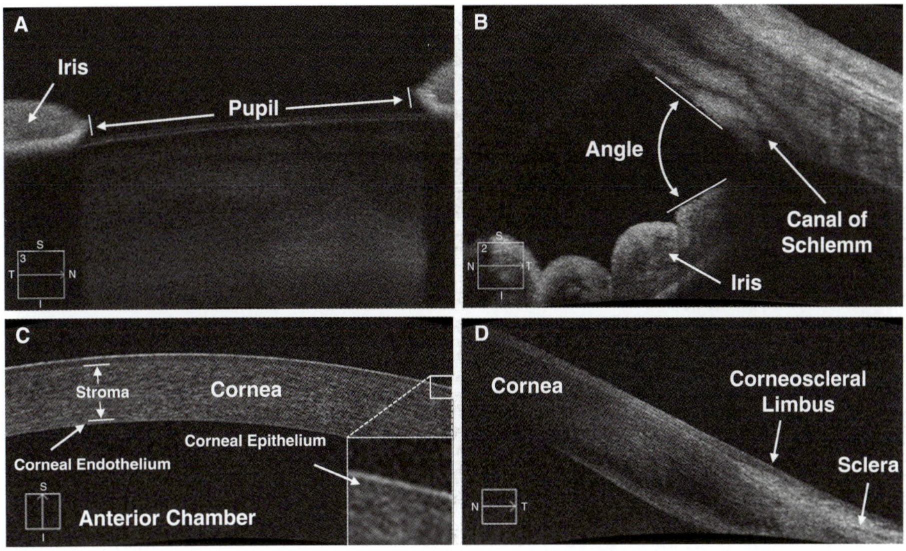

Figure 3.1 OCT of the anterior chamber. (A) Image of the pupil demarcated by the iris on either side. (B) Angle of the anterior chamber and canal of Schlemm. (C) Corneal endothelium, epithelium, stroma, and underlying anterior chamber. (D) The cornea and sclera meet at the corneoscleral limbus. Images courtesy of Rick Calderon, O.D.

(Figures 3.1D and 3.3). Its density and composition make it highly optically backscattering on OCT.

Iris

The iris divides the anterior from the posterior chamber (Figures 3.1A–B, 3.2, and 3.3). It is composed of sphincter and dilator muscles that control the size of the pupil and the amount of light entering the eye [3]. The iris is configured as a shallow cone that points anteriorly and is highly pigmented. Because the iris shadows deeper structures on OCT, images of the posterior parts of the eye must be obtained by focusing the OCT beam through the pupillary aperture.

Cornea

The corneal epithelium, Bowman's layer, and the corneal lamellae can be imaged using ultrahigh resolution OCT. Corneal adapter modules focus the OCT beam on the cornea, while post-processing algorithms correct for refraction of the OCT beam at the anterior corneal surface. The corneal epithelium is characterized by a low scattering layer on OCT (Figure 3.1C). The striated pattern seen in the corneal stroma is attributed to its collagen structure and organization [4]. Echo reflection artifacts appear in a plane through the center of the cornea, with a strong reflection present where the OCT beam is orthogonal to the air–cornea interface, and is reflected back into the instrument.

Lens

The lens is a normally transparent and avascular structure that focuses light on the retina with the help of its biconvex configuration (Figure 3.2). It is about 4 mm thick and 9 mm in diameter. Zonule fibers suspend the lens from the ciliary body, just behind the iris. Aqueous humor is present anterior to the lens, while vitreous humor is present posteriorly [3].

Posterior eye

Choroid and choriocapillaris

The choriocapillaris is a network of fenestrated choroidal capillaries located between the sclera and Bruch's membrane that provides nourishment to the nearby retinal pigment epithelium (RPE) and photoreceptors. In first-generation OCT images, a single layer described as the RPE-choriocapillaris complex was visible, and visualization of the individual layers of the outer retina beyond the photoreceptor inner segments was not possible. With improvements in axial image resolution, discernment of the components of the RPE-choriocapillaris complex became possible.

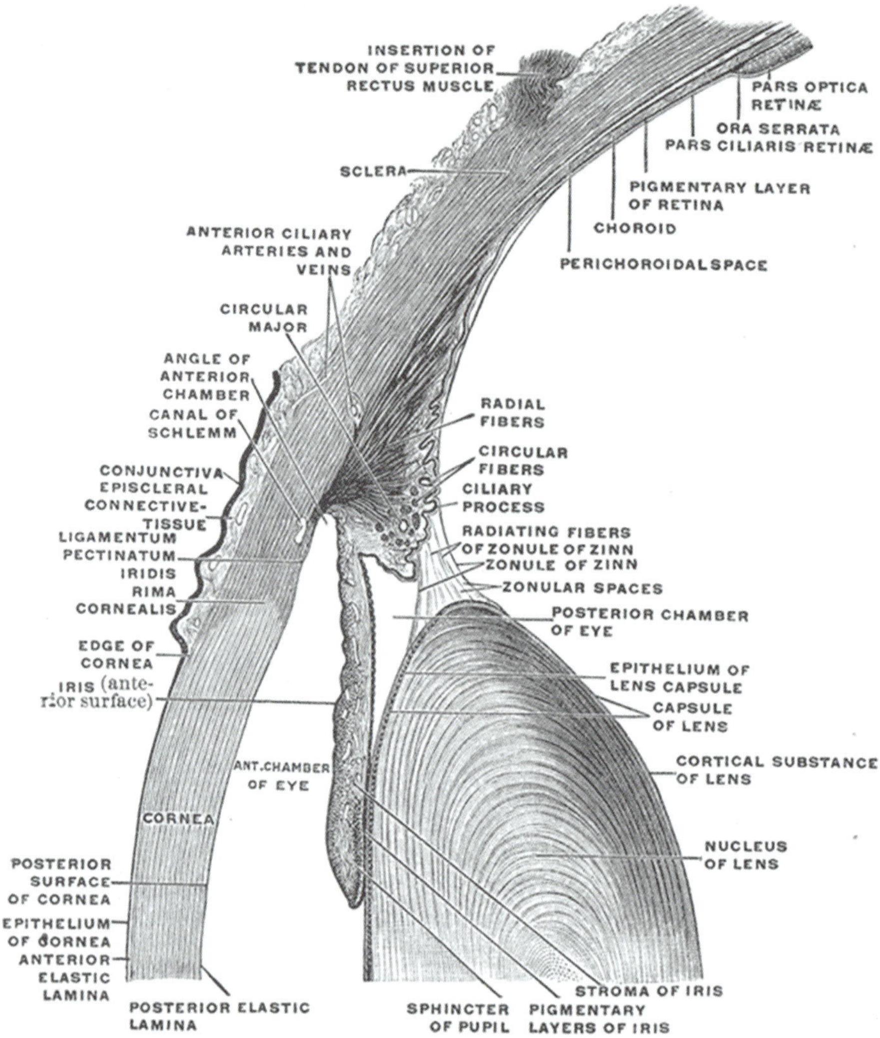

Figure 3.2 Detailed anatomy of the anterior segment of the eye and adjacent structures. Reproduced with permission from *Gray's Anatomy*.

Ultrahigh resolution OCT used for research purposes provides more detailed imaging of the choriocapillaris and choroid than standard commercially available OCT. While a standard ~800 nm light source can distinguish the major layers of the retina, the penetration of this wavelength to the choroid and choriocapillaris is limited by the optical scattering and absorbing properties of the RPE. The choriocapillaris is best visualized with ~1050 nm light, which undergoes less scattering and absorption by melanin and can provide additional diagnostic information despite a lower axial resolution [5]. The choriocapillaris appears on OCT as a highly backscattering layer with a mean thickness of 24 μm, with optical properties consistent with those of its blood-filled capillaries (Figure 3.4) [6].

Bruch's membrane

Bruch's membrane (BM) is positioned between the choriocapillaris and the RPE. It regulates the reciprocal exchange of nutrients and waste between the retina and general circulation. It normally increases in thickness with age [7]. According to some investigators, BM measures approximately 5 μm in thickness by OCT [8]. Others maintain that there is uncertainty

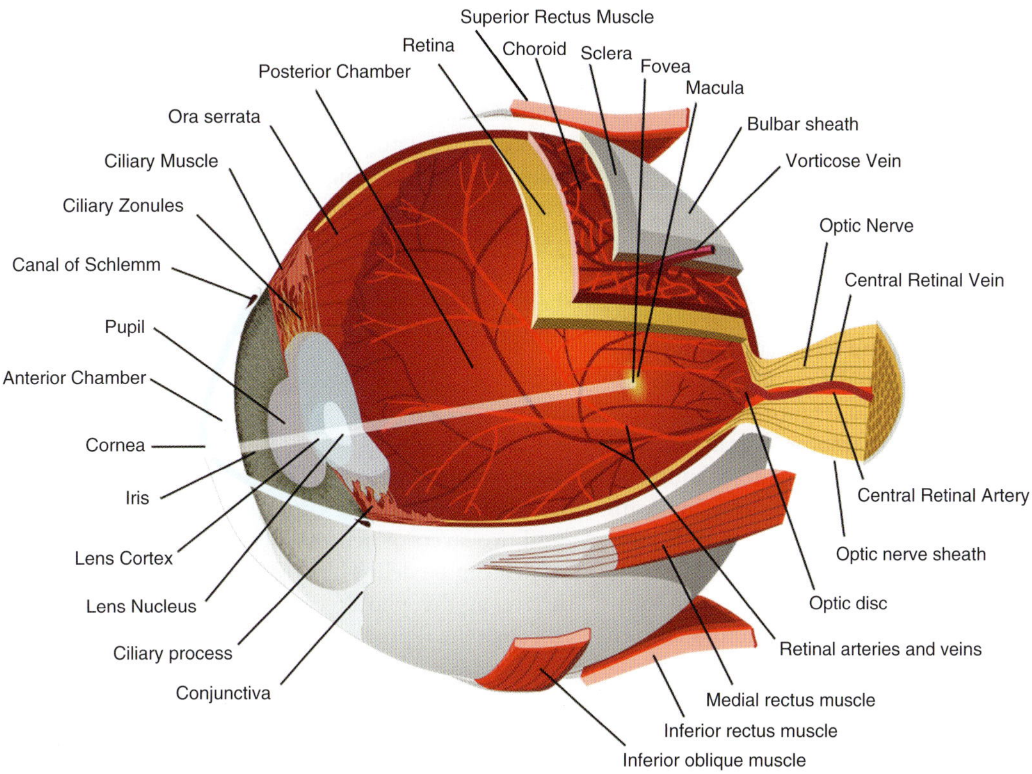

Figure 3.3 Anatomy of the human eye. Used with permission, Chabacano CC-SA 3.0.

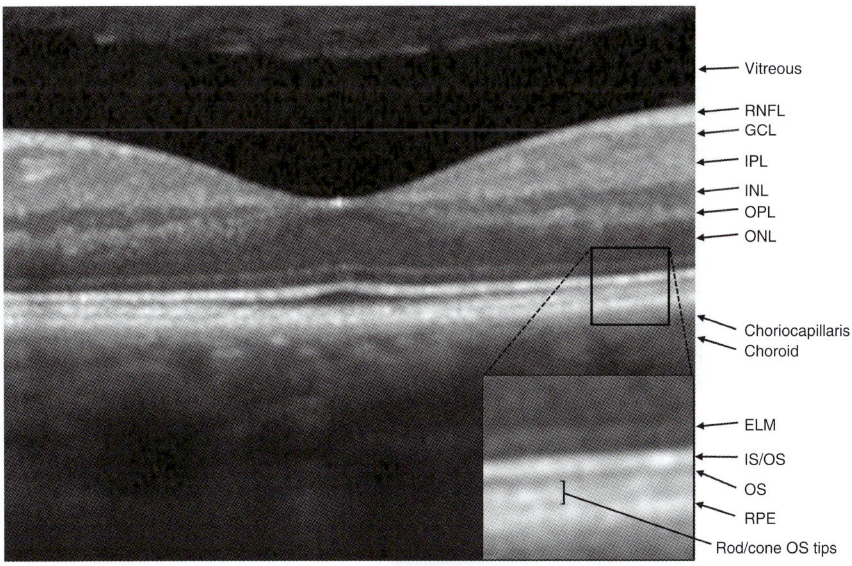

Figure 3.4 OCT of the fovea and identification of retinal layers. RNFL: Retinal nerve fiber layer; GCL: ganglion cell layer; OPL: outer plexiform layer; INL: inner nuclear layer; IPL: inner plexiform layer; ONL: outer nuclear layer; ELM: external limiting membrane; OS: photoreceptor outer segment; IS/OS: photoreceptor inner segment/outer segment junction; RPE: retinal pigment epithelium.

about the ability of OCT technology to resolve BM because its reported thickness is 1–5 μm and the axial resolution of ultrahigh resolution OCT is currently limited to 2–3 μm [9].

Retinal pigment epithelium (RPE)

The retinal pigment epithelium lies just below the photoreceptor layer in the retina, where its function is to provide metabolic and structural support for the photoreceptors. The RPE-choriocapillaris layer is present throughout the retina and terminates at the optic disc margin, where the choroidal circulation also terminates, at the lamina cribrosa (Figure 3.5). Light that is not absorbed by the photoreceptor layer is absorbed by the RPE, which contains the pigment melanin and prevents backscattered light from interfering with high-acuity vision in humans. The mean RPE layer thickness is 9 μm [6].

On first-generation OCT, the RPE and choriocapillaris were seen as indistinguishable components of a highly reflective layer (HRL) because these structures have similar optical properties and are in close proximity [10]. Later generations of OCT, however, demonstrated that the outer HRL has several components. The RPE may have a multilayer appearance on OCT due to differences in the length of cone and rod photoreceptor tips (Figure 3.4). Rods are longer and interdigitate with the RPE in the peripheral retina. Variation in the cone and rod distribution in the retina also influences the RPE's layered appearance [8]. The highly reflective nature of the RPE allows comparatively little light to pass through to the layers below. Below the choriocapillaris, the deep choroid and sclera are visible as weakly reflective layers.

Retina

Once light traverses the eye, it is focused on the neurosensory retina. The retina is traditionally divided into ten layers, including four cellular layers and two layers of neuronal interconnections, many of which can be delineated by OCT (Figure 3.4) [6]. To arrive at the photoreceptors, light must first pass through the retinal nerve fiber layer (RNFL), ganglion cell layer (GCL), inner plexiform layer (IPL), the amacrine, bipolar, and horizontal cells of the inner nuclear layer (INL), and the neuropil of the outer plexiform

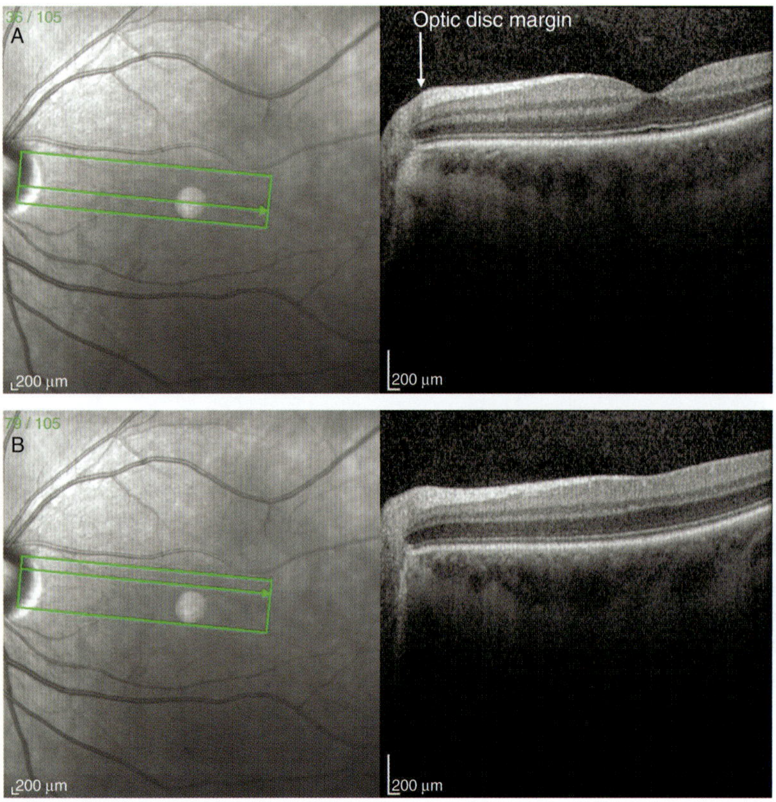

Figure 3.5 Papillomacular bundle OCT scan from the optic disc through the fovea (A) and perifoveal region (B). Note the increasing thickness of the retinal nerve fiber layer (RNFL) approaching the optic disc.

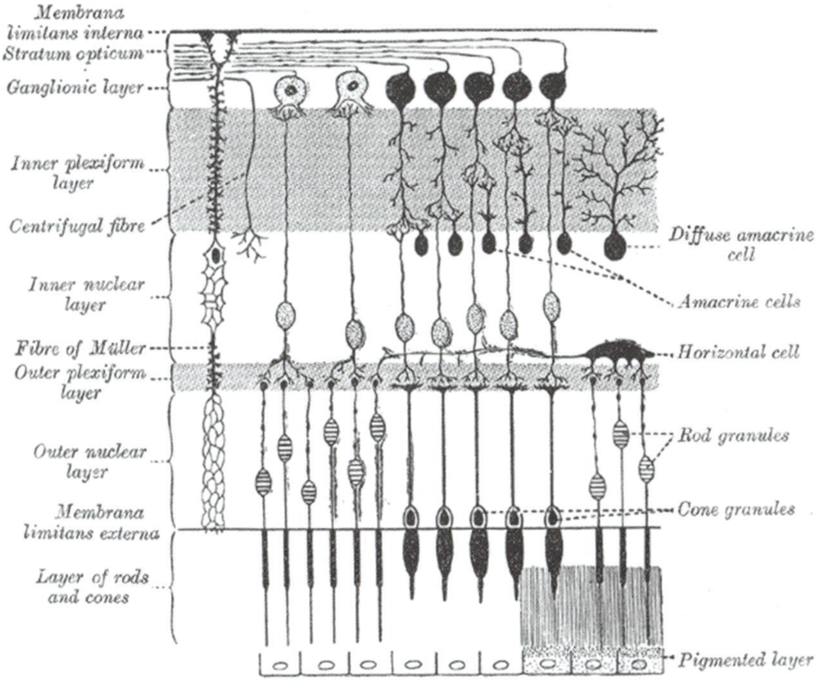

Figure 3.6 Schematic representation of retinal layers and their cellular components. The anterior retina, where light first reaches the retina, is at the top of the figure. Light passes through each of the layers before reaching the outer segments of the rod and cone photoreceptors, where the phototransduction cascade is initiated. Reproduced with permission from *Gray's Anatomy*.

layer (OPL) (Figure 3.6). The photoreceptors convert the electromagnetic energy of light into an electrochemical signal. Through a series of cellular connections, the signal is modified and relayed to ganglion cells, whose axons compose the retinal nerve fiber layer (RNFL) and serve as the final common output pathway of the retina.

The axial resolution of many commercially available OCT instruments is 4–7 μm. Generally, layers containing primarily cell bodies are weakly backscattering on OCT (dark), whereas layers containing primarily neuropil are highly backscattering (bright). In animal preparations, studies have demonstrated that many of the layers viewed on ultrahigh resolution OCT can be reliably correlated with histology [11]. The layers of the inner retina seen on OCT, extending from the vitreoretinal interface to the junction of the inner and outer photoreceptor segments (IS/OS junction), correlate well with histologic preparations of monkey retina [11].

Controversy persists, however, regarding the precise correlation between layers of the outer retina visualized on OCT (including the RPE, Bruch's membrane, and the choriocapillaris) and those demonstrated by histology [9]. For example, the strongest continuous backscattering signal in the outer retina on ultrahigh resolution OCT images has been interpreted as the RPE. While the optical properties of this backscattering layer are consistent with the RPE, some studies have reported that it appears thicker on OCT (up to 20–30 μm) [9] than on histologic sections (~9–12 ± 2 μm) [12]. On the other hand, other investigators report less of a discrepancy, with an average RPE thickness on OCT of 9 μm [6]. In the interpretation of retinal OCT images, it is important to recognize that OCT relies on differences in the optical properties of different retinal layers, whereas histology relies on postmortem tissue staining and light microscopy. While OCT provides extremely high spatial resolution, the correlation between these images and histology is likely to be imperfect.

Macula and fovea

The macula is located temporal to the optic nerve and measures approximately 5.5 mm in diameter. The macula is further divided into the fovea (1.5 mm in diameter) and foveola (0.35 mm). The fovea has up to 200,000 cones/mm^2 (nearly 15-fold higher than in peripheral retina) so that it can provide excellent visual acuity [13]. Furthermore, high-acuity vision is subserved by the unique synaptic configurations in the fovea, where each bipolar cell receives input from a single cone photoreceptor and each cone relays information to two ganglion cells [14]. The fovea contains an avascular center (0.4–0.6 mm in diameter) where photoreceptors can be densely packed without making provision for intervening capillaries. The foveal depression reaches its maximum depth at the center of the macula. Here, the inner layers of the retina, including the RNFL, GCL, OPL, INL, and IPL, taper and nearly disappear to allow light to directly stimulate the underlying cone photoreceptors without distortion. The ONL and photoreceptor outer segment layers become thicker in the foveal pit, reflecting this region's specialization for high spatial acuity. The fovea is readily identified using OCT and characterized by thinning of the anterior retina and dense aggregation of photoreceptors (Figure 3.4).

A map illustrating macular thickness in segments can be generated from a series of scans centered on the fovea. The thickness measurements are typically displayed in a segmented circular graph, with each segment colored to illustrate the relative thickness (Figure 3.10A and C).

Photoreceptors

After photons pass through the inner layers of the retina, including the GCL and INL and ONL layers, they reach the photoreceptors in the outer retina. There, they initiate a photochemical cascade that results in a change in the photoreceptor's firing rate. Humans possess four photoreceptor types: three cones and a rod. Each type of cone photoreceptor has a unique, optimal response to specific wavelengths of light, either short (blue), middle (green), or long (red). Rods, on the other hand, are saturated at natural light intensities and are incapable of discriminating colors; their higher sensitivity to light renders them effective for night vision (scotopic vision). The retinal photoreceptors are each made up of an outer segment, inner segment, nucleus, and synaptic ending. The membrane of the outer segment has a stacked-disc configuration that houses visual pigments, such as rhodopsin. The inner segment contains mitochondria and ribosomes, where opsin molecules are assembled to be relayed to the outer segment [15].

Ultrahigh resolution OCT has been able to characterize outer retinal morphology with impressive detail, even to the level of visualizing rod and cone outer segment tips [8]. A layer of minimal reflectivity (dark on OCT) just anterior to the RPE and choriocapillaris likely represents the outer segments (OS) of the retinal photoreceptors. This layer is thickest in the fovea, where there is an abundance of cone photoreceptors. Outside the fovea, the OS layer is less defined, because rods and cones with different outer segment lengths are mixed and give rise to a faintly layered appearance between the RPE and the inner segment/outer segment interface (IS/OS). The boundary between the inner and outer segments (IS/OS) is visible on OCT as a highly backscattering layer (bright on OCT) just anterior to the RPE (Figure 3.4). The backscattering nature of this layer suggests there is a difference in the refractive index of the outer and inner photoreceptor segments [8].

The distribution of cones and rods across the retina is highly skewed and directly reflects the specialized functions of the fovea and retinal periphery [16]. OCT demonstrates that the thickness of the photoreceptor layer is increased in the fovea, where there is a high concentration of cones with long outer segments to support high visual acuity. Photoreceptor inner and outer segment length both decrease with increasing distance from the foveola. The retinal periphery has lower concentrations of cones and is associated with lower visual acuity [8]. The tips of cone outer segments extend to the surface of the RPE in the foveola, but separate from the RPE with increasing distance from the foveal center.

Rods are virtually absent in the fovea; they are the dominant photoreceptor in the periphery, where they specialize in high sensitivity motion and light detection. Rod outer segment tips are longer than those of cones, extend to the RPE surface, and interdigitate with the RPE in the peripheral retina. The difference in outer segment length between rods and cones is demonstrated by bands visible on OCT just posterior to the IS/OS junction band, which correspond to the cone and rod outer segment tips (Figure 3.4). The distance between the IS/OS junction band and outer segment tips bands is believed to approximate the outer segment length [8].

Nuclear and plexiform layers

The neurosensory retina consists of three major layers: photoreceptors synapse with bipolar cells, which then relay their signal to ganglion cells. In addition, horizontal and amacrine cells form lateral connections between elements of these layers via direct excitatory or indirect inhibitory connections (Figure 3.6) [17]. While each bipolar cell receives input from a single photoreceptor in the fovea, bipolar cells in the retinal periphery summate the inputs from multiple photoreceptor cells to support more sensitive detection of light.

The nuclear layers of the retina exhibit an intermediate degree of backscattering of light and appear as varying shades of gray in grayscale OCT and as blue-black in false-color images. The three nuclear layers that can be discerned include the outer nuclear layer (ONL), inner nuclear layer (INL), and ganglion cell layer (GCL). The inner and outer plexiform layers, which contain mostly neuropil and dense synaptic connections, demonstrate greater optical backscattering.

The ONL is composed of cell bodies of rods and cones (Figure 3.5) and shares the optical properties of the other nuclear layers. The ONL increases in thickness at the fovea, despite reduced total retinal thickness. The external limiting membrane (ELM) is visualized with OCT as a thin, backscattering layer posterior to the ONL. It is not a physical membrane but probably represents a collection of junctions between photoreceptor cells and the supportive Müller cell processes. The membrane is situated between the photoreceptor cell body and the inner/outer segments of the photoreceptor.

The outer plexiform layer (OPL), also known as Henle's fiber layer, is somewhat thinner than the inner plexiform layer (IPL) and contains horizontal cell dendrites, bipolar cell dendrites, and photoreceptor axons (Figure 3.6). The synapses here represent the first integration of visual information in the retina. The OPL backscatters light to a moderate degree, resulting in a lighter gray layer on grayscale OCT and a mostly green layer in false-color images.

The inner nuclear layer (INL) is composed of the cell bodies of bipolar cells, amacrine cells, and horizontal cells (Figure 3.6). This layer is weakly backscattering, giving rise to a dark gray layer on grayscale OCT and a blue-black layer on false-color tomograms.

The inner plexiform layer (IPL) is found between the GCL and INL and contains neuropil made of ganglion cell dendrites, bipolar cell axons, and amacrine cell axons (Figure 3.6). The IPL is moderately backscattering on OCT images, producing a light gray layer on grayscale OCT and a blue-green layer on false-color images. The abundance of synapses in the IPL provides one of the last exchanges of visual information before being transmitted by the retinal ganglion cell axons to the lateral geniculate nuclei of the thalamus.

Ganglion cells serve as the final output pathway of visual information from the retina. There is a large convergence of information from the retinal photoreceptor cells, which include about 100 million rods and 4 million cones, to the approximately 1.2 million ganglion cells [14]. The majority of ganglion cell axons project to the lateral geniculate nucleus. There are three main types of ganglion cells, each with specialized functions in the detection of visual inputs. Anatomical differences underlie important physiological and functional differences in these types of cells. Eighty percent of ganglion cells are midget cells, 10% are parasol cells, and 10% are other types [15]. The fovea has a high concentration of midget ganglion cells. Via a narrow dendritic tree, these cells receive signals conveyed by a bipolar cell that has received inputs from a single cone. The GCL is made of ganglion cell bodies that lie just posterior to the retinal nerve fiber layer (RNFL). Like other nuclear layers in the retina, the GCL is weakly backscattering on OCT, giving rise to a dark gray layer on grayscale OCT and blue-black layer on false-color images. The GCL is thickest in the parafoveal region because of the high density of photoreceptors in the fovea, but decreases in thickness toward the optic disc (Figure 3.5A).

Retinal nerve fiber layer

The axons of ganglion cells travel in the retinal nerve fiber layer (RNFL), enter the optic nerve, travel through the chiasm and tract, and then finally synapse primarily in the lateral geniculate nucleus of the thalamus. Foveal ganglion cells send axons directly to the temporal aspect of the optic disc in the papillomacular bundle. The remaining temporal ganglion cell nerve axons are arranged on either side of the horizontal raphe and form arcuate bundles that course above and below the fovea and finally enter the superior and inferior portions of the optic nerve. Finally, axons

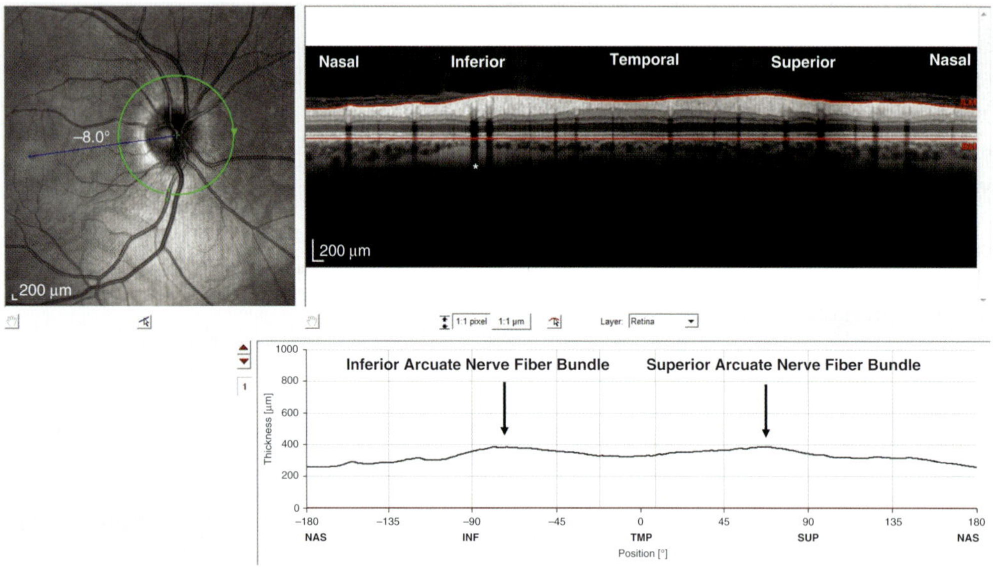

Figure 3.7 Circular peripapillary retina OCT scan. A scanning path with a 3.4 mm diameter (green circle) begins at the nasal retina (green arrowhead) and proceeds in a clockwise direction. The corresponding OCT image is displayed on the right with labeled retinal segments. Note the relative thickening of the retina superior and inferior to the optic disc, representing the superior and inferior arcuate nerve fiber bundles. The lower panel graphs the thickness of the peripapillary retina in a clockwise scan starting and ending in the nasal retina. The star (*) denotes an area of optical shadowing from an overlying blood vessel. NAS: nasal; INF: inferior; TMP: temporal; SUP: superior; INL: internal limiting membrane; BM: basement membrane.

originating nasal to the disc enter the nasal portion of the optic nerve.

The RNFL is highly backscattering, appearing as a bright layer on grayscale tomograms and as a red layer in false-color tomograms. It is the first layer of the retina encountered by the OCT beam and is found at the top of the computer-generated tomogram, immediately beneath the transparent vitreous. The RNFL varies in thickness with retinal location. As the axons of retinal ganglion cells travel toward the optic nerve head before forming the optic nerve, they accumulate and the RNFL thickness increases from the macula to the optic disc (Figure 3.5A) [4]. An increase in the slope of the retinal nerve fibers as they bend to form the optic nerve head causes a decrease in OCT signal. The retinal nerve fibers exhibit direction-dependent reflectance, with maximal reflectance observed when the nerve fibers are perpendicular to the OCT optical beam, as in the majority of the retina. In the macular region, the RNFL is thin because the bulk of the retina is occupied by densely packed photoreceptors.

Circular tomographs performed with a 1.5-disc diameter around the optic disc demonstrate a variation in RNFL thickness from 40 μm nasally to 230 μm superotemporally [10]. The superotemporal and inferotemporal bundling of nerve fibers are demonstrated by the increased RNFL thickness in these regions observed in circular tomographs (Figure 3.7).

OCT algorithms are capable of measuring the thickness of the RNFL. The standard for measurement of RNFL thickness is a circular scan around the optic disc (peripapillary region) (Figure 3.8). A diameter of 3.4 mm has been suggested as a standard size for the circle, as a diameter of 2.9 mm has been associated with lower reproducibility and a 4.5 mm circle captures a thinner part of the RNFL, which could potentially reduce the sensitivity of detection of small RNFL defects [18]. The normative database is also based upon 3.4 mm circular OCT scans. However, the optic disc margin is not perfectly circular, so a peripapillary scan path is not equidistant from the disc margin at all points, which is a potential source of error in these measurements. The RNFL is well known to increase in thickness approaching the optic disc, which may account for an increase in the RNFL thickness measured with a standard 3.4 mm circular scan in persons with larger optic discs [20]. OCT software facilitates RNFL comparisons between the two eyes, where even subtle asymmetries can be detected.

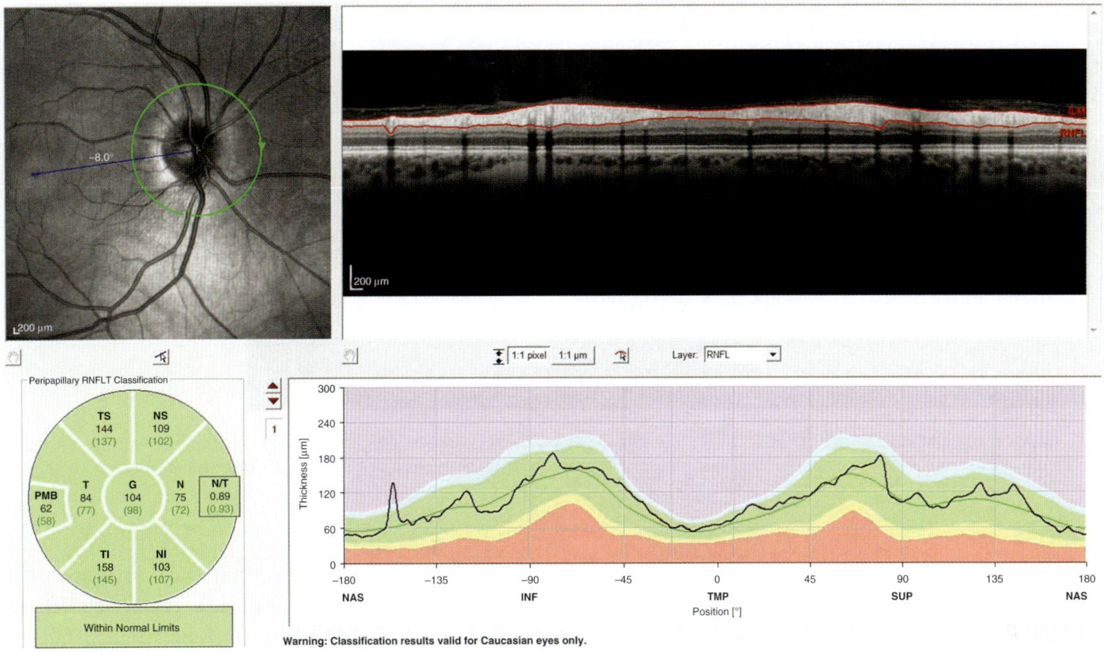

Figure 3.8 Measurement of peripapillary retinal nerve fiber layer (RNFL) thickness using OCT. Using a circular scan with a diameter of 3.4 mm centered in the optic disc (green line) measures one of the thickest regions of the RNFL, thereby increasing the scan's sensitivity. Thickness measurements can be plotted against age-matched normative data (bottom right). Purple: above normal limits ($p<0.01$); blue: borderline above normal limits ($p<0.05$); green: within normal limits ($p>0.05$); yellow: borderline below normal limits ($p<0.05$); red: below normal limits ($p<0.01$).

Retinal vasculature

The retinal blood supply is derived from the superior and inferior branches of the central retinal artery. Deoxygenated blood is collected from capillaries into venules that are posterior to the arteries and drain into the main retinal veins. These vessels travel on the anterior surface of the retina and are evident in tomographs as focal areas of increased backscatter that cast an optical shadow on deeper retinal structures (Figure 3.7, see star). Vascular structures found deeper in the optic nerve head are discussed below.

Optic nerve head complex

Each optic nerve is composed of approximately 1.2 million retinal ganglion cell axons (in contrast to the acoustic nerve, for example, which has only 31,000 axons) [21]. The intraocular segment of the optic nerve head (the optic disc) is typically located 3–4 mm nasal to the fovea and is 1 mm thick. The optic disc has a central depression, called the optic cup, which is typically 1/3 the size of the disc [22]. There are no retinal photoreceptors in the region of the optic disc, which gives rise to the monocular blind spot [23]. The optic nerve travels posteriorly through the lamina cribrosa to exit the back of the globe, where it abruptly increases in diameter from 3 mm to 4 mm.

The contour of the optic disc is easily visualized with OCT and demonstrates the normal optic cup and neuroretinal rim (Figure 3.9). The RPE, choriocapillaris, and photoreceptor layers terminate near the lamina cribrosa, and the site of termination can be used as a marker for the disc margin.

Because the retina is only about 0.5 mm thick, the axial dimension of OCT images is expanded to allow better visualization of the retinal layers (Figure 3.5). This expansion exaggerates the features of the optic nerve's head and cup, which must be interpreted with the appropriate axial and transverse scales. Disc diameter, cup diameter, neuroretinal rim area, and cup-to-disc ratio can be measured with OCT.

Detailed correlation between optic nerve head histology and SD-OCT images has been confirmed in monkeys [24]. Landmarks of the neural canal opening and the anterior lamina cribrosa were also

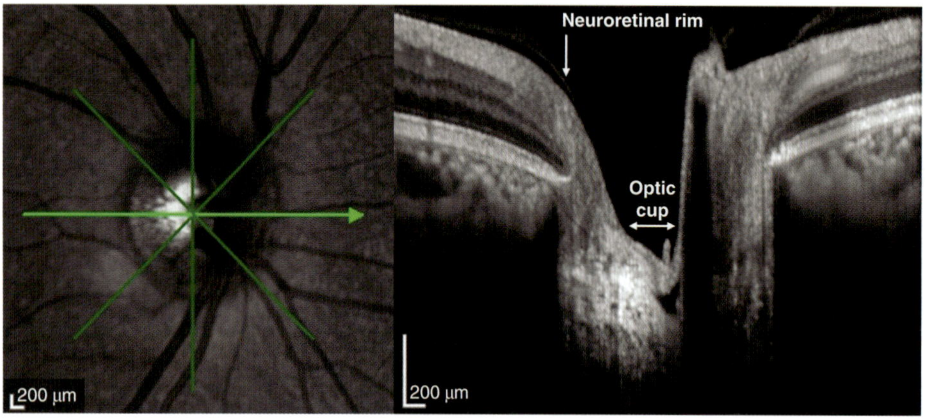

Figure 3.9 Optic nerve head appearance on OCT. The horizontal bold arrow depicts the scanning path used to obtain the image on the right. The abundance of vessels in the nasal half of the disc and the sharp increase in slope of the retinal nerve fibers entering the optic nerve cause a degradation of the OCT signal.

confirmed with histology, although deeper optic nerve head structures are not visualized as well by SD-OCT [24].

The lamina cribrosa (LC) is a mesh-like segment of the sclera with pores through which the retinal ganglion cell axons exit the eye to enter the optic nerve. SD-OCT imaging of the lamina cribrosa has recently been greatly improved by the use of adaptive optics (AO) and computer algorithms [25].

Deeper structures in the optic nerve complex have been traditionally difficult to image due in part to optical backscattering from the RPE. In addition, commercially available OCT machines are typically set up to preferentially image the retina. The sclera and deeper structures are visualized by a defocused, conical OCT imaging beam that widens after passing through the retina.

An imaging technique termed "enhanced depth imaging" (EDI) SD-OCT involves moving the OCT instrument closer to the eyes, allowing the focused OCT beam to image structures deep to the retina [26]. Deep vascular structures, such as the central retinal artery and vein and the short posterior ciliary arteries, can be identified using the EDI SD-OCT technique. The peripapillary choroid and sclera, and, less frequently, the subarachnoid space around the optic nerve, are also observed via EDI SD-OCT [27].

Automated quantitative retinal measurements

OCT is able to quantify retinal thickness by measuring the distance between retinal layers. There are highly reflective layers (HRL) on retinal OCT images at the inner and outer retinal boundaries. The first HRL, in the inner retina, represents the vitreoretinal surface or ILM, and the second HRL, in the outer retina, represents the RPE. The measurement between these layers is reported as the retinal thickness (Figure 3.10) [19].

Computer algorithms can automatically detect retinal layer boundaries to segment the internal structure of the retina and measure the thickness of some layers (Figure 3.8). Errors in boundary detection that occur with signal obscuration by vasculature or signal dropout are also corrected via computer algorithm [6]. In previous-generation OCT, errors in measuring the true anatomic retinal thickness were introduced by the software's inability to reliably distinguish between the RPE and the IS/OS junction as the outer retinal boundary [19]. However, the latest generation of ultrahigh resolution OCT is able to more reliably measure the actual retinal thickness from the RPE [28].

Computer algorithms are now able to reliably segment the retina into at least four layers at the macula: the RNFL, GCL + IPL, OPL + INL, and ONL + photoreceptor layers [29]. Although many of the individual component layers may be discerned by close visual inspection of OCT images, reliable segmentation algorithms are necessary to obtain standardized quantitative measurements for disease monitoring.

Three-dimensional OCT

Improvements in image acquisition speed with spectral-Fourier-domain (SD/FD) detection and

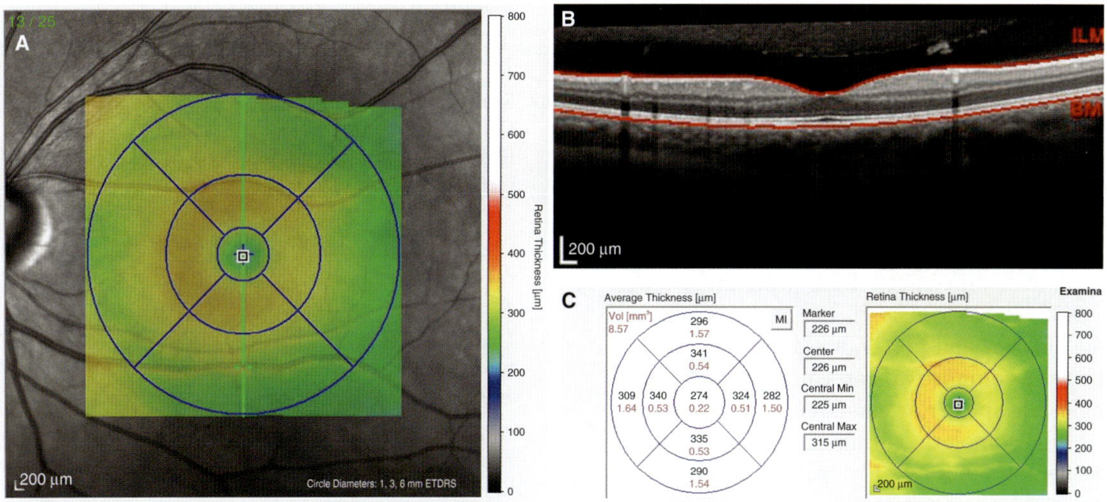

Figure 3.10 Measurement of retinal thickness using OCT. (A) A combination of vertical scanning paths (green line) are used to generate a map of the fovea and surrounding retina. (B) A segmentation computer algorithm measures the distance between the inner and outer boundaries of the retina: the basement membrane (BM) and the internal limiting membrane (ILM), respectively (red lines). (C) The data is used to generate a topographic map, with color coding of retinal thickness across various segments.

other advances in OCT technology have paved the way for three dimensional OCT images. The 50–100-fold increase in speed with SD/FD detection allows many closely spaced scans to be performed, which may cover the fovea, for example, and be used to assemble a volumetric map of the area imaged. Software programs enable 3-D renderings that can be rotated and viewed from any angle, or even dissected so that individual layers can virtually be removed. 3-D OCT can also provide data for quantitative mapping of individual retinal layers.

Future OCT applications

Variations of the application of OCT technology have allowed the extraction of functional information from the eye. One example is Doppler OCT, in which specialized techniques permit the calculation of the Doppler shift due to moving blood with flow sensitivities on the order of tens of micrometers/second. Arteries and veins can be distinguished and quantitative imaging of retinal blood flow can be performed, even of individual vessels [9]. The term "optical coherence angiography" has been given to the use of Doppler OCT to generate 3-D visualization of retinal vasculature [30]. Doppler OCT methods enable measurements of blood flow within the retinal vasculature, but they are unable to assess vascular permeability and leakage, as with traditional fluorescein angiography.

Some of the latest OCT techniques have demonstrated the ability to assess retinal physiology (termed "optophysiology") in addition to structure. Interestingly, physiologic processes that occur at the cellular level, such as depolarization and changes in cellular swelling, can cause small changes in a retinal cell's optical properties, which can be detected with OCT. For example, changes in the optical backscattering of the photoreceptor outer segment layer can be detected following a single flash of light [8]. The clinical application of this technology requires further research and validation.

Recent technological developments have introduced adaptive optics (AO), which allow for correction of chromatic aberrations inherent to the human eye that have limited the ability of OCT to resolve individual cells in the retina. AO restore the ability of OCT to see even the conic shape of the cone outer segments in some cases. Images using AO have estimated the width of a cone to be ~4 µm, as they are in histologic sections [9]. AO has also allowed visualization of the lamina cribrosa with commercially available OCT, although further research is needed to establish the utility of AO OCT for other clinical applications.

Conclusion

The anatomy of the anterior visual pathways is well-visualized using currently available OCT technology. Research has demonstrated good correlation between OCT retinal layers and retinal histopathology [11]. Nevertheless, as OCT relies on differences in optical properties and histopathology relies on light microscopy and fixed tissue staining to generate contrast, there are small differences. Even with these differences, OCT is able to discern important features of both the anterior and posterior segments of the eye, including the conjunctiva, cornea, anterior chamber and angle, lens, posterior chamber, retina, and optic nerve head complex. Ultrahigh resolution OCT approaches the ability of histopathology to resolve retinal details and approximates a "living biopsy" by which detailed anatomic information can be obtained. Beyond the ability to produce exquisite structural images, the adaptation of OCT technology to extract functional, physiologic information from the eyes suggests exciting future applications for OCT in anterior visual pathway imaging.

References

1. Huang D, Swanson EA, Lin CP, et al. Optical coherence tomography. *Science* 1991; **254**: 1178–81.
2. Kagemann L, Wollstein G, Ishikawa H. Visualization of the conventional outflow pathway in the living human eye. *Ophthalmology* 2012; **119**: 1563–8.
3. Riordan-Eva P. Chapter 1. Anatomy & embryology of the eye. In: Riordan-Eva P, Cunningham, Jr. ET, eds. *Vaughan & Asbury's General Ophthalmology*. 18th ed. New York: McGraw-Hill; 2011. http://www.accessmedicine.com/content.aspx?aID=55780501. Accessed May 22, 2013.
4. Wollstein G, Folio LS, Nevins JE, et al. Chapter 2. Interpretation of the optical coherence tomography image. In: Schuman JS, Puliafito CA, Fujimoto JG, Duker JS, eds. *Optical Coherence Tomography of Ocular Diseases*. 3rd ed. Thorofare, NJ: SLACK Incorporated; 2013.
5. Považay B, Herman B, Unterhuber A, et al. Three-dimensional optical coherence tomography at 1050 nm versus 800 nm in retinal pathologies: enhanced performance and choroidal penetration in cataract patients. *J Biomed Optics* 2007; **12**: 041211.
6. Drexler W, Morgner U, Ghanta RK, et al. Ultrahigh-resolution ophthalmic optical coherence tomography. *Nat Med* 2001; 7: 502–7 (Erratum in: *Nat Med* 2001; 7: 636).
7. Booij JC, Baas DC, Beisekeeva J, et al. The dynamic nature of Bruch's membrane. *Prog Retin Eye Res* 2010; **29**: 1–18.
8. Srinivasan VJ, Monson BK, Wojtkowski M, et al. Characterization of outer retinal morphology with high-speed, ultra-high resolution optical coherence tomography. *Invest Ophthalmol Vis Sci* 2008; **49**: 1571–9.
9. Drexler W, Fujimoto JG. State-of-the-art retinal optical coherence tomography. *Prog Ret Eye Res* 2008; **27**: 45–88.
10. Hee MR, Izatt JA, Swanson EA, et al. Optical coherence tomography of the human retina. *Arch Ophthalmol* 1995; **113**: 325–32.
11. Anger EM, Unterhuber A, Hermann B, et al. Ultrahigh resolution optical coherence tomography of the monkey fovea. Identification of retinal sublayers by correlation with semithin histology sections. *Exp Eye Res* 2004; **78**: 1117–25.
12. Spraul CW, Lang GE, Grossniklaus HE. Morphometric analysis of the choroid, Bruch's membrane, and retinal pigment epithelium in eyes with age-related macular degeneration. *Inv Ophth & Vis Sci* 1996; **37**: 2724–35.
13. Hirsch J,d Curcio CA. The spatial resolution capacity of human foveal retina. *Vision Res* **29**: 1095–101.
14. Rosenzweig MR, Breedlove SM, Leiman AL. *Biological Psychology* 3rd Edition, Sunderland, MA: Sinauer Associates, Inc. 2002; Chapter 10, pp. 288–93.
15. Prasad S, Galetta SL. Anatomy and physiology of the afferent visual system. *Handb Clin Neurol* 2011; **102**: 3–19.
16. Osterberg G. Topography of the layer of rods and cones in the human retina. *Acta Ophthalmol* 1935; **13**: 1–103.
17. Flores-Herr N, Protti DA, Wassle H. Synaptic currents generating the inhibitory surround of ganglion cells in the mammalian retina. *J Neurosci* 2001; **21**: 4852–63.
18. Schuman JS, Pedut-Kloizman T, Hertzmark E, et al. Reproducibility of nerve fiber layer thickness measurements using optical coherence tomography. *Ophthalmology* 1996; **103**: 1889–98.
19. Costa RA, Skaf M, Melo Jr LAS, et al. Retinal assessment using optical coherence tomography. *Prog Ret Eye Res* 2006; **25**: 325–53.
20. Savini G, Zanini M, Carelli V, et al. Correlation between retinal nerve fibre layer thickness and optic nerve head size: an optical coherence tomography study. *Br J Ophthalmol* 2005; **89**: 489–92.
21. Bruesch SR, Arey LB. The number of myelinated and unmyelinated fibers in the optic nerve of vertebrates. *J Comp Neurol* 1942; 77: 631–655.

22. Jonas JB, Gusek GC, Naumann GO. Optic disc, cup and neuroretinal rim size, configuration and correlations in normal eyes. *Invest Ophthalmol Vis Sci* 1988; **29**: 1151–8.

23. Mariotte LA. A new discovery touching vision. *Phil Trans R Soc Lond* 1668; **3**: 668–71.

24. Strouthidis NG, Grimm J, Williams GA, Cull GA, Wilson DJ, Burgoyne CF. A Comparison of optic nerve head morphology viewed by spectral domain optical coherence tomography and by serial histology. *Invest Ophthalmol Vis Sci* 2010; **51**: 1464–74.

25. Kim TW, Kagemann L, Girard MJ, et al. Imaging of the lamina cribrosa in glaucoma: perspectives of pathogenesis and clinical Applications. *Curr Eye Res* 2013; **38**: 903–909.

26. Spaide RF, Koizumi H, Pozonni MC. Enhanced depth imaging spectral-domain optical coherence tomography. *Am J Ophthalmol* 2008; **146**: 496–500.

27. Park SC, De Moraes CG, Teng CC, Tello C, Liebmann JM, Ritch R. Enhanced depth imaging optical coherence tomography of deep optic nerve complex structures in glaucoma. *Ophthalmology* 2012; **119**: 3–9.

28. Wojtkowski M, Srinivasan VJ, Fugimoto JG, et al. Three-dimension retinal imaging with high-speed ultrahigh-resolution optical coherence tomography. *Ophthalmology* 2005; **112**: 1734–46.

29. Walter SD, Ishikawa H, Galetta KM, et al. Ganglion cell loss in relation to visual disability in multiple sclerosis. *Ophthalmology* 2012; **119**: 1250–7.

30. Makita S, Hong Y, Yamanari M, et al. Optical coherence angiography. *Opt Express* 2006; **14**: 7821–40.

Chapter 4

Optical coherence tomography in acute optic neuritis

Andrew P. D. Henderson, S. Anand Trip, and David H. Miller

Background

Optic neuritis usually refers to a symptomatic attack of inflammatory demyelination of the optic nerve. This is usually of acute onset and presents with painful loss of vision, which worsens over several days, and recovers (partially or completely) over several months. In Western countries, the most common form of optic neuritis is that associated with multiple sclerosis (acute idiopathic optic neuritis), but there are other forms of optic neuritis (such as that associated with neuromyelitis optica (NMO), and chronic relapsing inflammatory optic neuropathy (CRION) [1, 2]). Optic neuritis is highly associated with multiple sclerosis. Approximately 50% of all patients with multiple sclerosis have optic neuritis at some point in the course of their disease, and for many patients, it is the first clinical episode.

The annual incidence of acute idiopathic optic neuritis in temperate climates is approximately 5 per 100,000. Although optic neuritis can occur at any age, the peak incidence is in the fourth decade of life, and women outnumber men approximately three to one [3, 4].

Most commonly, optic neuritis is unilateral. The usual symptoms of optic neuritis are periorbital pain (which may precede the onset of visual loss noted by the patient), pain on eye movement, and reduction in vision (both central and peripheral). Patients with optic neuritis may also experience positive visual phenomena (phosphenes), usually provoked by eye movement. Particularly in the recovery phase of the illness, patients may notice temporary worsening of vision accompanied by elevations in body temperature (a type of Uhthoff's phenomenon). The pain typically lasts only a few days, and the visual loss may worsen for up to two weeks before recovery ensues.

Visual acuity is nearly universally diminished by optic neuritis. The effect may range from mild to no perception of light, although moderate impairment is more common than either severe or mild impairment [5]. Color vision is almost always affected by optic neuritis, even after visual recovery. In the Optic Neuritis Treatment Trial (ONTT), 84% of patients had detectable abnormalities when using Ishihara pseudoisochromatic plates, and the Farnsworth-Munsell 100 Hue test was abnormal in 94% [6]. Although the typical description of the visual loss of optic neuritis is of a centrocaecal scotoma, any visual field deficit may occur. In the ONTT, the most common visual field defect noted by automated perimetry was a diffuse reduction in sensitivity in the affected eye, followed by altitudinal or other nerve fiber bundle defects. Central or centrocaecal scotomas were only seen in 8.2% of patients at presentation [7]. There is almost always a detectable relative afferent pupillary defect in acute optic neuritis [8]; the exceptions to this are if there has been a previous attack of optic neuritis in the fellow eye and the afferent arms of the pupillary light reflex are equally affected. Approximately one third of patients with optic neuritis will have detectable swelling of the optic disc on fundoscopy (i.e., pappilitis) [5].

The prognosis for visual recovery after optic neuritis is usually good. In the ONTT, the median visual acuity after twelve months was 20/16, and 95% of patients had a visual acuity of 20/40 or better. Even for patients with a visual acuity of 20/200 or worse at study entry, 84% had a visual acuity of 20/40 or better at one year [9]. Notwithstanding these favorable prognostic outcomes, we now know that many people with optic neuritis sustain significant and persistent loss of low contrast letter acuity, and retinal nerve fiber layer

Optical Coherence Tomography in Neurological Disease, ed. Peter A. Calabresi, Laura J. Balcer, and Elliot M. Frohman. Published by Cambridge University Press.

thickness (RNFL) reductions, both of which carry important ramifications for visual impairment in low light settings (e.g., driving at night; edge detection such as when walking stairs).

In adults, optic neuritis is usually unilateral, but approximately 10% of all optic neuritis is bilateral, either simultaneous or occurring in short succession [10]. The optic neuritis associated with neuromyelitis optica is more often bilateral. This should be distinguished from the phenomenon in unilateral acute optic neuritis (i.e., unilateral symptoms), where changes in the visual field can be identified on formal examination in the fellow eye; in the ONTT, 48% of patients had some abnormality detected in the fellow eye [11].

There are also chronic and subclinical forms of optic neuritis. The chronic form, which should not be diagnosed without excluding compressive lesions on neuroimaging, can occur as the presenting symptom of multiple sclerosis [12] or develop later in the course of the disease [13].

Retinal nerve fiber layer (RNFL) imaging using fundus photography

Hoyt and colleagues [14] identified visible nerve fiber layer defects in the symptomatic eye of a 30-year-old woman with probable optic neuritis. Following this, Frisén and Hoyt [15] were the first to identify changes in the retina in multiple sclerosis; they described two patients with evidence of retinal nerve fiber layer (RNFL) loss without evidence of clinically overt acute optic neuritis. They identified these now recognized cardinal features of optic neuropathy, while utilizing a hand-held ophthalmoscope using red-free illumination, and illustrated their findings in a paper using red-free photography.

Sharpe and Sanders [16] found that retinal nerve fiber layer defects, which were more conspicuous due to hypermyelination of the patient's retinal nerve fibers (the retinal axons that contribute to 80% of the composition of the retinal nerve fiber layer are typically unmyelinated, until they make their passage through the lamina cribrosa, at which point they achieve oligodendrocyte-derived myelination), in a patient with bilateral optic neuritis in the context of multiple sclerosis (see Figure 4.1). Elbøl and Work [17] examined red-free retinal photographs of 20 patients with multiple sclerosis, seven of whom had a prior history of optic neuritis. In the nine eyes with a past history of optic neuritis, eight had visible RNFL defects, and five eyes had visual field defects. MacFadyen and colleagues [18] described the retinal and electrophysiological findings in 57 patients with multiple sclerosis, half of whom had a history of optic neuritis. Of the 27 eyes with a clinical history of optic neuritis, 17 had detectable RNFL defects.

Unfortunately, although examination of the RNFL is possible with a hand-held ophthalmoscope, an approximately 50% loss of axons is required before RNFL changes are visible [19], and the loss is not readily quantifiable.

Retinal nerve fiber layer changes in optic neuritis using optical coherence tomography

Parisi and colleagues [20] examined 14 patients with multiple sclerosis, all of whom had a prior episode of optic neuritis with complete visual recovery. Using early generation optical coherence tomography (i.e., time-domain OCT), they found that peripapillary RNFL thickness was significantly reduced in eyes affected by optic neuritis when compared with healthy control eyes, and was also reduced in clinically unaffected fellow eyes but to a lesser extent. This study did not attempt to find an association with clinical tests of visual function and did not study the macula using OCT.

Trip and colleagues [21] used Stratus OCT (Carl Zeiss Meditech, Palo Alto, CA) to study 25 patients with a history of a single previous attack of optic neuritis and poor visual recovery, comparing their affected eye with their clinically unaffected fellow eye, and with the eyes of 15 healthy control subjects. They found significant reductions of RNFL thickness (68.7 μm in affected eyes vs 94.6 μm in fellow eyes vs 102.9 μm in control eyes) and macular volume (6.10 mm^3 in affected eyes vs 6.71 mm^3 in fellow eyes vs 6.83 mm^3 in control eyes) in the affected eyes of patients, when compared with both their clinically unaffected fellow eye and the eyes of control subjects. Reduced RNFL thickness was significantly correlated with worse visual function for LogMAR acuity, Humphrey visual field mean deviation, and color vision. Reduced macular volume correlated with reduced color vision, but not with reduced overall field sensitivity, nor with visual acuity.

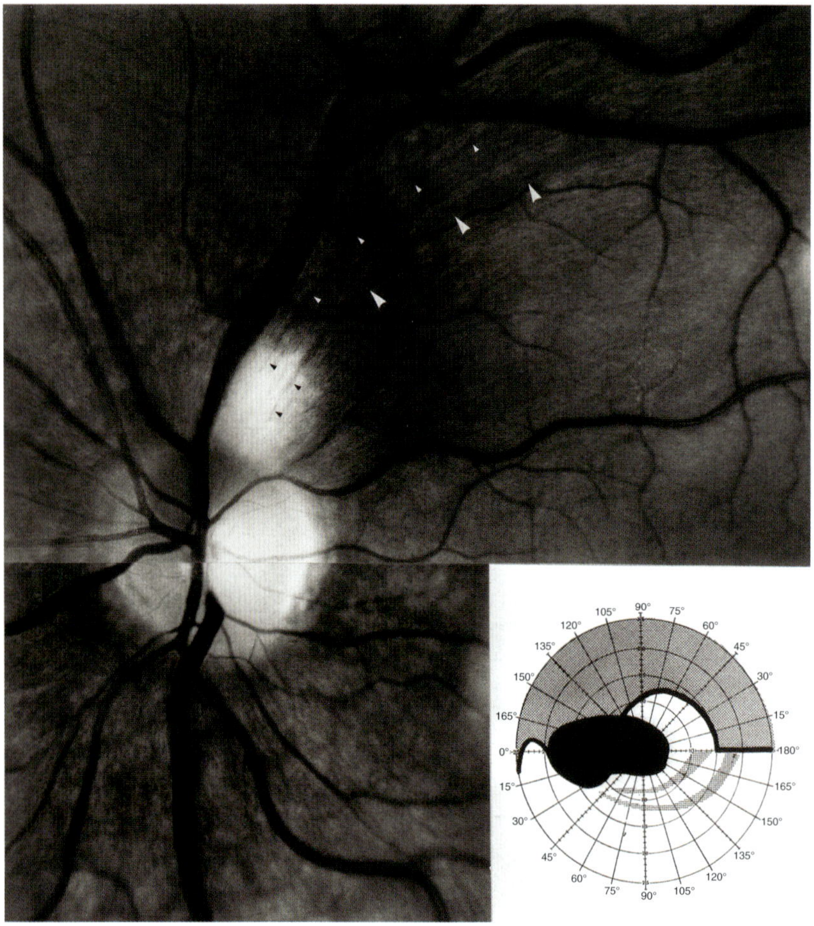

Figure 4.1 This image demonstrates RNFL defects visible on red-free photography in the left eye of a patient with optic neuritis in association with multiple sclerosis. There are visual field defects in areas of the visual field corresponding to the visible RNFL defects. From Sharpe and Sanders [16].

Costello and colleagues studied 54 patients recruited within one month of onset of an attack of optic neuritis and found reductions in the retinal nerve fiber layer of the affected eyes when compared with that of the fellow eyes of the same group (77.5 μm in the affected vs 99.8 μm for the fellow eye) [26]. Lower RNFL values were correlated with worse visual field mean sensitivity, and those patients with worse vision had significantly lower RNFL values. The authors hypothesized that the majority of the RNFL thinning would be evident by between three and six months after the acute attack, although they were not able to analyze their data to calculate the time to first detectable thinning.

Since these papers, several other authors have replicated the findings in the chronic stage, long after an attack of optic neuritis, when vision is stable (see Table 4.1 and Figure 4.2). Petzold and colleagues [2] have performed a meta-analysis of most of these studies. They found that the mean loss of RNFL thickness due to optic neuritis was 20.38 μm, using the fellow eye as a baseline comparator. This may be an overestimate due to ascertainment bias in early studies of acute optic neuritis, and some patients may have significantly less thinning.

In some patients, recurrent attacks of optic neuritis are associated with further reductions in RNFL thickness, and thereby depletion of optic nerve axons [22–24], suggesting that inflammation *per se* is involved in axonal degeneration, in addition to any effects mediated by compression of the optic nerve against the inelastic optic nerve sheath, or within the bony optic nerve canal.

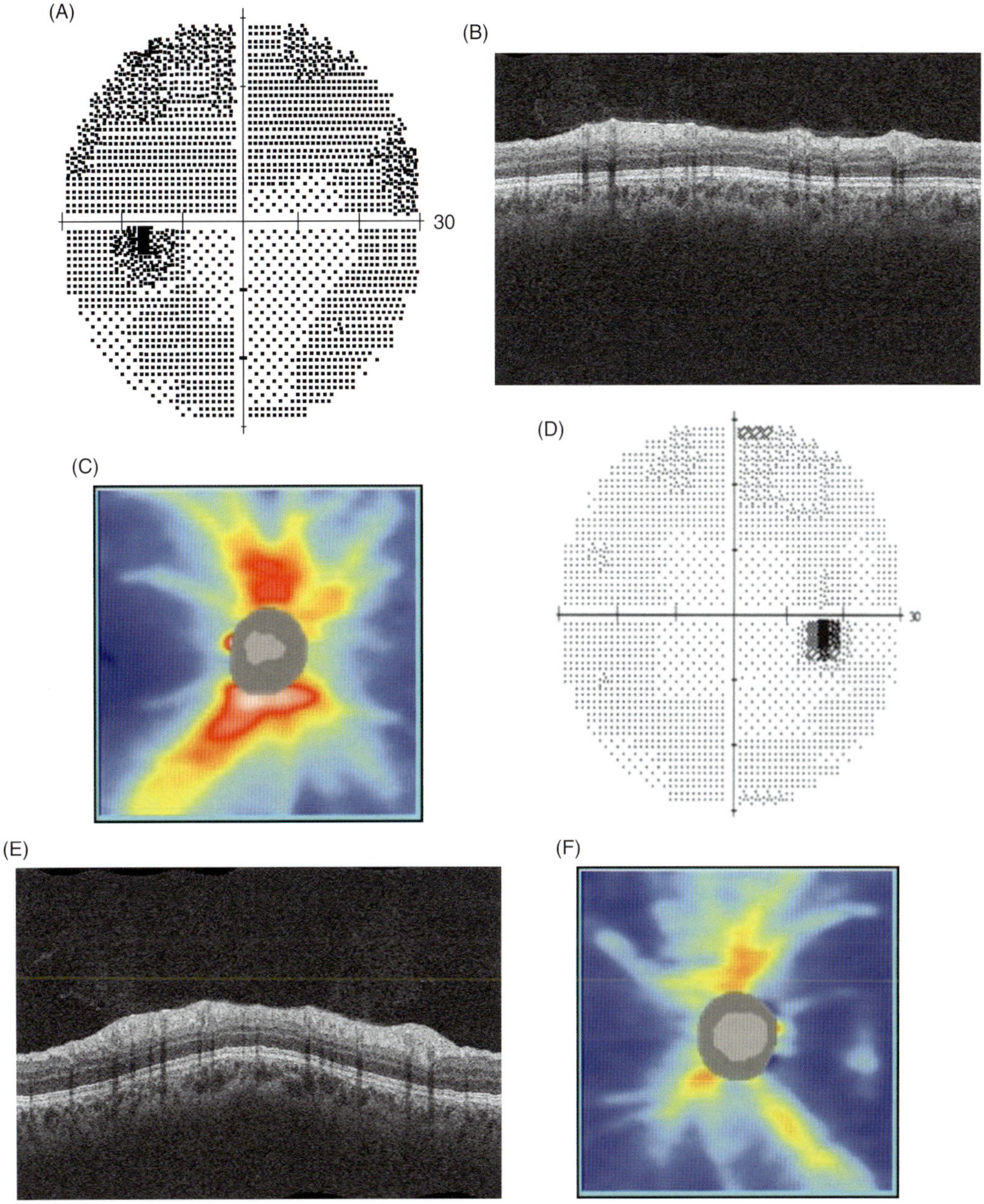

Figure 4.2 Visual fields (A. and D.), OCT images of the circumpapillary retina (B. and E.), and RNFL thickness maps of the peripapillary retina (C. and F.) in a 20-year-old woman four months after unilateral left-sided optic neuritis associated with multiple sclerosis.

The visual acuity in the right eye was 6/5 and in the left eye was 6/6. There is reduced RNFL thickness on the left (circumpapillary RNFL thickness 72 μm compared with 109 μm on the right), despite good visual recovery.

Changes in the macula and deep layers of the retina

Trip and colleagues [21], in their cohort of optic neuritis patients selected for poor recovery, found that the overall macular volume in the affected eye was reduced when compared to that of the fellow eye (6.10 mm^3 in affected eyes vs 6.71 mm^3 in unaffected patient eyes) and also when compared to that of healthy control eyes (6.83 mm^3). Pulicken and colleagues [28] found reduced macular volume in the eyes of subjects with a history of optic neuritis, in a cohort

Table 4.1 RNFL findings after optic neuritis

	Optic neuritis		Fellow eyes		Healthy control	
	Mean (SD)	**n**	**Mean (SD)**	**n**	**Mean (SD)**	**n**
Trip (2005) [21]	68.7 (18.8)	25	94.6 (14.9)	25	102.9 (14.6)	15
Fisher (2006) [25]	85 (17)	63	–*	–	105 (12)	72
Costello (2006) [26]	77.5	54	99.8	54	–	–
Albrecht (2007) [27]	74.47 (22.15)	21	–	–	103.4 (10.96)	11
Pulicken (2007) [28]	84.2 (14.7)	62	93.9 (13.1)	62	102.7 (11.5)	47
Pueyo (2008) [29]	84.46	25 (eyes)	94.2	75 (eyes)	104.97	25 (eyes)
Zaveri (2008) [30]**	81.8 (19.3)	41	95.6 (15.0)	48	104.6 (10.3)	43
Klistorner (2008) [31]	84.5 (15.1)	32	103.8 (10.8)	32	104.0 (9.2)	25
Siger (2008) [32]	83.9 (17.6)	20	91.08 (19.3)	20	100.3 (12.1)	12
Frohman (2009) [33]	70.3 (13.4)	12	101.8 (6.0)	12	101.9 (8.9)	8
Ratchford (2009) [34]	88.3 (2009)	155	–	–	102.4	77
Burkholder (2009) ** [35]	85.7 (19.0)	164 (328 eyes)	95.6 (14.5)	366 (730 eyes)	104.5 (10.7)	111
Bock (2010) {Bock:2010 da}	86.2 (16.2)	73 (eyes)	97.0 (13.1)	189 (eyes)	105.2 (9.4)	203
Garcia-Martin et al. (2011) [36]	81.2	34	94.9	34	–	–
Syc (2012) [37]	78.7 (11.7)	73 (eyes)	84.9 (12.2)	123 (eyes)	93.4 (10.4)	100
Costello et al. (2012) [38]	90.8 (16.9) Females 73.5 (14.0) Males	105 (Females) 39 (Males)	103.4 (14.0) Females 100.1 (13.8) Males	105 (F) 39 (M)	–	–
Monteiro et al. (2012) [39]	94.6 (19.0)	45 (eyes)	101.2 (11.6)	74 (eyes)	107.6 (9.4)	82 (eyes)

* Direct comparison between patients with one eye affected not published
** Some patients had bilateral optic neuritis; fellow eyes have no clinical history of optic neuritis but the whole cohort had confirmed multiple sclerosis.

of patients with multiple sclerosis, as did Ratchford and colleagues [34]. Macular volume encompasses the whole retina from the vitreoretinal interface to the retinal pigment epithelium, and a reduction in volume likely reflects loss of other components of the retina rather than simply the RNFL.

We have observed small degrees of whole macular swelling in patients in the early phases of acute idiopathic optic neuritis, to a lesser extent than is visible in the RNFL, and it is usually only notable when the affected eye is compared to the unaffected fellow eye.

Gelfland and colleagues [40] reported the appearance of macular microcysts in the retina of patients with multiple sclerosis. Of the 318 patients studied, 15 (3.8%) had small lucencies in the deep layers of the retina. The microcysts, which they termed microcystic macular edema, occurred principally in the inner nuclear layer of the retina and were more common in eyes with a past history of optic neuritis, and were associated with greater thinning of the RNFL, and with a lower visual acuity. Microcystic macular edema was also associated with greater disability and more rapid progression. Saidha and colleagues [41] reported cystic changes in the macula of some of their patients (10/164, 6% of patients had microcysts evident on OCT). These changes were also associated with worse visual function and higher MS severity scores (although not higher disability as measured by the Expanded Disability Status Scale; EDSS). The presence of NMO is associated with worse vision, and in multiple sclerosis, with markers of increased disease activity such as increased contrast enhancing and T2 lesion formation. It is not clear what microcystic macular edema represents pathologically or pathophysiologically, as it is seen in other inflammatory optic neuropathies [42,43] and non-inflammatory optic neuropathies [44]. It may be that it represents only a marker of severity, perhaps related to trans-synaptic degenerative mechanisms [45]. Kaushik and colleagues [46] found inner nuclear layer thickening and retinal ganglion cell layer thinning to be inversely proportional, and proposed that inner nuclear layer thickening was on a spectrum which included microcysts of the inner nuclear layer at the more severe end.

Pathologic studies of the retina in patients with multiple sclerosis demonstrate that, in addition to atrophy of the RNFL, there is thinning of the ganglion cell layer and inner nuclear layers [47, 48]. Early forms of OCT lacked sufficient tissue penetration properties to quantify these changes, whereas spectral-domain OCT allows examination of the outer retinal layers such as the ganglion cell layer and the inner nuclear layer. Syc and colleagues [37] examined patients with multiple sclerosis, patients with neuromyelitis optica, and healthy controls, and they found reductions in a combined measure of the ganglion cell layer and inner plexiform layer (GCL/IPL) in eyes with a history of optic neuritis in their cohort of patients with multiple sclerosis when compared to control eyes and to eyes without a history of optic neuritis. They also serially studied a group of patients with acute optic neuritis and found that GCL/IPL thinning was evident at three months after the onset of symptoms. There was no swelling apparent in these layers of the retina, raising the possibility that atrophy of these layers of the retina might be detectable earlier than in the RNFL, where edema confounds early detection of tissue atrophy.

The time course of changes to RNFL and macula

In the early phases of optic neuritis there may be swelling of the RNFL [31,49,50] (see Figure 4.3). Although RNFL swelling is not evident in all cases of optic neuritis, RNFL measurement by OCT is more sensitive for the detection of RNFL swelling than fundoscopy, and is in keeping with the optic nerve swelling observed on MRI [51]. Studies using scanning laser polarimetry, which utilizes the birefringent properties of the RNFL to calculate its thickness, suggest that there is axonal loss evident in the RNFL in the early stages of acute optic neuritis [52], which is not detectable using conventional OCT because swelling of the axons of the RNFL obscures early axonal loss.

The swelling is most commonly followed by loss of RNFL thickness (Figure 4.2). The majority of RNFL thinning occurs in the first three months after symptom onset, and is near complete by six months [22,26]. Using modeled data from a cohort of patients with acute optic neuritis, we would predict that approximately half the RNFL loss will occur within one month of symptom onset and 99% of the loss will have occurred by 4.75 months [50].

Atrophy of the RNFL is detectable only after partial resolution of early edema and is likely to be detectable 1.5 to 2 months after the onset of symptoms [50] (see Figure 4.4). The time taken for loss of macular volume (our modeling suggests that 99% of the loss takes place by approximately 11 months) seems to be longer than that of RNFL thickness, suggesting that perhaps thinning of deeper layers, such as thinning of the ganglion cell layer, or different mechanisms, such as trans-synaptic retinal degeneration, are at play in the macula.

Predictors of severity of RNFL loss

The eventual degree of axonal loss in the RNFL is variable after a single attack of optic neuritis, ranging from little or minor RNFL loss to significant loss

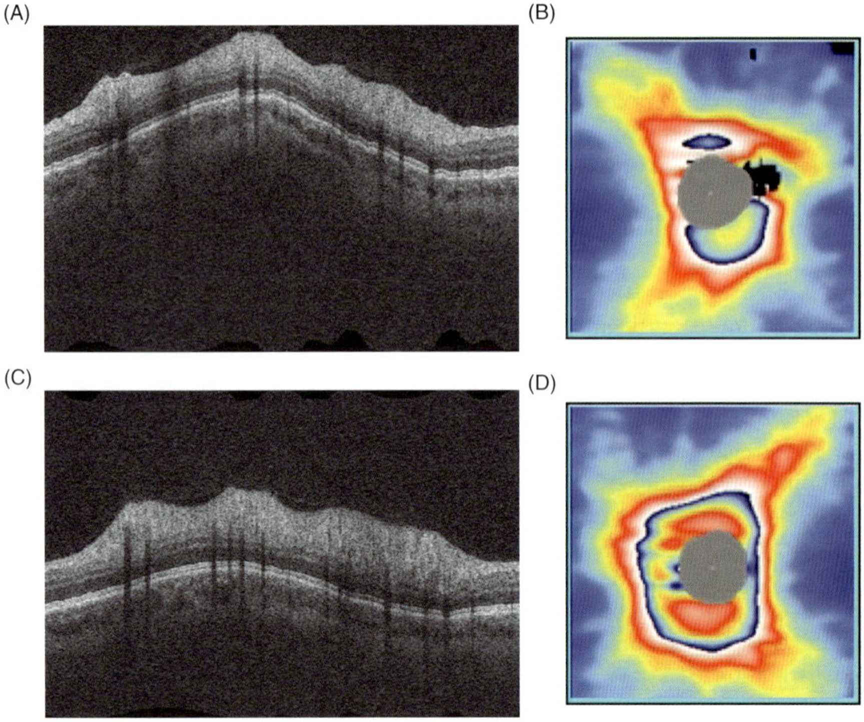

Figure 4.3 Asymmetric swelling of the RNFL in a patient with chronic relapsing inflammatory optic neuropathy (CRION[1]). The images were taken ten days after the onset of bilateral eye pain, pain on eye movement, and development of bilateral reduced visual acuity and visual field sensitivity. There is significant swelling of both RNFL, which is more marked on the left (average circumpapillary RNFL thickness 146 μm right and 223 μm left). A. and C. are circumpapillary OCT images of the retina of the left and right eye, respectively; the highly reflective RNFL at the top of the retinal image is markedly swollen. B. and D. are peripapillary thickness maps of the RNFL, again demonstrating marked swelling of the RNFL.

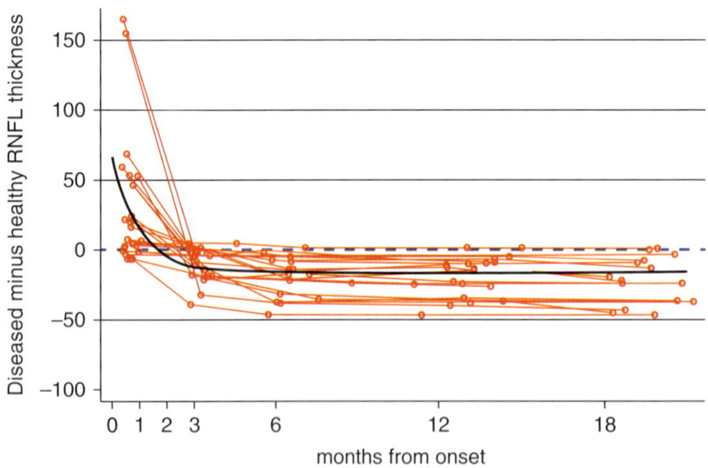

Figure 4.4 Model predicting the time course of RNFL thinning following a single episode of optic neuritis. Red lines indicate individual patient courses; the overall model is indicated in black; and the dashed line represents the time at which atrophy would be detectable using the fellow eye as comparison.

with associated poor visual recovery. In our cohort of patients, we found baseline visual evoked potential (VEP) latency and amplitude, and baseline measures of visual function (full- and low-contrast visual acuity, and whole field mean deviation) were associated with later RNFL loss. Of these measures, full-field VEP latency and a measure of color vision, the Farnsworth-Munsell 100 Hue test, best predicted eventual RNFL loss [53], suggesting that initial axonal dysfunction is associated with later axonal death. Somewhat unexpectedly, the degree of initial RNFL edema is not strongly associated with the eventual RNFL atrophy.

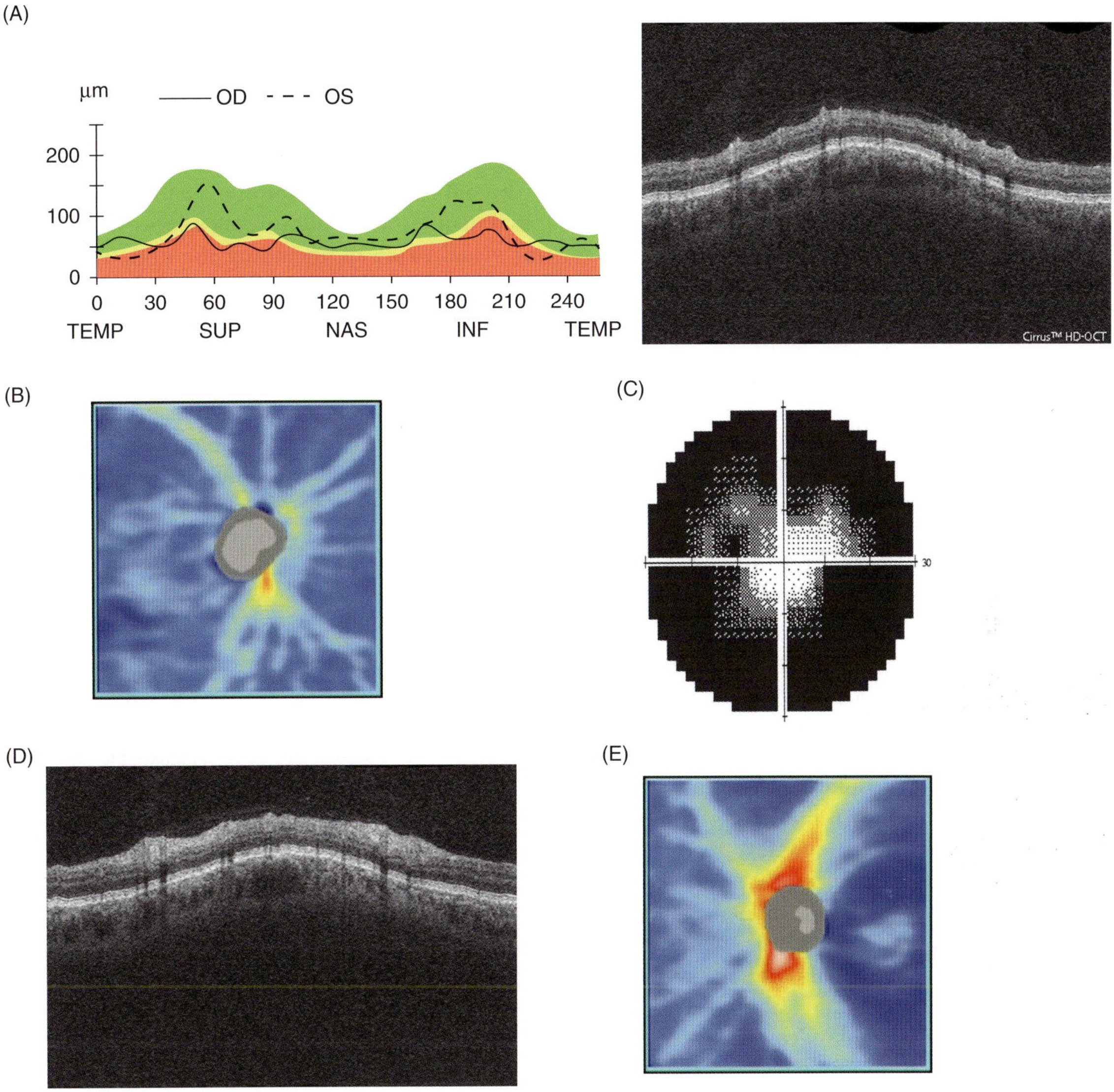

Figure 4.5 Left eye visual field (C.right eye not shown as NPL), OCT images of the circumpapillary retina (A. and D.) and RNFL thickness maps (B. and D.) from a 45-year-old man with neuromyelitis optica after multiple episodes of bilateral optic neuritis. A. shows circumpapillary RNFL thickness plotted against a normative database (95%, 5%, and 1% of normal eyes lie within the green, yellow, and red range as indicated).

The right eye had no perception of light and an unreactive pupil, and the corrected visual acuity in the left eye was 6/18.

Costello and others [38] studied a group of patients with optic neuritis and found there were sex-specific differences in the degree of RNFL loss after optic neuritis. Male subjects experienced greater RNFL loss in their affected eye. The authors suggested that the mechanism underlying this difference in outcome between genders might be related to the differences that underlie poorer outcome (in terms of destructive lesion load and overall disability) for men when compared with women with multiple sclerosis [54,55].

Changes in the retina in neuromyelitis optica

Neuromyelitis optica (NMO) is an inflammatory demyelinating disease in which the pathology is most often concentrated in the optic nerves and spinal cord. It is pathologically distinct from multiple sclerosis [56], with greater loss of both oligodendrocytes and neurons, and characteristic abnormalities of astrocytes [57]. In the majority of patients, it is associated with the presence of antibodies to aquaporin-4 [58,59]. Neuromyelitis may present with either optic neuritis (both bilateral and unilateral) or transverse myelitis, or both [60].

The optic neuritis associated with NMO is often severe and is associated with poor recovery. Of the 12 patients documented in O'Riordan and colleagues' case series [61], 10 had count fingers or worse vision in one or more eyes. Of these 12 patients, 10 had a bilateral optic neuropathy due either to recurrence in the fellow eye or simultaneous optic neuritis. At the nadir of vision in neuromyelitis associated optic neuritis, visual acuity is usually count fingers or worse [60,62], and recovery is typically not as complete as in acute idiopathic optic neuritis. Recurrent attacks are associated with further reductions in vision [23, 60, 63–65].

Ratchford and colleagues [34] studied a small cohort of patients with NMO. When compared with patients with multiple sclerosis, optic neuritis in NMO resulted in more severe RNFL thinning and macular volume loss, and there was more visual loss than in multiple sclerosis-associated optic neuritis. Using multivariate linear regression, they estimated that the initial attack of optic neuritis caused, on average, a 31μm reduction in the nerve fiber layer thickness, and each further attack resulted in approximately 10 μm of thinning.

Fernandes and colleagues [66] studied a group of patients with optic neuritis due to NMO, and compared them to a group of patients with optic neuritis due to multiple sclerosis and healthy controls. Although RNFL and ganglion cell layer atrophy were evident in both multiple sclerosis and in NMO, only patients with neuromyelitis optica had swelling of the inner nuclear layer. Sotirchos and colleagues [67] examined 39 patients with NMO and a group of healthy controls. They found microcystic macular edema was present in patients with a history of acute optic neuritis and was associated with more severe thinning of the RNFL and ganglion cell layer, and with poorer vision. Both Sotirchos and colleagues and Gelfand and colleagues found microcystic macular edema to be more prevalent in their cohorts of patients with neuromyelitis optica (26% and 20%, respectively) than in previously reported cohorts of patients with multiple sclerosis (where it is seen in approximately 5% [40,41]).

Optic neuritis as a model of relapse in multiple sclerosis

The optic nerve is part of the central nervous system, and, as such, can be considered a white matter tract. Optic neuritis resulting from a demyelinating lesion of the optic nerve is a common and characteristic initial manifestation of multiple sclerosis. The anterior visual pathway, including the optic nerve and RNFL, can be studied functionally (with quantitative tests of vision), structurally (with optic nerve and retinal imaging), and electrophysiologically (by measuring the visual evoked potential). Study of optic neuritis can give insights into the mechanisms of demyelination and remyelination, and loss and return of function in the demyelinating lesion in multiple sclerosis [73, 74]. The other significant advantage in favor of using optic neuritis as a model of acute inflammatory demyelination in proof of principle trials of neuroprotective agents is that the events of optic neuritis are complete within six months of the onset of symptoms, significantly curtailing the length of time taken to conduct phase II studies.

For the purposes of clinical trials, sample size estimates have been generated for both RNFL thickness, and also for a composite of the ganglion cell layer and inner plexiform layer (GCL\IPL). For a six-month trial with 80% power, aiming to detect a 50% treatment effect, the per-arm sample size using RNFL as an endpoint would be 36 [50]. This assumes that patients with no prior history of optic neuritis are recruited, so the unaffected fellow eye can be used as a comparator to assess visual loss. If the fellow eye is previously affected, or is not used as a comparator, then per-arm sample size rises to approximately 58 if RNFL loss is used as an endpoint. For a similar trial using GCL\IPL as an endpoint sample size would be 44 per-arm [37]. Because there does not appear to be any swelling of the GCL\IPL complex in optic neuritis, sample sizes are not dependent on using the fellow eye as a comparator. Given that RNFL and GCL\IPL complex measures can be acquired on Fourier-domain OCT, it is likely that both measures will be used to evaluate the efficacy of putative treatments, although some devices do not possess the segmentation algorithm to do so. The utility of a treatment that preserved retinal ganglion cells but not their axons is questionable.

Sühs and colleagues assessed the efficacy of erythropoietin as a neuroprotective agent in acute optic

Table 4.2 Studies of optic neuritis associated with neuromyelitis optica, and comparative studies with multiple sclerosis-associated optic neuritis

	NMO		NMO eyes without optic neuritis		Multiple sclerosis		Healthy control	
	Mean (SD)	n	Mean (SD)	n	Mean (SD)	n	Mean (SD)	n
de Seze et al. (2008) [68]	77.9 (22.6)	32	–	–	–	–	102.3	7.4
Merle et al. (2008) [69]	65.4 (25.2)	15	–	–	83.9 (24.1)	15	106.2 (24.5)	23
Naismith et al. (2009) [70]	70.5 (26.2)	22	–	–	80.7 (19.3)	47	–	–
Ratchford et al. (2009) [34]	63.6 (20.3) (NMO) 96.3 (14.3 (LETM)	26	–	–	88.3 (16.5) (past ON) 96.3 (14.3) (No prior ON)	378	102.4 (11.0)	77
Green and Cree (2009) [71]	59.2 (16.2)	16	–	–	82.0 (17.6)	20	–	–
Nakamura et al. (2010) [64]	63.8 (23.5)	18	106.4 (14.5)	8 (eyes)	84.3 (14.2)	14	–	–
Monteiro et al. (2012) [39]	82.7 (22.4) (NMO) 97.9 (10.7) (LETM)	33	97.9 (10.7)		94.6 (19.0) (past ON) 101.2 (11.6) (No prior ON)	60	107.6 (9.4)	41
Bouyon et al. (2013) [72]	87.4 (23.3) (baseline) 79.7 (22.4) (follow up)	30	–	–	–	–	–	–
Lange et al. (2013) [23]	63.7 (18.3) (one episode) 50.7 (8.1) (>1 episode)	26 6	97.0 (11.1)	18	73.9 (15.2) (prior ON) 93.2 (15.2) (no prior ON)	13 37	98.4 (14.4)	100
Bichuetti et al. (2013) [65]	65.3 (18.3) one episode 47.0 (6.1) two episodes	8 7	85.7 (20.5)	3	92.4 (14.0) (no prior ON) 80.1 (14.8) (one episode ON) 61.7 (7.1) (two episodes ON) 81.3(17.5)(three episodes ON)	63 28 4 3	–	–

neuritis, using RNFL thickness measured with OCT as the primary endpoint. They found that it was effective in reducing the RNFL atrophy following optic neuritis: in the treated group the median reduction in RNFL thickness was 7.5 μm whereas in the untreated group the median reduction in affected eye RNFL thickness was 16.0 μm. The trial required only 40 patients in total, and the primary outcome was measured at 16 weeks after randomization. Esfahani and colleagues [75] measured the effect of memantine given for two weeks after a first-ever attack of optic neuritis. Sixty patients were randomized 1:1 to either memantine (given as 5 mg daily for one week followed by 10 mg daily for two weeks) or a placebo. There was a significant difference in eventual RNFL thickness in the memantine treated group (91.3 μm vs. 78.9 μm in the placebo group) but no significant effect upon vision or neurophysiological measures of optic nerve function. Tsakiri and colleagues [76] evaluated the effect of simvistatin (80 mg daily for six months) upon the visual and neurophysiological measures of optic nerve function, and they found a beneficial effect on visual evoked potential latency and amplitude, but it did not quite ($p = 0.06$) reach the primary outcome of improving contrast sensitivity using Arden plates.

Several other trials using acute optic neuritis as a model of relapse and OCT as a primary or secondary endpoint are in the recruitment phase as this chapter is being written. The RENEW study (ClinicalTrials.gov Identifier: NCT01721161) is a trial of an anti-LINGO compound, BIIB-033. LINGO is an inhibitor of remyelination [77], and inhibition of LINGO promotes remyelination in animal models [78]. The primary endpoint is the change in optic nerve conduction, but RNFL thickness measured by OCT is a secondary outcome measure. The Amiloride Clinical Trial In Optic Neuritis (ACTION) study (ClinicalTrials.gov Identifier: NCT01802489) is a placebo-controlled trial of amiloride in acute optic neuritis. Amiloride blocks the acid-sensing ion channel and inhibits the influx of calcium, which can be associated with neuronal death [79]. The primary outcome measure is measurement of the RNFL thickness with scanning laser polarimetry; however, measurement of RNFL thickness by optical coherence tomography is a secondary outcome measure. There is also a phase II, double-blind, randomized controlled trial of phenytoin in acute optic neuritis (ClinicalTrials.gov Identifier: NCT01451593), which is using mean RNFL thickness as the primary outcome measure. Phenytoin, which blocks voltage-gated sodium channels, reduces the severity of, and preserves axonal integrity in, experimental allergic encephalomyelitis [80]. This study aims to recruit 90 patients and has a primary outcome measure that is measured at six months. The Fingolimod in Acute Demyelinating Optic Neuritis trial (ClinicalTrials.gov Identifier: NCT01757691) is assessing the neuroprotective effect of fingolimod in acute optic neuritis as measured using OCT of the retinal nerve fiber layer.

Optical coherence tomography has given considerable insight into the pathophysiology and clinical characteristics of acute optic neuritis. It also allows acute optic neuritis to be used as a model of the acute relapse in trials of neuroprotection, which require relatively small numbers and are quick to reach the final time point.

References

1. Kidd D, Burton B, Plant GT, Graham EM. Chronic relapsing inflammatory optic neuropathy (CRION). *Brain.* February 2003; **126**(Pt 2): 276–84.
2. Petzold A, Pittock S, Lennon V, Maggiore C, Weinshenker BG, Plant GT. Neuromyelitis optica-IgG (aquaporin-4) autoantibodies in immune mediated optic neuritis. *J Neurol Neurosurg Psychiatr.* January 2010; **81**(1): 109–11.
3. Rodriguez M, Siva A, Cross SA, O'Brien PC, Kurland LT. Optic neuritis: a population-based study in Olmsted County, Minnesota. *Neurology* [Internet]. February 1995; **45**(2): 244–50. Available from: http://www.neurology.org/content/45/2/244.short?sid=5d3bc217-394e-46d0-a720-df8704457287//www.neurology.org
4. Beck RW, Cleary PA, Anderson MM, Keltner JL, Shults WT, Kaufman DI, et al. A randomized, controlled trial of corticosteroids in the treatment of acute optic neuritis. *The Optic Neuritis Study Group. N Engl J Med.* February 27, 1992; **326**(9): 581–8.
5. Optic Neuritis Study Group. The clinical profile of optic neuritis. Experience of the Optic Neuritis Treatment Trial. *Arch Ophthalmol.* December 1991; **109**(12): 1673–8.
6. Trobe JD, Beck RW, Moke PS, Cleary PA. Contrast sensitivity and other vision tests in the optic neuritis treatment trial. *Am J Ophthalmol.* May 1996; **121**(5): 547–53.
7. Keltner JL, Johnson CA, Spurr JO, Beck RW. Baseline visual field profile of optic neuritis. The experience of the optic neuritis treatment trial. Optic Neuritis Study Group. *Arch Ophthalmol.* February 1993; **111**(2): 231–4.
8. Cox TA, Thompson HS, Corbett JJ. Relative afferent pupillary defects in optic neuritis. *Am J Ophthalmol.* November 1, 1981; **92**(5): 685–90.
9. Beck RW, Cleary PA. Optic neuritis treatment trial. One-year follow-up results. *Arch Ophthalmol.* June 1993; **111**(6): 773–5.
10. la Cruz de J, Kupersmith MJ. Clinical profile of simultaneous bilateral optic neuritis in adults. *British Journal of Ophthalmology.* May 2006; **90**(5): 551–4.
11. Beck RW, Kupersmith MJ, Cleary PA, Katz B. Fellow eye abnormalities in acute unilateral optic neuritis. Experience of the optic neuritis treatment trial. *Ophthalmology.* May 1993; **100**(5): 691–8.
12. Ormerod IE, McDonald WI. Multiple sclerosis presenting with progressive visual failure. *J Neurol Neurosurg Psychiatr.* September 1, 1984; **47**(9): 943–6.

13. Ashworth B. Chronic retrobulbar and chiasmal neuritis. *British Journal of Ophthalmology*. October 1967; **51**(10): 698–702.
14. Hoyt WF, Schlicke B, Eckelhoff RJ. Fundoscopic appearance of a nerve-fibre-bundle defect. *British Journal of Ophthalmology*. August 1972; **56**(8): 577–83.
15. Frisén L, Hoyt WF. Insidious atrophy of retinal nerve fibers in multiple sclerosis. Funduscopic identification in patients with and without visual complaints. *Arch Ophthalmol*. August 1, 1974; **92**(2): 91–7.
16. Sharpe JA, Sanders MD. Atrophy of myelinated nerve fibres in the retina in optic neuritis. *British Journal of Ophthalmology*. Aprl 1, 1975; **59**(4): 229–32.
17. Elbøl P, Work K. Retinal nerve fiber layer in multiple sclerosis. *Acta Ophthalmology*. August 1, 1990; **68**(4): 481–6.
18. MacFadyen DJ, Drance SM, Douglas GR, Airaksinen PJ, Mawson DK, Paty DW. The retinal nerve fiber layer, neuroretinal rim area, and visual evoked potentials in MS. *Neurology* [Internet]. September 1, 1988; **38**(9): 1353–8. Available from: http://neurology.org/content/38/9/1353.short
19. Quigley HA, Addicks EM. Quantitative studies of retinal nerve fiber layer defects. *Arch Ophthalmology*. May 1982; **100**(5): 807–14.
20. Parisi V, Manni G, Spadaro M, Colacino G, Restuccia R, Marchi S, et al. Correlation between morphological and functional retinal impairment in multiple sclerosis patients. *Invest Ophthalmol Vis Sci*. October 1999; **40**(11): 2520–7.
21. Trip SA, Schlottmann PG, Jones SJ, Altmann DR, Garway-Heath DF, Thompson AJ, et al. Retinal nerve fiber layer axonal loss and visual dysfunction in optic neuritis. *Ann Neurol*. September 2005; **58**(3): 383–91.
22. Costello F, Hodge W, Pan Y, Eggenberger E, Coupland S, Kardon R. Tracking retinal nerve fiber layer loss after optic neuritis: a prospective study using optical coherence tomography. *Multiple Sclerosis*. June 23, 2008; **14**(7): 893–905.
23. Lange AP, Sadjadi R, Zhu F, Alkabie S, Costello F, Traboulsee AL. Spectral-domain optical coherence tomography of retinal nerve fiber layer thickness in NMO patients. *J Neuroophthalmol* [Internet]. September 2013; **33**(3): 213–9. Available from: http://eutils.ncbi.nlm.nih.gov/entrez/eutils/elink.fcgi?dbfrom=pubmed&id=23863782&retmode=ref&cmd= prlinks
24. Bichuetti DB, Oliveira EML, Souza NA, Rivero RLM, Gabbai AA. Neuromyelitis optica in Brazil: a study on clinical and prognostic factors. *Multiple Sclerosis*. May 2009; **15**(5): 613–9.
25. Fisher J, Jacobs D, Markowitz C, Galetta S, Volpe N, Nanoschiavi M, et al. Relation of Visual Function to Retinal Nerve Fiber Layer Thickness in Multiple Sclerosis. *Ophthalmology*. February 2006; **113**(2): 324–32.
26. Costello F, Coupland S, Hodge W, Lorello GR, Koroluk J, Pan YI, et al. Quantifying axonal loss after optic neuritis with optical coherence tomography. *Annals of Neurology*. June 1, 2006; **59**(6): 963–9.
27. Albrecht P, Fröhlich R, Hartung H-P, Kieseier BC, Methner A. Optical coherence tomography measures axonal loss in multiple sclerosis independently of optic neuritis. *J Neurol*. November 9, 2007; **254**(11): 1595–6.
28. Pulicken M, Gordon-Lipkin E, Balcer LJ, Frohman E, Cutter G, Calabresi PA. Optical coherence tomography and disease subtype in multiple sclerosis. *Neurology*. November 27, 2007; **69**(22): 2085–92.
29. Pueyo V, Martin J, Fernandez J, Almarcegui C, Ara J, Egea C, et al. Axonal loss in the retinal nerve fiber layer in patients with multiple sclerosis. *Multiple Sclerosis*. June 2008; **14**(5): 609–14.
30. Zaveri MS, Conger A, Salter A, Frohman TC, Galetta SL, Markowitz CE, et al. Retinal imaging by laser polarimetry and optical coherence tomography evidence of axonal degeneration in multiple sclerosis. *Arch Neurol*. July 2008; **65**(7): 924–8.
31. Klistorner A, Arvind H, Nguyen T, Garrick R, Paine M, Graham S, et al. Axonal loss and myelin in early ON loss in postacute optic neuritis. *Ann Neurol*. September 2008; **64**(3): 325–31.
32. Siger M, Dziegielewski K, Jasek L, Bieniek M, Nicpan A, Nawrocki J, et al. Optical coherence tomography in multiple sclerosis: thickness of the retinal nerve fiber layer as a potential measure of axonal loss and brain atrophy. *J Neurol*. October 2008; **255**(10): 1555–60.
33. Frohman EM, Dwyer MG, Frohman T, Cox JL, Salter A, Greenberg BM, et al. Relationship of optic nerve and brain conventional and non-conventional MRI measures and retinal nerve fiber layer thickness, as assessed by OCT and GDx: a pilot study. *J Neurol Sci*. July 15, 2009; **282**(1–2): 96–105.
34. Ratchford JN, Quigg ME, Conger A, Frohman T, Frohman E, Balcer LJ, et al. Optical coherence tomography helps differentiate neuromyelitis optica and MS optic neuropathies. *Neurology*. July 28, 2009; **73**(4): 302–8.
35. Burkholder BM, Osborne B, Loguidice MJ, Bisker E, Frohman TC, Conger A, et al. Macular volume determined by optical coherence tomography as a measure of neuronal loss in multiple sclerosis. *Arch Neurol*. November 2009; **66**(11): 1366–72.
36. Garcia-Martin E, Pueyo V, Ara J, Almarcegui C, Martin J, Pablo L, et al. Effect of optic neuritis on progressive axonal damage in multiple sclerosis patients. *Mult Scler* [Internet]. June 20, 2011 Jun 20; **17**(7): 830–7. Available from: http://eutils.ncbi.

nlm.nih.gov/entrez/eutils/elink.fcgi?dbfrom=pubmed&id=21300734&retmode=ref&cmd=prlinks

37. Syc SB, Saidha S, Newsome SD, Ratchford JN, Levy M, Ford E, et al. Optical coherence tomography segmentation reveals ganglion cell layer pathology after optic neuritis. *Brain*. February 2012; **135**(Pt 2): 521–33.

38. Costello F, Hodge W, Pan YI, Burton JM, Freedman MS, Stys PK, et al. Sex-specific differences in retinal nerve fiber layer thinning after acute optic neuritis. *Neurology*. October 2012; **79**(18): 1866–72.

39. Monteiro MLR, Fernandes DB, Apóstolos-Pereira SL, Callegaro D. Quantification of retinal neural loss in patients with neuromyelitis optica and multiple sclerosis with or without optic neuritis using Fourier-domain optical coherence tomography. *Invest Ophthalmol Vis Sci* [Internet]. June 2012; **53**(7): 3959–66. Available from: http://eutils.ncbi.nlm.nih.gov/entrez/eutils/elink.fcgi?dbfrom=pubmed&id=22589446&retmode=ref&cmd=prlinks

40. Gelfand JM, Nolan R, Schwartz DM, Graves J, Green AJ. Microcystic macular edema in multiple sclerosis is associated with disease severity. *Brain*. June 2012; **135**(Pt 6): 1786–93.

41. Saidha S, Sotirchos ES, Ibrahim MA, Crainiceanu CM, Gelfand JM, Sepah YJ, et al. Microcystic macular edema, thickness of the inner nuclear layer of the retina, and disease characteristics in multiple sclerosis: a retrospective study. *Lancet Neurol*. October 4, 2012; **11**(11): 963–72.

42. Balk LJ, Killestein J, Polman CH, Uitdehaag BMJ, Petzold A. Microcystic macular edema confirmed, but not specific for multiple sclerosis. *Brain*. December 18, 2012; **135**(12): e226–6.

43. Kaufhold F, Zimmermann H, Schneider E, Ruprecht K, Paul F, Oberwahrenbrock T, et al. Optic neuritis is associated with inner nuclear layer thickening and microcystic macular edema independently of multiple sclerosis. *PLoS ONE*. 2013; **8**(8): e71145.

44. Abegg M, Zinkernagel M, Wolf S. Microcystic macular degeneration from optic neuropathy. *Brain*. December 18, 2012; **135**(12): 225–5.

45. van Buren JM. Trans-synaptic retrograde degeneration in the visual system of primates. *J Neurol Neurosurg Psychiatr*. October 1963; **26**: 402–9.

46. Kaushik M, Wang CY, Barnett MH, Garrick R, Parratt J, Graham SL, et al. Inner nuclear layer thickening is inversley proportional to retinal ganglion cell loss in optic neuritis. *PLoS ONE*. 2013; **8**(10): e78341.

47. Kerrison JB, Flynn T, Green WR. Retinal pathologic changes in multiple sclerosis. *Retina (Philadelphia, Pa)*. 1994; **14**(5): 445–51.

48. Green AJ, McQuaid S, Hauser SL, Allen IV, Lyness R. Ocular pathology in multiple sclerosis: retinal atrophy and inflammation irrespective of disease duration. *Brain*. June 2010; **133**(Pt 6): 1591–601.

49. Pro MJ, Pons ME, Liebmann JM, Ritch R, Zafar S, Lefton D, et al. Imaging of the optic disc and retinal nerve fiber layer in acute optic neuritis. *J Neurol Sci*. December 1, 2006; **250**(1–2): 114–9.

50. Henderson APD, Altmann DR, Trip AS, Kallis C, Jones SJ, Schlottmann PG, et al. A serial study of retinal changes following optic neuritis with sample size estimates for acute neuroprotection trials. *Brain*. September 2010; **133**(9): 2592–602.

51. Hickman SJ, Toosy AT, Jones SJ, Altmann DR, Miszkiel KA, MacManus DG, et al. A serial MRI study following optic nerve mean area in acute optic neuritis. *Brain*. November 2004; **127**(Pt 11): 2498–505.

52. Garas A, Simó M, Holló G. Nerve fiber layer and macular thinning measured with different imaging methods during the course of acute optic neuritis. *European Journal of Ophthalmology*. October 22, 2010.

53. Henderson APD, Altmann DR, Trip SA, Miszkiel KA, Schlottmann PG, Jones SJ, et al. Early factors associated with axonal loss after optic neuritis. *Ann Neurol*. December 21, 2011; **70**(6): 955–63.

54. Khaleeli Z, Ciccarelli O, Manfredonia F, Barkhof F, Brochet B, Cercignani M, et al. Predicting progression in primary progressive multiple sclerosis: a 10-year multicenter study. *Ann Neurol*. June 2008; **63**(6): 790–3.

55. Koch M, Kingwell E, Rieckmann P, Tremlett H, UBC MS Clinic Neurologists. The natural history of secondary progressive multiple sclerosis. *J Neurol Neurosurg Psychiatr*. September 2010; **81**(9): 1039–43.

56. Lucchinetti CF, Mandler RN, McGavern D, Brück W, Gleich G, Ransohoff RM, et al. A role for humoral mechanisms in the pathogenesis of Devic's neuromyelitis optica. *Brain*. July 2002; **125**(Pt 7): 1450–61.

57. Parratt JD, Prineas JW. Neuromyelitis optica: a demyelinating disease characterized by acute destruction and regeneration of perivascular astrocytes. *Mult Scler*. September 30, 2010; **16**(10): 1156–72.

58. Lennon VA, Wingerchuk DM, Kryzer TJ, Pittock SJ, Lucchinetti CF, Fujihara K, et al. A serum autoantibody marker of neuromyelitis optica: distinction from multiple sclerosis. *Lancet*. November 2004; **364**(9451): 2106–12.

59. Lennon VA, Kryzer TJ, Pittock SJ, Verkman AS, Hinson SR. IgG marker of optic-spinal multiple sclerosis binds to the aquaporin-4 water channel. *J Exp Med*. August 15, 2005; **202**(4): 473–7.

60. Wingerchuk DM, Hogancamp WF, O'Brien PC, Weinshenker BG. The clinical course of neuromyelitis optica (Devic's syndrome). *Neurology*. 1999; **53**(5): 1107–14.

61. O'Riordan JI, Gallagher HL, Thompson AJ, Howard RS, Kingsley DP, Thompson EJ, et al. Clinical, CSF,

and MRI findings in Devic's neuromyelitis optica. *J Neurol Neurosurg Psychiatr.* April 1996; **60**(4): 382–7.

62. Papais-Alvarenga RM, Carellos SC, Alvarenga MP, Holander C, Bichara RP, Thuler LCS. Clinical course of optic neuritis in patients with relapsing neuromyelitis optica. *Arch Ophthalmol.* January 2008; **126**(1): 12–6.
63. Rivera JF, Kurtzke JF, Booth VJA, Corona T V. Characteristics of Devic's disease (neuromyelitis optica) in Mexico. *J Neurol.* May 2008; **255**(5): 710–5.
64. Nakamura M, Nakazawa T, Doi H, Hariya T, Omodaka K, Misu T, et al. Early high-dose intravenous methylprednisolone is effective in preserving retinal nerve fiber layer thickness in patients with neuromyelitis optica. *Graefes Arch Clin Exp Ophthalmol.* December 2010; **248**(12): 1777–85.
65. Bichuetti DB, de Camargo AS, Falcão AB, Gonçalves FF, Tavares IM, de Oliveira EML. The retinal nerve fiber layer of patients with neuromyelitis optica and chronic relapsing optic neuritis is more severely damaged than patients with multiple sclerosis. *J Neuroophthalmol* [Internet]. September 2013; **33**(3): 220–4. Available from: http://eutils.ncbi.nlm.nih.gov/entrez/eutils/elink.fcgi?dbfrom=pubmed&id=23917443&retmode=ref&cmd=prlinks
66. Fernandes DB, Raza AS, Nogueira RGF, Wang D, Callegaro D, Hood DC, et al. Evaluation of inner retinal layers in patients with multiple sclerosis or neuromyelitis optica using optical coherence tomography. *Ophthalmology.* February 2013; **120**(2): 387–94.
67. Sotirchos ES, Saidha S, Byraiah G, Mealy MA, Ibrahim MA, Sepah YJ, et al. In vivo identification of morphologic retinal abnormalities in neuromyelitis optica. *Neurology* [Internet]. April 8, 2013; **80**(15): 1406–14. Available from: http://eutils.ncbi.nlm.nih.gov/entrez/eutils/elink.fcgi?dbfrom=pubmed&id=23516321&retmode=ref&cmd=prlinks
68. de Seze J, Blanc F, Jeanjean L, Zéphir H, Labauge P, Bouyon M, et al. Optical coherence tomography in neuromyelitis optica. *Arch Neurol.* July 2008; **65**(7): 920–3.
69. Merle H, Olindo S, Donnio A, Richer R, Smadja D, Cabre P. Retinal peripapillary nerve fiber layer thickness in neuromyelitis optica. *Invest Ophthalmol Vis Sci.* October 2008; **49**(10): 4412–7.
70. Naismith RT, Tutlam NT, Xu J, Klawiter EC, Shepherd J, Trinkaus K, et al. Optical coherence tomography differs in neuromyelitis optica compared with multiple sclerosis. *Neurology.* March 24, 2009; **72**(12): 1077–82.
71. Green AJ, Cree BAC. Distinctive retinal nerve fibre layer and vascular changes in neuromyelitis optica following optic neuritis. *J Neurol Neurosurg Psychiatr.* September 2009; **80**(9): 1002–5.
72. Bouyon M, Collongues N, Zéphir H, Ballonzoli L, Jeanjean L, Lebrun C, et al. Longitudinal follow-up of vision in a neuromyelitis optica cohort. *Mult Scler* [Internet]. August 30, 2013; **19**(10): 1320–2. Available from: http://eutils.ncbi.nlm.nih.gov/entrez/eutils/elink.fcgi?dbfrom=pubmed&id=23413296&retmode=ref&cmd=prlinks
73. Compston A. Mechanisms of axon-glial injury of the optic nerve. *Eye.* November 2004; **18**(11): 1182–7.
74. Kolappan M, Henderson APD, Jenkins TM, Wheeler-Kingshott CAM, Plant GT, Thompson AJ, et al. Assessing structure and function of the afferent visual pathway in multiple sclerosis and associated optic neuritis. *J Neurol.* March 2009; **256**(3): 305–19.
75. Esfahani MR, Harandi ZA, Movasat M, Nikdel M, Adelpour M, Momeni A, et al. Memantine for axonal loss of optic neuritis. *Graefes Arch Clin Exp Ophthalmol.* June 2012; **250**(6): 863–9.
76. Tsakiri A, Kallenbach K, Fuglø D, Wanscher B, Larsson H, Frederiksen J. Simvastatin improves final visual outcome in acute optic neuritis: a randomized study. *Mult Scler.* January 2012; **18**(1): 72–81.
77. Jepson S, Vought B, Gross CH, Gan L, Austen D, Frantz JD, et al. LINGO-1, a transmembrane signaling protein, inhibits oligodendrocyte differentiation and myelination through intercellular self-interactions. *J Biol Chem.* June 22, 2012; **287**(26): 22184–95.
78. Mi S, Pepinsky RB, Cadavid D. Blocking LINGO-1 as a therapy to promote CNS repair: from concept to the clinic. *CNS Drugs.* July 2013; **27**(7): 493–503.
79. Canessa CM, Horisberger JD, Rossier BC. Epithelial sodium channel related to proteins involved in neurodegeneration. *Nature.* February 4, 1993; **361**(6411): 467–70.
80. Black JA, Waxman SG. Phenytoin protects central axons in experimental autoimmune encephalomyelitis. *J Neurol Sci.* November 15, 2008; **274**(1–2): 57–63.

Chapter 5

Optical coherence tomography and visual outcomes in acute optic neuritis

Fiona Costello

Introduction

Optic neuritis (ON) is generally viewed as an inflammatory optic nerve injury, which is strongly associated with multiple sclerosis (MS). Optical coherence tomography (OCT) provides a reliable means of capturing neuronal and axonal structural deficits in the afferent visual pathway (AVP), which can be compared to tests of visual function, to devise a structural–functional paradigm of brain injury. In this respect, the eye provides a unique view into the effects of central nervous system (CNS) inflammation, which may enhance our understanding of disease mechanisms that contribute to neurological disability in MS. This chapter addresses the published experience with OCT in the diagnosis and management of acute ON, with particular emphasis on visual outcomes in patients presenting with this condition.

Optic neuritis

Optic neuritis represents the first clinical manifestation of MS in approximately 20% of cases and is, therefore, one of the most commonly encountered clinically isolated syndromes (CIS) that is a harbinger of the disease [1, 2]. In addition to its being the clinical inception for many, an additional 30% to 70% of affected individuals develop ON over time [3]. Hence, the anterior visual pathway is a frequent target in MS, and much of what we have come to understand about ON has been derived from the long term follow-up of the Optic Neuritis Treatment Trial (ONTT) [4]. This randomized, multicenter study was initially designed to compare the benefits of treatment with either intravenous methylprednisolone (250 mg every 6 hours for 3 days followed by oral prednisone (1 mg/kg/day] for 11 days), oral prednisone (1 mg/kg/day for 14 days), or oral placebo (for 14 days) in 457 patients with acute ON [4]. From the ONTT, we learned that most ON patients are young (mean age: 32 years), Caucasian (85%), and predominantly women (77%) [3]. Ninety-two percent of patients report pain at the onset of vision loss, which is often characterized as an "ache" made worse with eye movement [4]. Vision loss is generally subacute, progressing over hours to days. The severity of vision loss in ON may range from mild to no light perception initially. In patients with unilateral or asymmetric optic nerve involvement, a relative afferent pupil defect (RAPD) can be detected in the affected eye, or, in cases of bilateral involvement, in the more severely affected eye. Bilateral involvement of the anterior visual system, with the magnitude of pathology being equivocal, can represent the setting where sluggish pupillary responses are observed, but without evidence of a RAPD. We have yet to elucidate a validated method by which we can detect "non-relative" APDs; an important goal in studying the relationship between structural and physiologic measures of tissue injury and cross-correlation.

Dyschromatopsia, or decreased color vision, is also common in patients with optic neuritis. This finding can be particularly helpful in localizing the diagnosis in patients with mild central vision loss, who have disproportionate deficits in color vision function. In cases of retrobulbar ON, the fundus examination is initially normal, whereas patients with anterior ON or "papillitis" may manifest optic disc swelling acutely (in conjunction with a corresponding compromise in visual acuity, contrasting with the disc swelling associated with true papilledema, where a relative preservation of acuity is maintained until later in the course, and more severe field suppression) [2]. The initial period of visual recovery occurs within weeks, and further improvement

Optical Coherence Tomography in Neurological Disease, ed. Peter A. Calabresi, Laura J. Balcer, and Elliot M. Frohman. Published by Cambridge University Press.

Table 5.1 Atypical features of acute optic neuritis

Age greater than 50
Optic atrophy at acute presentation
Orbital signs (proptosis)
Severe optic disc edema
Prominent vitreous cell
Hemorrhage affecting the optic nerve or surrounding retina
Bilateral simultaneous loss of vision at onset
Lack of recovery after one month
Lack of pain at onset or pain that persists more than two weeks
Systemic symptoms and signs (fever, weight loss, rash)

Table 5.2 Clinical conditions mimicking optic neuritis

Neuromyelitis optica
Steroid responsive optic neuropathies (including sarcoidosis)
Optic perineuritis
Neuroretinitis
Compressive lesions (pituitary lesions, meningiomas, aneurysms)
Infectious optic neuropathies (syphilis, tuberculosis, Lyme)
Ischemic optic neuropathies
Leber's hereditary optic neuropathy
Big blind spot syndromes

in vision is seen up to a year after the acute episode [4, 5]. Atypical features of ON (Table 5.1), such as bilateral involvement at presentation, optic disc hemorrhages, vitreous reaction, absence of pain, and poor clinical recovery, should prompt investigations for possible clinical mimics (Table 5.2).

In the post-acute phase, most ON patients develop optic disc pallor as a "footprint" of the original injury. The prognosis for recovery after typical ON is generally good, with approximately 95% of patients achieving a visual acuity of 20/40 vision in their affected eye a year after clinical presentation [2, 5, 6, 7]. Despite regaining "normal" vision, however, many ON patients report persistent problems, including fatigue and heat-induced (Uhthoff's phenomenon) vision loss, altered motion and depth perception, and decreased spatial vision at low contrast levels. There is, therefore, discordance between what patients report versus what is captured with standardized ophthalmic testing in the setting of post-acute ON, indicating a need for more sensitive measures of vision loss in this patient population.

Optic neuritis and the afferent visual pathway: designing a clinical model of MS

Attitudes continue to evolve from viewing MS as a demyelinating disease to a broader perspective in which the relative contributions of inflammation, axonal loss, and neurodegeneration are weighed in the balance [2]. Yet the pathogenesis of MS, and by extension the factors that underpin disability in the disease, remain unknown. Accordingly, there is a need for a clinical model amenable to noninvasive imaging that captures different mechanisms of tissue injury contributing to disability progression. As a putative model of MS, the AVP model, with ON as its relapse "prototype" lesion, offers several potential advantages:

1. *Localization – Defining Where the Problem Is*: In the setting of acute ON, the AVP model provides objective evidence of a symptomatic lesion, which can be precisely localized in the CNS [2]. Given a typical history, the presence of an RAPD in the affected eye, pain on movement, a visual field defect that follows the topography of the retinal nerve fiber layer (RNFL), color vision loss, and, in some cases, optic disc hyperemia in the absence of hemorrhage or vitreous cell production, is highly suggestive of ON. Because the cardinal clinical manifestations have been so well established, ON is the best characterized CIS affecting MS patients [1].
2. *Time of Onset – Defining When the Problem Starts:* As foveating animals, humans are "hard-wired" to seek high-resolution images in the world around them. In light of the highly specialized nature of the AVP, any perturbation in the system that interferes with visual perception, particularly central vision, will generally be noticed and reported by affected individuals [2]. Because ON is both clinically relevant and prevalent, functional recovery can be monitored from a relatively precise point of onset in the AVP model of MS.
3. *Quantifiable – Defining the Relation between Structure and Function:* The AVP is a functionally

eloquent system and deficits can be captured with highly reproducible measures of visual function including high- and low-contrast visual acuity, automated perimetry, and color vision testing. Furthermore, OCT provides structural measures of neuronal and axonal integrity in the AVP. By pairing OCT measures with quantitative visual outcomes, we can devise a structural-functional paradigm to elucidate the temporal evolution and relative contributions of inflammation, axonal loss, neuronal damage, and cortical compensation to post-ON recovery in the AVP model of MS [2].

4. *The Back of the Eye Is the Front of the Brain:* Previous pathological studies have shown that tissue specific injury in the AVP mirrors global CNS effects in MS patients [8]. During an acute ON event, cytokine release induces transient conduction block, likely induced by nitric oxide [9]. When myelination and axonal integrity are intact, recovery ensues with the removal of inflammatory mediators. During recovery from ON, remyelination improves saltatory conduction through sodium channels, which are distributed along the demyelinated optic nerve segment [9].

In conjunction with the characteristic mechanisms described above, cortical plasticity is also believed to play a role in optimizing function in the more chronic phases of recovery, albeit the timeline and mechanisms involved therein are not well understood. The AVP model can be used to detect and monitor tissue injury, in association of specific factors that underpin injury. Further, this very same approach may be germane to our ability to identify preventative, protective, and perhaps even restorative properties of neurotherapeutic strategies [2].

The role of optical coherence tomography in acute ON: quantifying the structural consequences of an inflammatory injury in the afferent visual pathway

> "*Form and function should be one, joined in a spiritual union.*" [10] — *Frank Lloyd Wright*

Frank Lloyd Wright was referring to architecture with his iconic comment, but this principle applies equally well to the visual system in which anatomical integrity and clinical function are tightly linked, allowing precise topographic localization of pathological lesions [2]. Since Hemholtz's invention of the ophthalmoscope in 1851, the structural consequences of optic nerve injury have been visualized acutely as optic disc edema, followed by the insidious evolution of optic disc pallor over weeks to months after the onset of symptoms, and corresponding defects in the retinal nerve fiber layer (RNFL) [2, 7]. The RNFL has the distinct feature of being an unmyelinated region of the CNS and represents an accessible substrate through which we can sample neuro-axonal integrity in the CNS. In the current ocular imaging era, measure of changes in the peripapillary RNFL, retinal ganglion cell layer plus inner plexifom layer (GCL+IPL), and deeper neuronal layer in the retina can be quantified with OCT to provide an in vivo "optical biopsy" [3] of the AVP. From these OCT measures of structural integrity we can potentially interpret the temporal evolution and functional impact of axonal and neuronal damage in the CNS.

Optical coherence tomography in acute and chronic ON

At the time of an acute ON event, when vision loss is at its nadir, patients often manifest peripapillary RNFL measurements that are either comparable to or increased in their affected eye (ON eye) relative to their fellow eye (non-ON eye) [2, 7]. Correspondingly, the optic nerve in the ON eye may be mildly edematous or hyperemic secondary to axoplasmic flow stasis **(Case 1)**. In contrast, OCT-measured macular volume (MV) and GCL + IPL values are similar between ON eyes and fellow eyes in patients with acute ON [2, 7, 11]. In the ensuing two to three months, optic disc pallor and RNFL thinning evolve, with earliest signs of significant RNFL atrophy manifesting in the temporal RNFL region [2, 7]. The RNFL, MV, and GCL+ IPL values continue to decrease for six to 12 months after symptom onset, plateauing thereafter [2, 7,11–13]. From studies to date, the inner and outer nuclear layers are unaffected in acute ON and do not differ between ON eyes and fellow eyes of ON patients during longitudinal follow-up [11]. Visual recovery 12 months after ON is not related to the extent of peripapillary RNFL swelling seen acutely, but ultimately is

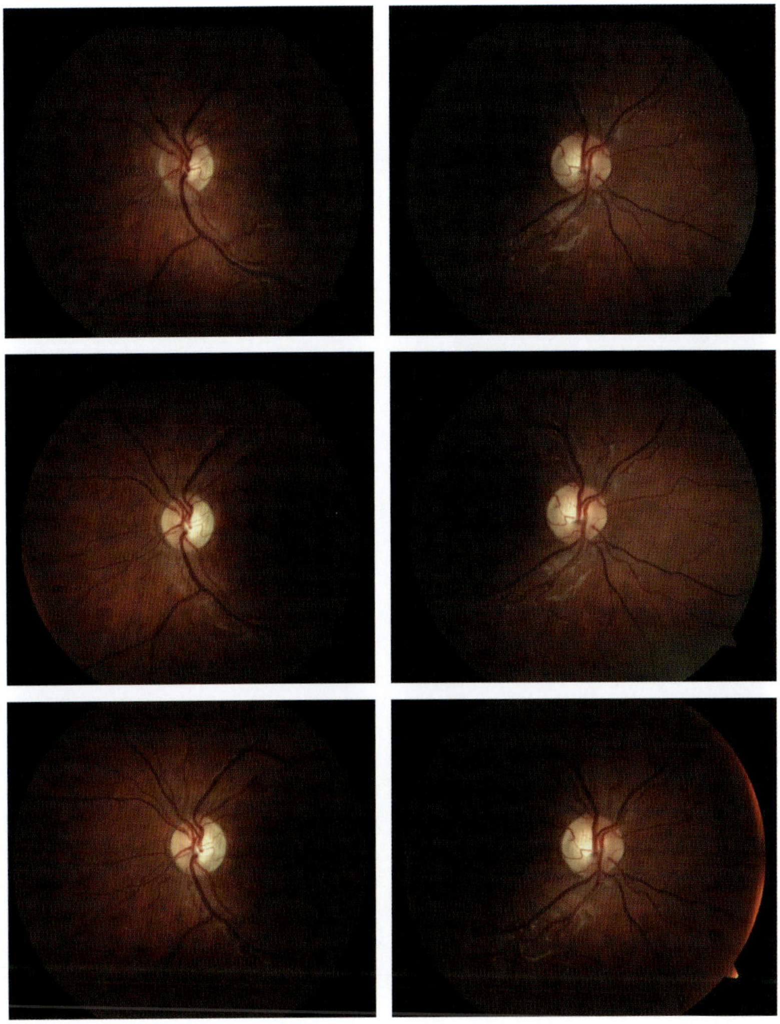

Figure 5.1

associated with the amount of RNFL, MV, and GCL+IPL thinning observed 6–12 months following the inception of the ON related clinical syndrome [2, 7, 11–13].

Interpreting RNFL changes in patients with recurrent ON

It can be difficult to detect RNFL changes in the setting of recurrent ON, because the extent of cumulative RNFL atrophy can be severe and the corresponding visual outcomes dire. In a recent OCT study of 193 MS patients, peripapillary RNFL values were compared between 29 eyes affected by two or more ON events, 125 eyes affected by a single ON event, and 232 eyes without ON. The mean RNFL values were significantly lower in recurrent ON eyes (64 μm) relative to single ON eyes (86 μm) and eyes without ON (100 μm) [14]. Yeh and colleagues [15] noted that average RNFL thickness decreased with an increasing number of ON episodes in pediatric patients with demyelinating syndromes, which supports the premise that recurrent inflammatory events have a cumulative impact in the AVP. This creates a practical challenge to using OCT in the diagnosis and management of acute ON in a patient with preexisting RNFL/MV/GCL+IPL atrophy, because increments of change in OCT measures decrease over time and may be subtle in the context of a new ON event.

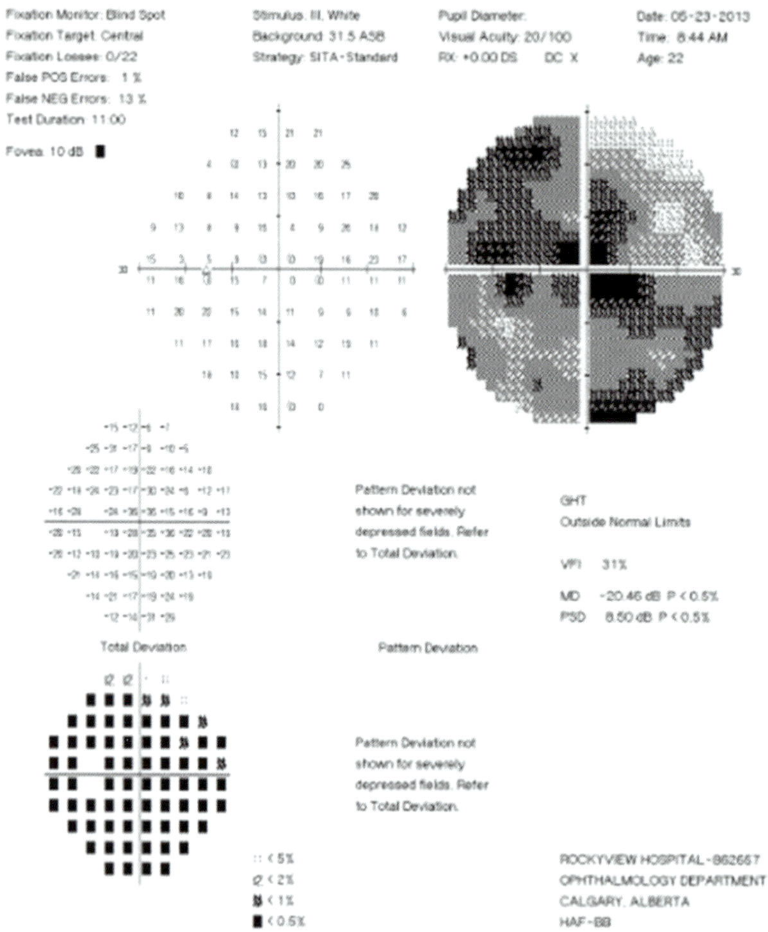

Figure 5.1 (cont.)

Comparing RNFL changes in ON associated with neuromyelitis optica to RNFL changes in ON associated with MS

Neuromyelitis optica (NMO) is a severe inflammatory process of the optic nerves and spinal cord (with occasional brain involvement) that is generally associated with poor clinical recovery. Not surprisingly, RNFL atrophy tends to be extensive in ON eyes of patients with NMO. Several studies have explored the role of OCT in distinguishing ON associated with NMO from that associated with MS. Naismith [16] reported lower RNFL values in ON eyes of 22 NMO patients compared to ON eyes of 47 MS patients and noted that the superior and inferior RNFL quadrants were more severely affected in the former. In this study, the odds of falling into the NMO group increased by 8% for every 1-μm decrease in peripapillary RNFL thickness [16]. In a related study, there was significantly worse RNFL thinning in NMO ON eyes (64 μm) relative to RRMS ON eyes (88 μm) and control eyes (102 μm) [17]. Ratchford [17] reported that a first episode of ON was estimated to cause 24 μm more RNFL loss in NMO eyes relative to RRMS ON eyes. Nakamura [18] described lower RNFL values in NMO ON eyes than in MS ON eyes (64 μm versus 84 μm; $p = 0.0006$) and noted that the frequency of ON relapses and the time to initiate treatment with high-dose intravenous methylprednisolone significantly affected the preservation of RNFL thickness in NMO patients. Syc [11] evaluated 22 NMO patients and reported that GCL+ IPL thickness was decreased in NMO ON eyes compared to NMO non-ON eyes, and that NMO eyes with and without remote ON history had reduced GCL+ PIL thicknesses compared with

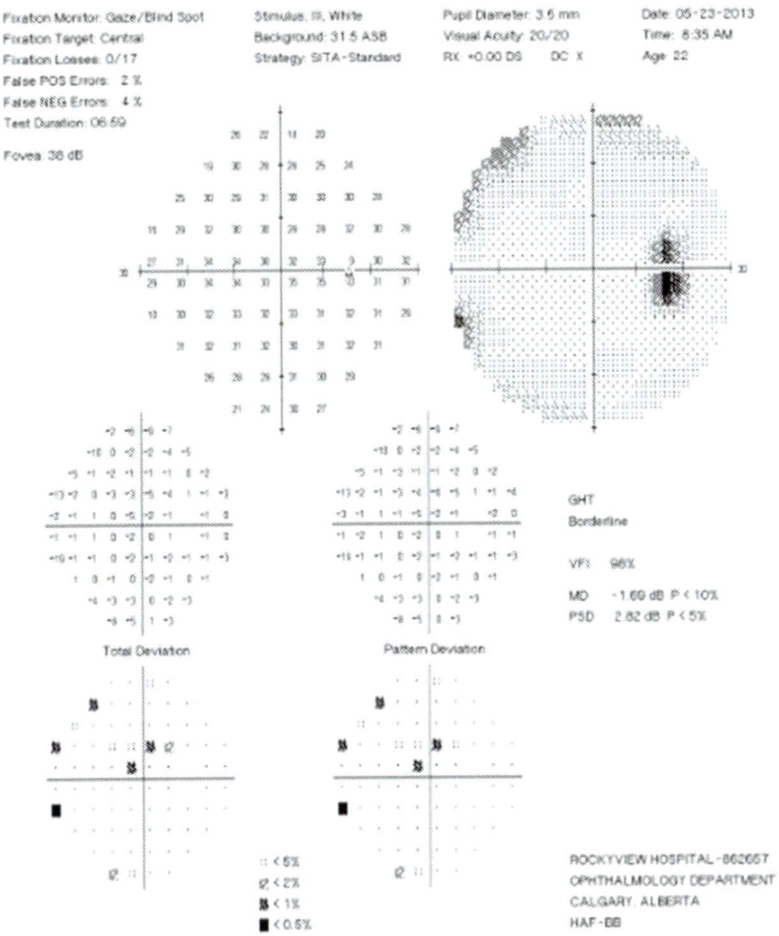

Figure 5.1 (cont.)

those of healthy controls. The importance of diagnosing NMO early cannot be overstated because the natural history of ON associated with this disorder is poor and long-term immunosuppressive therapy is needed. It is noteworthy that patients who manifest an inter-eye asymmetry in RNFL thickness of 15 μm or greater have been deemed more likely to have the diagnosis of NMO (75%) than RRMS (24%) [17]. Yet in studies showing significantly more RNFL thinning in NMO ON eyes relative to MS ON eyes, there has been considerable overlap in the distribution of RNFL values. Hence, in using OCT to differentiate ON associated with NMO from ON associated with MS, it is important to be mindful of issues that could affect RNFL values in either group, including recurrent ON in the same eye and bilateral optic nerve involvement.

Optical coherence tomography and visual outcomes in acute optic neuritis

Optical coherence tomography has been viewed as a putative marker of neuronal and axonal integrity in the afferent visual pathway. If axonal and neuronal damage contribute to neurological disability, one would infer that OCT-measured changes in peripapillary RNFL, MV, and GCL + IPL should correspond to visual deficits in patients with acute ON. In this context, OCT would be a useful ancillary test that could be used to construct a structural–functional paradigm, by which factors influencing injury and repair might be better understood in MS patients.

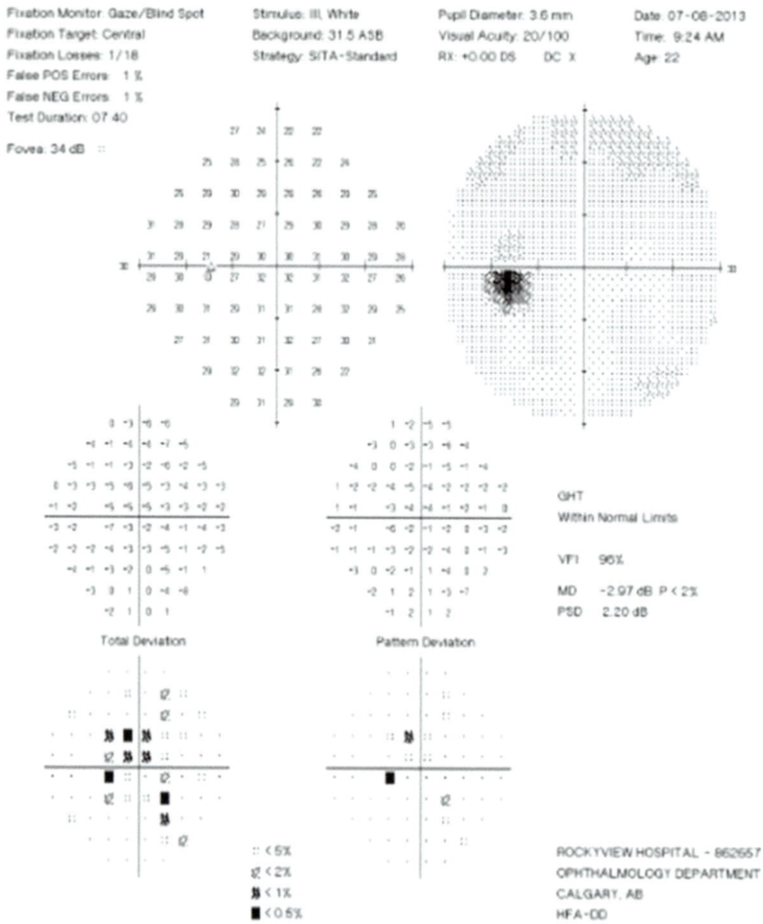

Figure 5.1 (cont.)

High-Contrast Visual Acuity: High-Contrast Visual Acuity (HCVA) refers to the spatial resolving ability of the eye and has long been the mainstay of visual standard testing. The most common HCVA charts employed in clinical research studies include the Snellen and Early Treatment Diabetic Retinopathy Study (ETDRS) charts. The Snellen chart has letters of different sizes arranged from largest at the top to smallest at the bottom, which are read, one eye at a time, at a distance of six meters (20 feet). Snellen visual acuity is usually expressed as a fraction with the numerator equal to the distance from the chart and the denominator being the size of the smallest line that can be read. Because there are numerous limitations to Snellen visual acuity charts [2, 19], the ETDRS method has become the "gold standard" HCVA test for most current clinical trials. The ETDRS charts are superior to Snellen charts because interpatient differences are more accurately measured and longitudinal follow-up measurements have had more consistent precision, regardless of whether the patients had mild or severe vision loss. [19]. In the ETDRS charts, best corrected visual acuity can be converted to logMAR HCVA, which converts the geometric sequence of a traditional chart to a linear scale [19]. In logMAR notation, lower scores correspond to better vision, and as acuity becomes worse, the value of the logMAR increases.

In the setting of acute ON, HCVA impairment is generally maximal at onset, and the deficit in HCVA at one month can predict long-term recovery. Kupersmith and colleagues [20] used the ONTT database to evaluate various "cut points" for baseline and 1-month vision levels that predicted abnormal

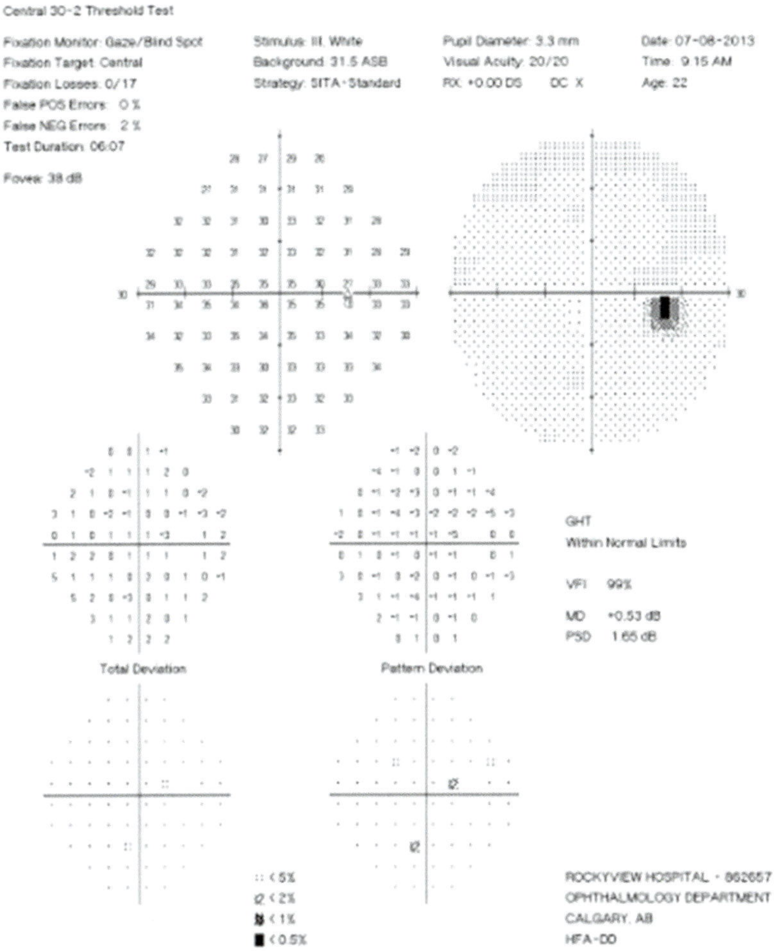

Figure 5.1 (cont.)

six-month vision. Based on their findings, failure to reach a one-month HCVA cut off of 20/50 correlated with having moderate-to-severe loss in this domain of function after six months [20]. On a practical level, if HCVA has not improved by one month, it should also prompt the physician to consider alternate diagnoses or ON mimics (Table 5.2).

At initial presentation, OCT-measured peripapillary RNFL values may be elevated, reflecting optic disc edema in patients with acute ON. In contrast, MV and GCL +IPL thickness maybe normal (in the case of a CIS patient), or perhaps slightly reduced (in the case of MS patients with preexisting damage to the AVP). Initially, there is generally poor concordance between OCT measures of structural integrity and functional outcomes in patients with acute ON. In the post-acute phase, however, lower RNFL, MV, and GCL + IPL values correlate with worse visual function [2, 7, 11–13]. In a prior prospective OCT study, measures of RNFL thickness were compared with logMAR HCVA scores for 54 patients observed a minimum of three months after acute ON [12]. Regression analyses showed that the predictive value for RNFL thickness was significant only for patients with RNFL measures less than 70 μm; lower RNFL values correlated with worse visual acuity outcomes after ON [12]. Not surprisingly, HCVA is worse in the post-acute phase of ON for NMO patients [17]. In their study of 26 NMO patients, Ratchford and colleagues [17] reported a threshold of RNFL thickness measuring 60 μm, below which visual acuity outcomes were poor in the setting of NMO.

Low-Contrast Letter Acuity: While HCVA has been used as the primary outcome in clinical trials

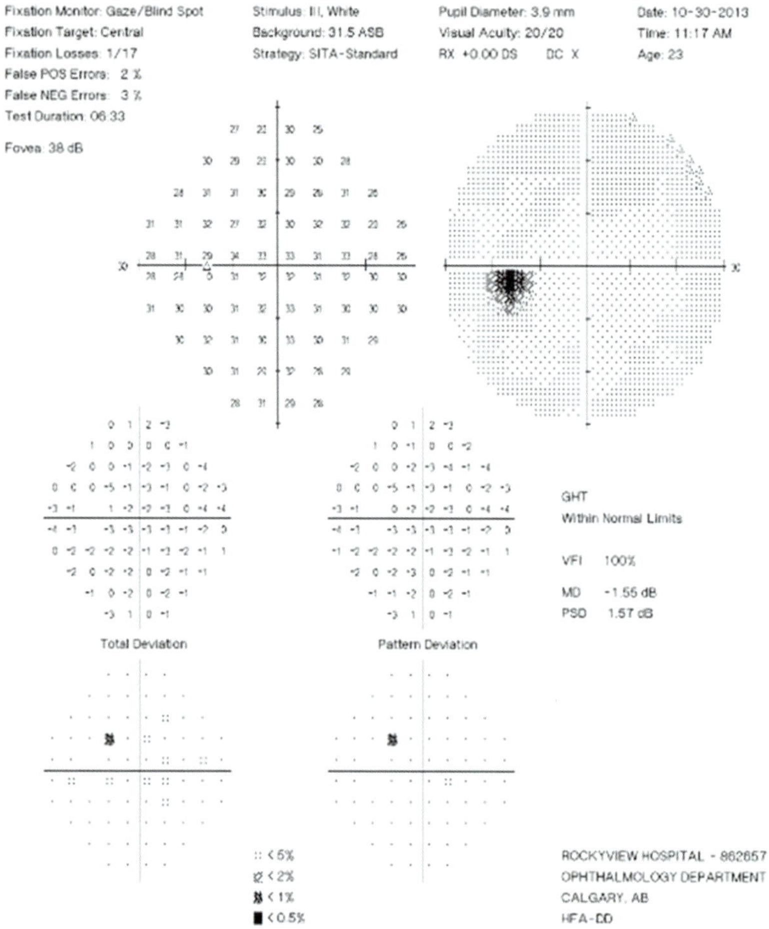

Figure 5.1 (cont.)

in ophthalmology, it is a relatively crude measure of afferent visual function in MS. In fact, many patients will report significant vision problems after acute ON, even in the setting of 20/20 HCVA [21]. High-contrast visual acuity is determined under optimal circumstances of high contrast and high luminance, and it is therefore not surprising that HCVA tends to manifest the most obvious early improvement in acute ON patients. Yet the real visual world is one of varying spatial and temporal frequencies, contrast, color, luminance, and glare [2]. Over the past decade, Balcer and colleagues have spearheaded the implementation of low-contrast letter acuity (LCLA) testing in MS clinical research with the use of Sloan charts [22]. Sloan charts have a standardized format based on the ETDRS HCVA charts and employ three contrast levels: 100% (high-contrast), 2.5%, and 1.25% (lowest contrast level) [22]. Charts are scored letter by letter, and numbers of letters identified correctly constitute the score for each chart. Recently, visual improvement and loss by the LCLA chart has been defined as a seven-letter change in score [22]. In the IMPACT trial and in heterogeneous MS cohorts LCLA testing has been shown to be a highly reliable and practical means of identifying MS-related visual loss compared to other available tests [22]. Low-contrast letter acuity scores have also been shown to correlate with quality-of-life outcomes [22], and, in many respects, to capture the many shades of gray that represent visual perception in our day-to-day lives. In clinical practice, measuring LCLA can be hampered in acute ON patients who present with severe vision loss (worse than 20/200) because they will not be able to visualize the charts [21]. However,

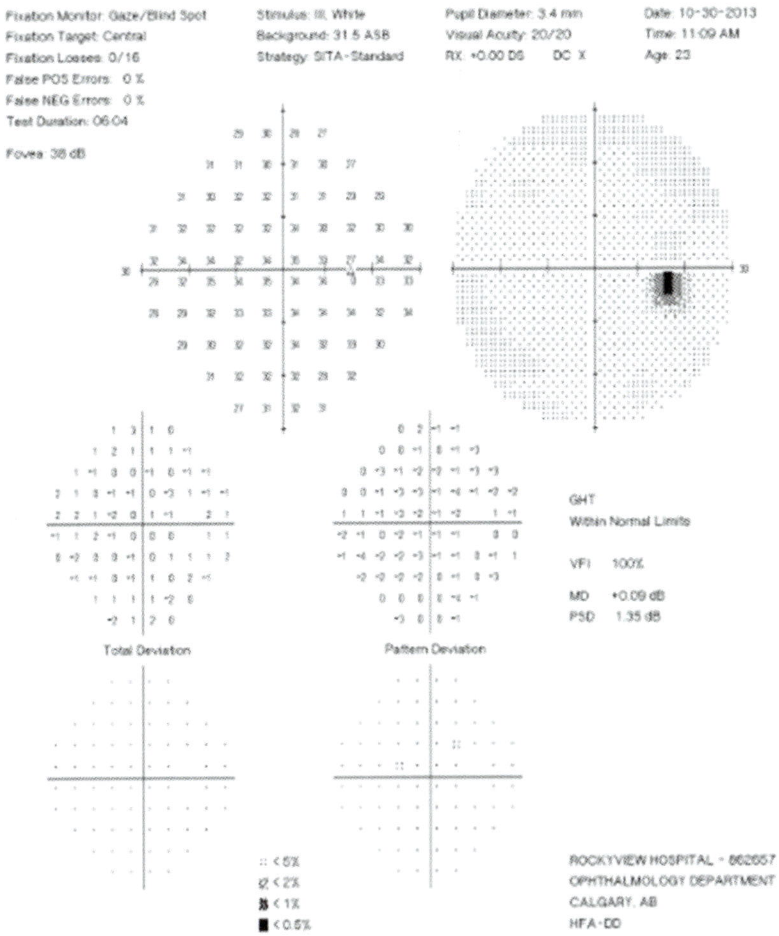

Figure 5.1 (cont.)

post-acutely, LCLA can be used to detect persistent visual deficits that may otherwise be missed in patients who have regained "normal" vision on standard HCVA and visual field testing. Previous studies have shown robust correlations between OCT-measured RNFL, MV, and LCLA outcomes in ON and MS patients [2, 7, 21]. In 2006, Fisher [21] conducted a cross-sectional study comparing RNFL thickness among MS eyes with a history of ON (MS ON eyes), MS eyes without a history of ON (MS non-ON eyes), and disease-free controls. They noted that RNFL thickness was reduced significantly among MS patients (92 μm) relative to controls (105 μm) and that RNFL values were particularly reduced in MS ON eyes (85 μm) [21]. Furthermore, for every one-line decrease in LCLA or contrast sensitivity score, the mean RNFL thickness decreased by 4 μm [21]. More recently, Syc [11] followed 20 acute ON patients with serial HCVA, LCLA, and OCT testing at baseline (within four weeks), three months, and six months of initial presentation. Low-contrast visual acuity at three months improved in ON eyes compared with baseline (2.5% $p = 0.006$; 1.25%, $p = 0.02$) [11]. In this same study, 22 NMO/NMO-spectrum patients were studied in cross-sectional fashion. Ganglion cell layer + IPL, RNFL, and macular thickness values were decreased in NMO ON eyes compared to NMO non-ON eyes, and both NMO eyes with and without remote ON compared with those of healthy controls. Ganglion cell layer+ IPL thickness was significantly associated with 1.25% LCLA in NMO eyes, and 1.25% and 2.5% LCLA in NMO non-ON eyes [11]. Hence, LCLA testing is more sensitive in detecting visual deficits than

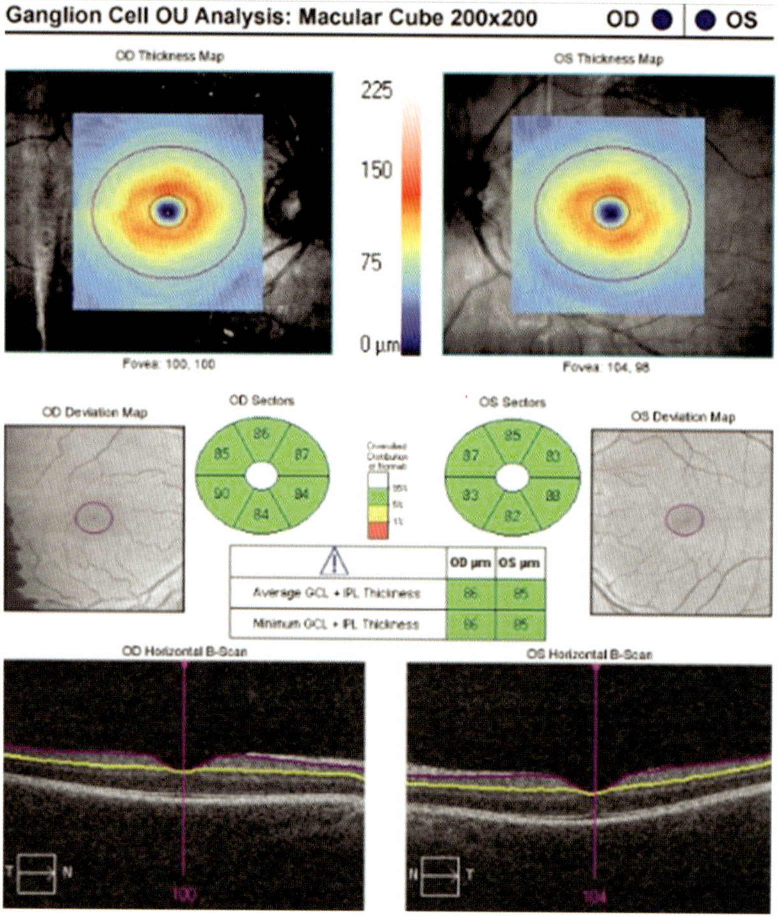

Figure 5.1 (cont.)

HCVA testing in MS, and inclusion of these functional outcomes in the AVP model will better capture deficits that impact quality of life and day-to-day function in these patients.

Color Vision: Dyschromatopsia or loss of color vision is common in the setting of acute ON, and improves weeks to months after initial presentation. Indeed, the detection of disproportionate color vision loss can be key to making the diagnosis in patients with acute ON who manifest mild deficits in HCVA function. One of the challenges in interpreting color vision outcomes is that various modalities are used, and there is less standardization relative to HCVA, LCLA, and perimetry testing. Raz and colleagues [23] followed 21 patients with new-onset acute ON with serial HCVA, perimetry, color vision (Ishikawa pseudoisochromatic plates), visual evoked potentials (VEP), contrast sensitivity, motion perception, and OCT testing. In ON eyes, HCVA, visual field, and color perception were significantly impaired at initial presentation and recovered completely after one month [23]. Contrast sensitivity recovered after four months [23]. After 12 months, the RNFL values in both ON eyes and non-ON eyes were reduced when compared to the normal controls. The VEP amplitudes of ON eyes were decreased in the acute phase but not subsequently [23]. Both ON eyes and non-ON eyes of ON patients had significantly prolonged VEP latencies at all testing phases. This study demonstrated that functional recovery occurs at different time points, depending on the testing modality used to follow ON patients.

Various other testing techniques have been used effectively to capture color vision deficits in ON and

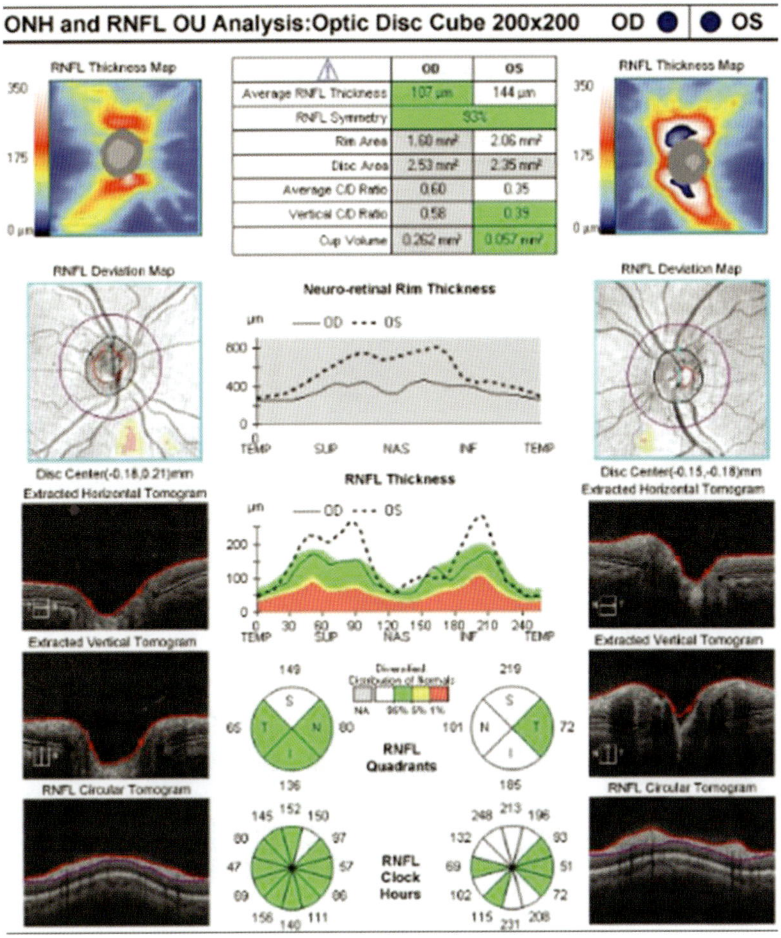

Figure 5.1 (cont.)

MS patients. Hardy-Rand-Rittler (HRR) pseudoisochromatic color plates have demonstrated an advantage over the Ishihara method, because the former are more sensitive to red–green and blue–yellow deficits caused by neuro-ophthalmic disorders [2]. Recently Villoslada and colleagues [24] studied 213 MS patient and 47 healthy controls to determine the relationship between HCVA, LCVA, color vision (HRR pseudoisochromatic plates and Lanthony D15 tests), and OCT measures in MS patients. Multiple sclerosis patients showed HCVA and LCLA deficits but exhibited even more profound abnormalities in color discrimination relative to controls [24]. Moura and colleagues [25] assessed chromatic discrimination in 35 MS patients (with and without ON) and 74 age-matched controls using the Cambridge color test (CCT) to determine the magnitude and chromatic axes of color vision loss in both patient groups. They also endeavored to evaluate age-related changes in chromatic discrimination in both patient groups compared to normal control subjects. Color thresholds for both ON eyes and non-ON eyes in MS patients were significantly higher than controls' along the protan and tritan axes [25]. In addition, the ON and non-ON groups differed significantly along all three-color axes [25]. Multiple sclerosis patients manifested progressive color discrimination impairment with age (along the deutan and tritan axes) that was almost two times faster than controls, even in the absence of ON [25]. In a seminal OCT study, Trip [26] selected 25 ON patients in the post-acute phase with incomplete visual recovery, and performed cross-sectional analyses comparing OCT measured peripapillary RNFL thickness and MV, VEP, HCVA, perimetry, and color vision testing (Farnsworth–Munsell). In this study, RNFL thickness

Approximately six weeks later the RNFL values have decreased in the left eye (103 μm) along with the evolution of temporal pallor in this eye. Note the RNFL thickness in the temporal quadrant has decreased in the left eye (yellow) relative to the right eye. In contrast to the left eye, RNFL values in the right eye remain stable (106 μm). There is evident thinning of the ganglion cell analysis measurements in the left eye (numbers in red) as compared to the right eye (numbers in green)

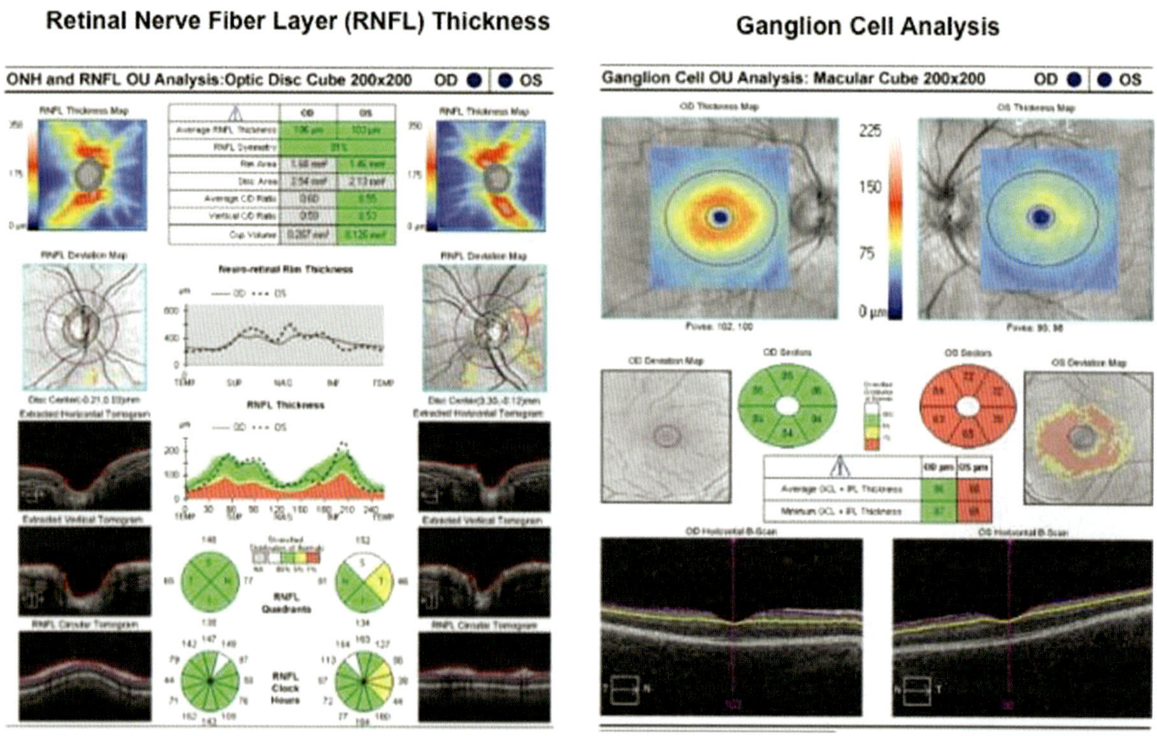

Figure 5.1 (cont.)

was reduced by 33%, and macular volume by 11% in ON eyes relative to control eyes [26]. Interestingly, in ON eyes lower MV values were associated with color vision loss. The authors highlighted that axons originating in the macula pass in the papillomacular bundle to the temporal side of the optic disc; consistent with this, MV values were related to the thickness of the temporal RNFL quadrant in this study [26].

Given that NMO patients have generally more severe ON than that seen in MS patients, RNFL values are reduced in NMO ON eyes, and they correlate with more severe color vision deficits than their MS counterparts. In a cross-sectional study of 15 NMO patients, 15 MS patients, and 23 controls, Merle and colleagues [27] reported lower RNFL values in NMO patients (65 μm) relative to MS (84 μm) and control (106 μm) eyes. This group employed OCT, HCVA, LCLA (1.25% and 2.5%), perimetry, and Farnsworth 100 Hue color vision testing. There was a significant correlation between the average peripapillary RNFL thickness, HCVA, LCLA, and visual field scores [27]. Yet, there was no correlation between OCT measures and color vision testing. These investigators did not use temporal RNFL or MV measurements in their study, which may in part explain the differences in their results as compared to the findings by Trip et al. [27]. Future studies could further explore the optimal color vision test to use in patients with acute ON, and determine whether GCL+ IPL thickness as a marker of neuronal integrity correlates with color vision deficits in various phases of recovery.

Visual Field Testing: Visual field testing has been described as the "cornerstone" of the sensory visual examination and provides invaluable information about the integrity of afferent visual pathway function from the retina to the visual cortex [28]. Perimetry has evolved through stages since original

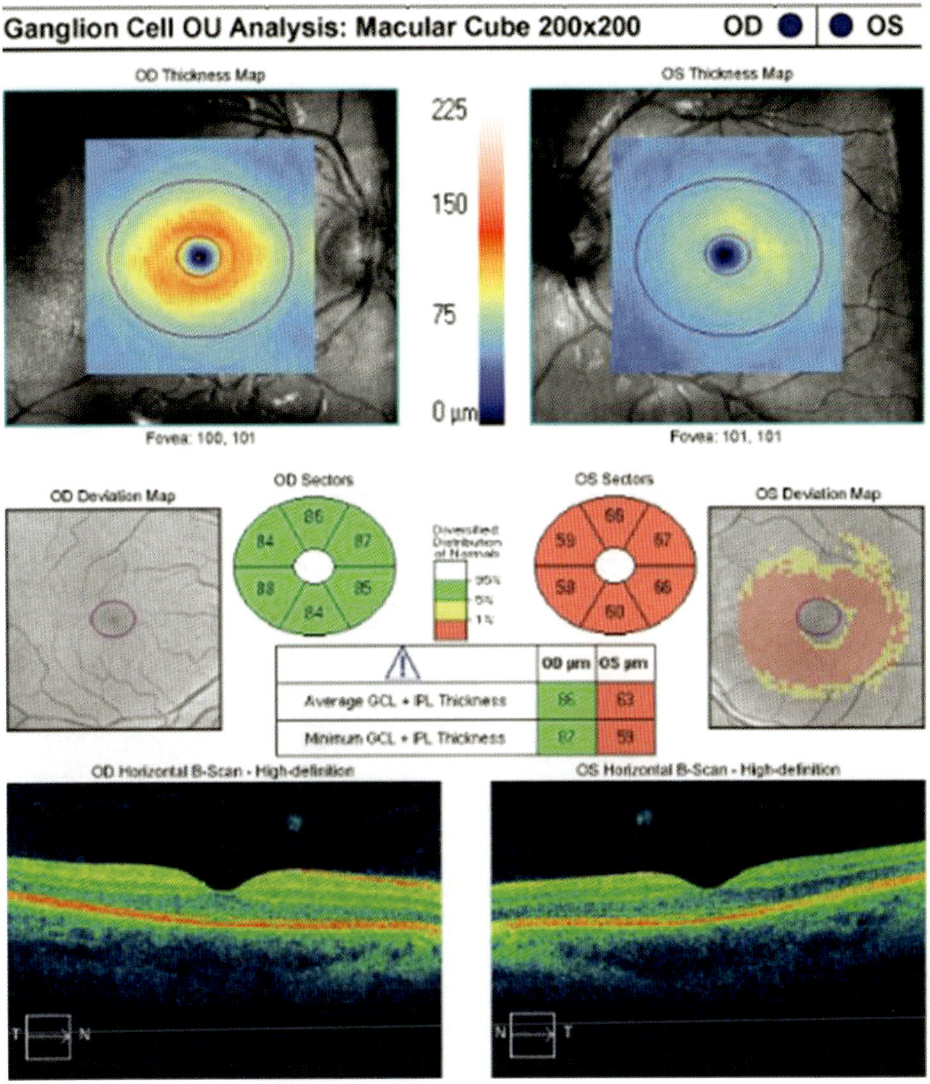

Figure 5.1 (cont.)

confrontation-based techniques to allow quantification and statistical analysis in its currently used computerized forms. This provides critical information about visual function, including both central and peripheral channels. Moreover, many of the perimeters in common use today are readily available in most cities around the developed world, allowing for standardization between centers, and easier comparisons across offices over time. In the recent 15-year follow-up from the ONTT, Keltner [29] defined visual field characteristics and classifications for the entire cohort, from baseline through 15 years (10,443 visual fields). At initial presentation, 100% of the visual fields from the ON eyes and 75% of the visual fields from the fellow (non-ON) eyes in patients were abnormal [29]. After year one of the study, 50% of the visual fields were abnormal in ON eyes, whereas the abnormal visual field frequency in non-ON eyes ranged between 34% and 40% [29]. Diffuse and central visual field losses were more prominent in ON eyes than non-ON eyes at baseline. Retinal nerve fiber bundle defects (partial arcuate, paracentral, and arcuate) were the most prominent localized abnormalities in ON and non-ON eyes during the study [29]. After 15 years, 40% of abnormalities in the ON eyes and 26% in the non-ON eyes consisted of localized defects [29]. Foveal threshold, as measured by Humphrey perimetry,

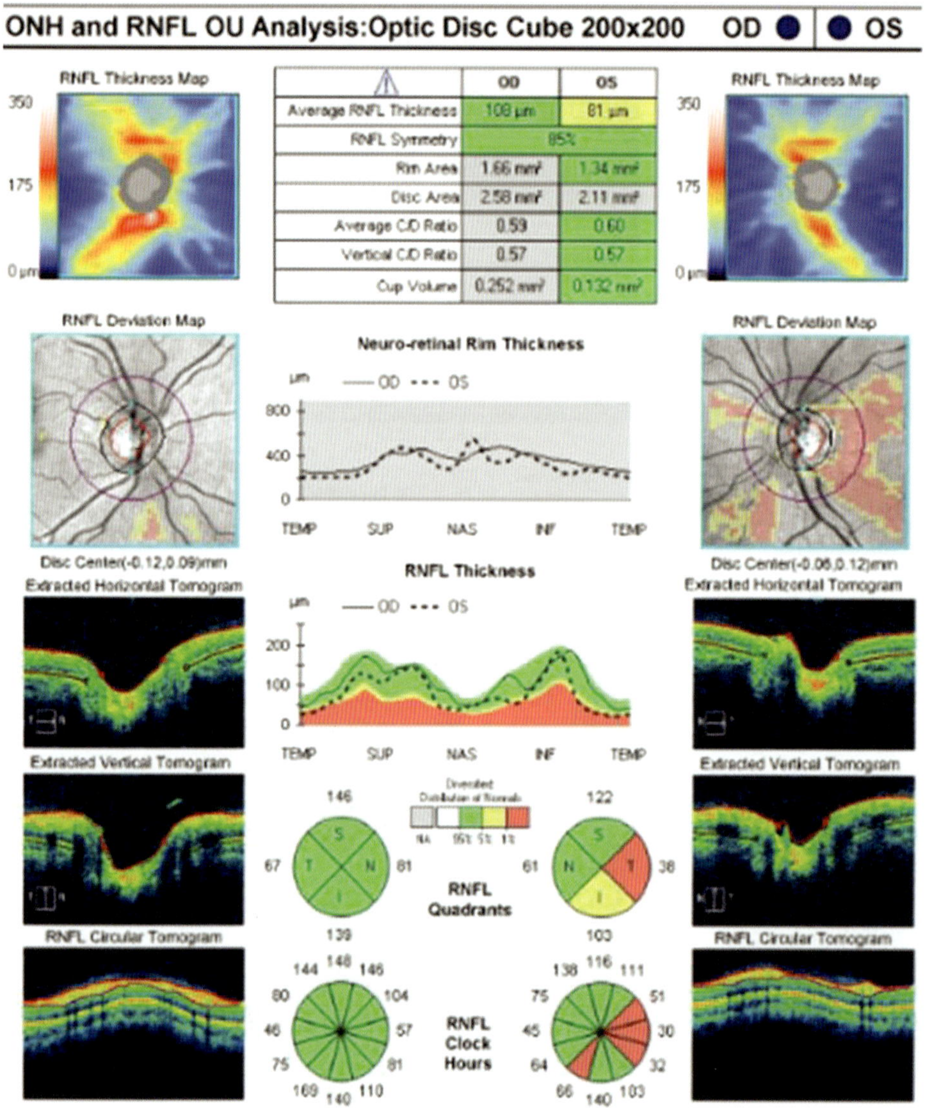

Figure 5.1 (cont.)

correlated with HCVA and contrast sensitivity in ON eyes at baseline, six months, and one year [29].

For all of the established advantages of automated perimetry, there are potential pitfalls with this testing modality in a patient population that is subject to fatigue-related visual dysfunction. Wall and colleagues [30] followed 17 patients with ON and ten healthy control subjects with repeat intra-day and interday automated perimetry testing (five Humphrey 30–2 tests were administered during a seven-hour period on the same day and at the same period on five separate days). Optic neuritis patients demonstrated variations in visual field sensitivity outside the entire range of variability for normal controls [30]. These variations occurred for multiple tests performed on the same day, at specific times, and for tests performed at specific times on different days [30]. Thus, when using automated perimetry, or for that matter any subjective psychophysical test to follow ON and MS patients, distinguishing true change from variability remains a challenge. In the case of automated perimetry, this requires more than comparing a current visual field test with the most recent previous visual field test; rather, trends should be observed over time.

In 2006, our group followed 54 patients with acute ON prospectively over a 12-month period with serial OCT, HCVA, and automated perimetry testing [12]. Thinning of the RNFL was seen in the majority of patients (74%), and it tended to occur within 3 to 6 months of symptom onset [12]. The average peripapillary RNFL values were thinner in ON eyes (78 μm) than in non-ON eyes (100 μm) [12]. Patients with incomplete visual recovery demonstrated worse RNFL loss after ON. Regression analyses revealed a threshold of RNFL thickness (75 μm), below which RNFL measurements predicted persistent visual field dysfunction [12]. In this same study, measures of RNFL thickness were compared with log MAR visual acuity for 54 patients observed a minimum of three months after acute ON. The predictive value for RNFL thickness was significant only for patients with measures less than 70 μm, below which RNFL values were associated with worse HCVA outcomes after ON [12]. Interestingly, in subsequent work, an OCT-measured RNFL threshold of 80 μm was found to distinguish patients with persistent LCLA deficits after acute ON [22]. Given that LCLA, automated perimetry techniques, and HCVA are variably sensitive to persistent visual deficits after acute ON, OCT testing may reveal a range of RNFL (and MV and GCL+IPL) thresholds that predict visual recovery, depending on visual outcome used.

Visual Evoked Potential Testing: The VEP is a response of the brain to repeated visual stimulation and has traditionally been recorded when visual field is stimulated with a single checkerboard pattern in the full-field (ff-VEP). The VEP is known to be generated at the level of striate cortex. The magnitude of the VEP is interpreted to reflect the number of functional afferent fibers reaching this region [31, 32]. In ON patients, the number of functional afferent fibers is believed to be determined by the severity of the inflammation and axonal degeneration along the visual pathway [31, 32]. Therefore, diminished VEP amplitude indicates inflammation-induced conduction block, axonal atrophy, or a combination of both [31, 32]. Subsequently, an increase in VEP amplitude is a consequence of resumed conduction in previously blocked fibers, due to resolution of inflammation and edema, or possibly expansion of synaptic activity along the visual pathway [31, 32]. Delayed VEP conduction is recognized as one of the earliest features of acute ON, with the subsequent shortening of latency thought to represent remyelination [31, 32]. Because it is a summation of a large number of neuronal elements, the ffVEP is greatly dominated by the macular region due to its cortical overrepresentation [31, 32]. Moreover, the waveform of the ffVEP is prone to cancellation and distortion, which sometimes leads to apparent, rather than real, latency delay [31, 32]. In contrast, the multifocal VEP (mfVEP) allows stimulation of small areas of the visual field. The result is a detailed topographical assessment of small groups of axons within the optic nerve and visual cortex, which is resistant to waveform distortion [31, 32]. In a recent study, Klistorner and colleagues [31] used mfVEP and OCT testing to study 25 subjects with acute unilateral ON. While mfVEP amplitude asymmetry at baseline varied significantly among the patients, it was, on average, very high, indicating considerable reduction of amplitude in ON eyes [31]. The inter-eye asymmetry in mfVEP amplitude decreased over time, indicating functional recovery [31]. There was a negative correlation between the inter-eye asymmetry of OCT-measured RNFL thickness and that of mfVEP amplitude at one month, consistent with vasogenic edema in the acute phase (causing an increase in RNFL thickness with a corresponding reduction in mfVEP amplitude) [31]. Over the course of recovery, the correlation became progressively more robust, suggesting the diminishing role of optic nerve edema in measured RNFL thickness and unmasking the association between RNFL atrophy and low mfVEP amplitude [31]. The potential correlation between OCT-measured RNFL values and mfVEP measures of anterior visual pathway damage was demonstrated by the same group, who evaluated 32 patients with unilateral ON and 25 control subjects with mfVEP and OCT testing [32]. The mean RNFL thickness in ON eyes (85 μm) was reduced by 19% compared with control eyes (104 μm). There was a 40% reduction in the amplitude of the mfVEP in ON eyes relative to control eyes [32]. In addition to demonstrating the utility of mfVEP in tracking optic nerve injury in ON patients, this study further confirmed the significant correlations between structural and functional measures of optic nerve integrity, and showed that demyelination contributes to axonal loss. It may, therefore, be feasible to pair mfVEP and OCT testing to capture the synergistic effects of acute demyelination and axonal loss over time in ON/MS patients. Furthermore, the putative relationship between the VEP latency and axonal loss encourages the notion that therapeutic interventions aimed at reducing the effects of demyelination or enhancing remyelination may be given a trial in the AVP model.

Motion Perception Testing: Standard tests of visual function generally interrogate our perception of "form," and tend to ignore perception of motion, which has an enormous impact on the day-to-day function. In the convalescent phase, many ON patients report the "Pulfrich phenomenon" (a binocular perception that a small target moving in a frontal plane is traveling in an elliptical path) and describe difficulties tracking moving objects. The hypothesis that ON can have prolonged effects on visual motion processing, which may persist after there has been an objective return to normal "form" perception, was further explored by Raz and colleagues in a series of elegant papers [23, 33]. They prospectively followed 21 ON patients over one year with tests of spatial and dynamic visual function including: HCVA, perimetry, contrast sensitivity, color vision, VEP, and OCT testing [23, 33]. In addition, the authors developed a novel set of motion perceptual tasks to test dynamic visual deficits as part of their protocol [23, 33]. In ON eyes, visual acuity, visual field, and color vision deficits were significantly impaired in the acute phase, and subsequently improved after one month [23]. Contrast sensitivity deficits tended to persist somewhat longer, improving four months after symptom onset [23]. As compared to tests of spatial visual function, motion perception was impaired during the full follow-up period of one year [23]. Thus, motion perception testing revealed the most significant and prolonged impairment after ON and was independent of contrast sensitivity levels [23].

In a follow-up study, the same group aimed to identify mechanisms underpinning the sustained deficits in dynamic visual functions following ON. They hypothesized that motion perception may be more vulnerable to slowed conduction in the optic nerve, which could be measured with VEP testing [33]. To explore this theory further, they did serial motion perception and ffVEP testing at presentation, one month, four months, and twelve months after acute ON [33]. The VEP amplitudes in ON eyes were significantly reduced compared to fellow eyes in the acute phase, but these differences resolved in later phases of recovery [33]. As has been previously reported, visual performance with HCVA, contrast sensitivity, and motion perception at one month was highly predictive of visual recovery a year after acute ON [33]. Intact VEP amplitudes were associated with recovered visual acuity and contrast sensitivity after ON, suggesting that these visual functions depend on a sufficient amount of visual information reaching the cortex [33]. Yet motion perception was impaired even in patients with intact VEP amplitudes, indicating that an intact amount of visual projection alone does not impact dynamic visual function [33]. Instead, while the magnitude of contrast sensitivity improvement related to the extent of VEP amplitude restoration, the magnitude of motion perception improvement depended on the extent of VEP latency reduction post-ON [33]. From these findings, it was inferred that there is a need for rapid transmission of visual input to perceive motion. Moreover, motion perception testing in concert with VEP may serve to assess the processes of demyelination and remyelination in the AVP model of MS.

Binocular Summation: Binocular summation refers to the improved visual function observed when patients perform threshold tasks such as contrast detection with a binocular view as compared to monocular vision [34]. Conversely, binocular inhibition refers to worse outcomes for visual threshold tasks obtained with binocular vision as compared to the monocular view obtained when patients use their better seeing eye [34]. The phenomena of binocular summation and inhibition are not well understood, but appear to be related to neural input from both eyes within the post-geniculate visual pathway [34]. Given that binocular summation is most likely processed at the cortical level, MS and ON patients may experience functional limitations due to interruptions in normal cortical signaling. In a recent study of 1,007 patients with MS and 324 disease-free controls, binocular summation was substantial for LCLA at the 2.5% and 1.25% levels [34]. With HCVA, only 3% of patients showed similar degrees of summation [34]. Increasing age, greater interocular differences in acuity, and prior ON were factors associated with lower magnitudes of binocular summation and worse binocular inhibition [34]. Greater degrees of binocular summation were predictive of better quality-of-life outcomes, indicating that the capacity to use both eyes together is an important factor in determining how well patients with MS perform daily activities [34]. In future studies, the effects of binocular summation and inhibition could potentially be compared to OCT (as a structural measure of neuronal and axonal damage), VEP (as a demyelination and remyelination marker), and functional MRI (as a means of detecting cortical activation).

In this way, the relative contribution of cortical compensation to visual recovery, and the factors that govern the potential for cortical plasticity, may be determined after acute ON in patients with CNS demyelinating disorders.

Summary

The AVP model offers an exciting opportunity to explore disease mechanisms that contribute to neurological disability in MS patients. Monitoring the acute and chronic consequences of clinically overt ON events may shed light on factors that the govern injury and repair in acute inflammatory relapse in the CNS. Highly sensitive and standardized tests of vision can be paired with high-resolution imaging measures of structural integrity in the AVP pathway to develop a structural–functional paradigm of CNS injury. In the future, the AVP model may allow us to determine how remyelination contributes to axonal and neuronal repair. Furthermore, this model may also help us determine whether retinal damage in MS arises from retrobulbar optic nerve pathology or primary neuronal pathology.

References

1. Miller D, Barkhof F, Montalban X, Thompson A, Filippi M. Clinically isolated syndromes suggestive of multiple sclerosis, Part 1: natural history, pathogenesis, diagnosis and prognosis. *Lancet Neurol.* 2005; **4**: 281–88.
2. Costello F. The afferent visual pathway: designing a structural-functional paradigm of multiple sclerosis. *ISRN Neurol* 2013; doi:10.1155/2013/134858.
3. Frohman EM, Fujimoto JG, Frohman TC, Calabresi PA, Cutter G, Balcer LJ. Optical coherence tomography: a window into the mechanisms of multiple sclerosis. *Nat Clin Pract Neurol.* 2008; **4**: 664–75.
4. Beck RW, Cleary PA, Anderson MM, et al. A randomized, controlled trial of corticosteroids in the treatment of acute optic neuritis. The Optic Neuritis Study Group. *N Engl J Med.* 1992; **326**: 581–8.
5. Hickman SJ, Dalton CM, Miller DH, Plant GT. Management of acute optic neuritis. *Lancet.* 2002; **360**: 1953–62.
6. Beck RW, Cleary PA, Optic Neuritis Study Group. Optic Neuritis Treatment Trial one year follow-up results. *Arch Ophthalmol.* 1993; **111**: 773–5.
7. Costello F, Klistorner A, Kardon R. Optical coherence tomography in the diagnosis and management of optic neuritis and multiple sclerosis. *Ophthalmic Surg Lasers Imaging.* 2011; **48**: S28-S40.
8. Green AJ, McQuaid S, Hauser SL, Allen IV, Lyness R. Ocular pathology in multiple sclerosis: retinal atrophy and inflammation irrespective of disease duration. *Brain* 2010; **133**: 1591–1.
9. Miller D, Barkhof F, Montalban X, Thompson A, Filippi M. Clinically isolated syndromes suggestive of multiple sclerosis, part 2: non-conventional MRI, recovery processes, and management. *Lancet Neurol.* 2005; **4**: 341–8.
10. http://www.guggenheim.org/new-york/education/school-educator-programs/teacher-resources/arts-curriculum-online?view=item&catid=730&id=120
11. Syc S, Saidha S, Newsome SD, et al. Optical coherence tomography segmentation reveals ganglion cell layer pathology after optic neuritis. *Brain.* 2012; **135**: 521–33.
12. Costello F, Coupland S, Hodge W, et al. Quantifying axonal loss after optic neuritis with optical coherence tomography. *Ann Neurol.* 2006; **59**: 963–9.
13. Henderson APD, Altmann DR, Trip SA, Kallis C, Jones SJ, Schlottmann PG, et al. A serial study of retinal changes following optic neuritis with sample size estimates for acute neuroprotection trials. *Brain* 2010; **133**: 2592–602.
14. Costello F, Hodge W, Pan YI, Metz L, Kardon RH. Retinal nerve fiber layer and future risk of multiple sclerosis. *Can J Neurol Sci.* 2008; **35**: 482–7.
15. Yeh EA, Weinstock-Guttman B, Lincoff N, et al. Retinal nerve fiber thickness in inflammatory demyelinating diseases of childhood onset. *Mult Scler.* 2009; **15**: 802–10.
16. Naismith RT, Tutlam NT, Xu J, et al. Optical coherence tomography differs in neuromyelitis optica compared with multiple sclerosis. *Neurology.* 2009; **72**: 1077–82.
17. Ratchford JN, Quigg ME, Conger A, et al. Optical coherence tomography helps differentiate neuromyelitis optica and MS optic neuropathies. *Neurology.* 2009; **73**: 302–8.
18. Nakamura M, Nakazawa T, Doi H, et al. Early high-dose intravenous methylprednisolone is effective in preserving retinal nerve fiber layer thickness in patients with neuromyelitis optica. *Graefes Arch Clin Exp Ophthalmol.* 2010; **248**: 1777–85.
19. Kaiser PK. Prospective Evaluation of Visual Acuity Assessment: A Comparison of Snellen versus ETDRS Charts in Clinical Practice (An AOS Thesis). *Trans Am Ophthalmol Soc.* 2009; **107**: 311–24.
20. Kupersmith MJ, Gal RL, Beck RW, et al. Optic Neuritis Study Group. Visual function at baseline and 1 month in acute optic neuritis: predictors of visual outcome. *Neurology.* 2007 Aug 7; **69**(6): 508–14.
21. Fisher JB, Jacobs DA, Markowitz CE, et al. Relation of visual function to retinal nerve fiber layer

thickness in multiple sclerosis. *Ophthalmology*. 2006; **113**: 324–32.

22. Sakai RE, Feller DJ, Galetta KM, Galetta SL, Balcer LJ. Vision in Multiple Sclerosis: The Story, Structure–Function Correlations, and Models for Neuroprotection. *Journal of Neuro-Ophthalmology* 2011; **31**: 362–73.
23. Raz N, Dotan S, Benoliel T, et al. Sustained motion perception deficit following optic neuritis. Behavioral and cortical evidence. *Neurology;* 2011; **76**: 2103–11.
24. Villoslada P, Cuneo A, Gelfand J, Hauser SL, Green A. Color vision is strongly associated with retinal thinning in multiple sclerosis. *Mult Scler*. 2012; **18**(7): 991–9.
25. Moura AL, Teixeir RA, Oiwa NN, et al. Chromatic discrimination losses in multiple sclerosis patients with and without optic neuritis using the Cambridge Colour Test. *Vis Neurosci Vis*. 2008; **25**(3): 463–8.
26. Trip SA, Schlottmann PG, Jones SJ, et al. Retinal nerve fiber layer axonal loss and visual dysfunction in optic neuritis. *Ann Neurol*. 2005; **58**: 383–91.
27. Merle H, Olindo S, Donnio A, Richer R, Smadja D, Cabre P. Retinal Peripapillary Nerve fiber layer thickness in neuromyelitis optica. *Invest Ophthalmol Vis Sci*. 2008; **49**: 4412–7.
28. M. Wall. Choice and interpretation of visual field testing. In: Levin LA, Arnold AC. *Neuro-Ophthalmology the Practical Guide*. Chapter 4, Thieme Medical Publishers, 2005.
29. Keltner JL, Johnson CA, Cello KE. Visual field profile of optic neuritis: A final follow-up report from the Optic Neuritis Treatment Trial from baseline through 15 years. *Arch Ophthalmol*. 2010; **128**(3): 330–7
30. Wall M, Johnson CA, Kutzko KE, Nguyen R, Brito C, Keltner JL. Long- and short-term variability of automated perimetry results in patients with optic neuritis and healthy subjects. *Arch Ophthalmol* 1998; **116**(1): 53–61.
31. Klistorner A, Arvind H, Nguyen T, et al. Axonal loss and myelin in early ON loss in postacute optic neuritis. *Ann Neurol*. 2008; **64**: 325–31.
32. Klistorner A, Arvind H, Nguyen T, et al. Multifocal VEP and OCT in optic neuritis: a topographical study of the structure-function relationship. *Doc Ophthalmol*. 2009; **118**: 129–37.
33. Raz N, Dotan S, Chokron S, Ben-Hur T, Levin N. Demyelination Affects Temporal aspects of perception: An optic neuritis study. *Ann Neurol*. 2012; **71**: 531–8.
34. Pineless SL, Birch EE, Talman LS. One eye or two: A comparison of binocular and monocular low-contrast acuity testing in multiple sclerosis. *Am J Ophthalmol* 2011; **152**: 133–40.

Chapter 6

Optical coherence tomography and low-contrast acuity

Shin C. Beh and Laura J. Balcer

Introduction

Multiple sclerosis (MS) is perhaps the quintessential neurologic disorder for which the structure–function correlations provided by optical coherence tomography (OCT) have allowed the visual system to serve as a model for understanding the disorder and testing new therapies. Low-contrast letter acuity testing has provided a sensitive and reliable measure of visual function that completes this model in conjunction with OCT. However, it was low-contrast letter acuity that first emerged in the line of investigation that brought vision to a prominent place within MS research and clinical trials.

In the 1990s, in a quest for a more sensitive outcome measure, the National MS Society Clinical Outcomes Assessment Task Force developed the MS Functional Composite (MSFC) [1]. Not yet included in the MSFC at that time, however, was a measure of visual function; this was the case since high-contrast visual acuity, measured most frequently using Snellen charts, did not show sufficient sensitivity to change over time in the clinical trial datasets used to develop the MSFC. The ability of low-contrast sensitivity testing to detect visual abnormalities that would otherwise be missed with Snellen charts in the Optic Neuritis Treatment Trial (ONTT) spurred the use of low-contrast vision as an exploratory outcome measure in MS clinical trials. Even prior to the identification of low-contrast letter acuity as a potential visual component for the MSFC and test of function for MS research, an extensive literature on various forms of low-contrast vision testing provided evidence supporting its role in MS.

What is low-contrast vision?

Spatial contrast can be understood as the light–dark transition at the border or edge of an image that delineates the existence of a pattern or object [2]. More specifically, contrast is defined as the ratio of the difference in the luminance of these two adjacent areas to the lower or higher of these luminance values [2]. The amount of contrast can be quantified using the Weber (used when background luminance remains constant) or Michelson (used when both light and dark components change) formulas [3, 4].

The minimum amount of contrast needed to visualize a target is referred to as the contrast threshold [2, 3]. In clinical research, it is typically expressed as contrast sensitivity, where sensitivity is simply the reciprocal, or inverse, of contrast threshold [2, 3]. Contrast sensitivity is expressed on a logarithmic_{10} scale, to make the values linear and permit comparison at low- and high-contrast levels [2, 3].

The size of a target influences how much contrast is required to distinguish it from its background. Any target size may be depicted by lines of appropriate spacing, subtending a specific visual angle. The number of adjacent dark and light lines (cycles) within a defined visual angle is defined as the spatial frequency. A high spatial frequency (or high number of cycles per degree) consists of more densely packed lines, while a low spatial frequency is displayed as sparsely packed lines [3]. The contrast-sensitivity function represents the relationship between contrast sensitivity and spatial frequency [3, 4].

On the other hand, visual acuity (VA) refers to a measure of the spatial-resolving ability of the visual system, typically under conditions of high contrast (black on white, or at least 85% contrast); all the targets are presented at the same contrast level, but their sizes vary during the test [2].

Optical Coherence Tomography in Neurological Disease, ed. Peter A. Calabresi, Laura J. Balcer, and Elliot M. Frohman. Published by Cambridge University Press.

The neural substrate for low-contrast vision

In the retina, rod photoreceptors specialize in scotopic (low-light-level) vision, while cone photoreceptors mediate chromatic vision in photopic (high-light-level) conditions. Beyond the level of the photoreceptors, there are predominantly two parallel but morphologically and physiologically distinct neuronal populations – the large type A (or phasic) retinal ganglion cells (RGC) and the smaller type B (or tonic) RGCs [5–7].

The type A RGCs form the magnocellular (M– or dorsal) pathway that projects to the magnocellular layers (via thick axons in the optic nerve) of the lateral geniculate nucleus (LGN), and subsequently the 4C-alpha layer of the striate cortex [8–11]. Making up 10% of the total RGC population, almost all these M cells have large receptive fields, have high-contrast sensitivity but poor chromatic sensitivity, and are responsible for detection of low and medium spatial frequencies, motion, and fast flicker [12–17]. In other words, M-cells are more sensitive achromatic stimuli of higher temporal, and lower spatial, frequencies [7, 18, 19]. The M-pathway has been shown to be responsible for frequency-doubling technology (FDT) contrast sensitivity [20, 21].

The type B RGCs, making up the parvocellular (P– or ventral) pathway, project via thinner optic nerve axons to the four parvocellular layers of the LGN, and subsequently to the 4C-beta layer of the striate cortex [9–11, 22]. About 80% of the RGC population consists of these P cells. Almost all P cells receive antagonistic input from red and green cones and, therefore, possess high chromatic sensitivity (particularly red–green color selectivity) but far lower contrast sensitivity and smaller receptive fields compared to the M-cells [13, 14, 17, 23, 24]. P-cells are more sensitive to stimuli of lower temporal and higher spatial frequencies [18, 19].

More recently discovered, the koniocellular (K) pathway conveys information regarding blue–yellow opponency to cortical layers above 4C, and it is both morphologically and functionally distinct from the M- and P-pathways [25–29]. The precise role of the K-pathway in vision has yet to be elucidated.

Measuring contrast sensitivity

When initially introduced into clinical practice and research, contrast-sensitivity testing consisted of computer-generated visual images as test targets (usually vertically oriented sine-wave gratings) with software-controlled threshold measurement protocols [2]. The use of these devices in a busy clinical setting was impractical due to a number of factors, including high cost, a difficult calibration process, the lack of normative data, and time-consuming testing protocols [2].

As a result, chart-based methods of assessing contrast sensitivity grew more popular in the 1980s [2]. The cycles per degree of the gratings or size of the letters on these charts determine the spatial frequency being evaluated [3]. Historically, the first commercially available, printed contrast-sensitivity tests for clinical use were the Arden plates, a booklet consisting of seven plates, with sine-wave grating printed on each [2]. Early on, there were observations that Arden plate contrast sensitivity was abnormal in various disorders, even in the presence of normal high-contrast VA [2]. However, its weaknesses are that the testing method does not involve a forced-choice method and the results are contingent on the speed of the examiner exposing the contrast images [3].

The VisTech chart and its later incarnation, the Functional Acuity Contrast Test (FACT) are wall-mounted grating charts [2, 3]. Problems with these charts include poor test–retest reliability, redundant information, and a high probability of correct guessing (since only three answer choices were available) [2, 3]. The Sine-Wave Contrast Test (SWCT) is almost identical to the VisTech charts, and it suffers from similar limitations [2]. The CSV-1000 is another distance, grating-based chart that utilizes an internal retroillumination system and is mounted on the wall or a stand [2]. Retroillumination is advantageous, since it eliminates variation resulting from lighting conditions, but having only two answer choices creates a 50% chance of guessing correctly [3].

There are various commercially available letter charts, including Pelli-Robson, the most widely used contrast sensitivity letter chart [30]. Consisting of letters of a single large size and varying contrast, the Pelli-Robson chart estimates the peak of the contrast-sensitivity function. It is a wall-mounted chart consisting of eight rows of letters, with two triplets of letters per row, placed at 1 meter testing distance. The contrast in each successive triplet decreases by a factor of 0.15 log units, from near 100% at the top to less than 1% at the bottom. During testing, the patient reads from the top of the chart and proceeds down until he or she can read no more. The Pelli-Robson charts demonstrate high test–retest reliability, are relatively unaffected by background luminance, have a normative database, and are easy and efficiently administered. As a result, they are a frequent choice for epidemiologic studies [2, 3]. Pelli-Robson charts are good measures of medium to low spatial frequencies [31]. However, since the letters are of uniform size, this method can only detect contrast sensitivity loss at a single spatial frequency [32]. This may be problematic in neurologic or ophthalmic disorders that impair contrast sensitivity for intermediate spatial frequencies, referred to as "notch" loss of contrast [33–36].

Measuring low-contrast letter acuity

Low-contrast letter acuity charts provide diagnostic information qualitatively similar to that of contrast sensitivity tests, and they possess comparable sensitivity [37, 38]. However, their format differs from that of contrast sensitivity because they include lines of letters of progressively smaller size and a single contrast level. The Low-Contrast Sloan Letter Charts (LCSLC) were first used as an exploratory MS clinical trial outcome in the IMPACT (International MS Progressive Avonex Clinical Trial) study of interferon beta-1a for secondary progressive MS. While the LCSLC were initially chosen for investigation in MS due to a difficulty obtaining the Pelli-Robson contrast sensitivity charts commercially, the LCSLC charts actually have several advantages for a clinical trial outcome [1, 39]. In addition to potentially capturing "notch" loss of contrast that could theoretically be missed by contrast-sensitivity testing, the LCSLC have a standardized format based on that of the Bailey-Lovie and ETDRS (Early Treatment Diabetic Retinopathy Study) charts, the standard charts used for acuity measurement in ophthalmology clinical trials (Figure 6.1) [40–42]. The charts are designed for distance measurement (thus, minimizing the effects of presbyopia), and the varying letter sizes allow for the testing of multiple spatial frequencies [1, 32]. Three contrast levels are typically used: 100% (high-contrast), 2.5%, and 1.25% [1]. The number of letters identified (from a maximum of 70 per chart) is recorded; this letter-by-letter scoring system is similar to the continuous scale of the logMAR (log minimal angle of resolution), but it is quantitative and reliable (important

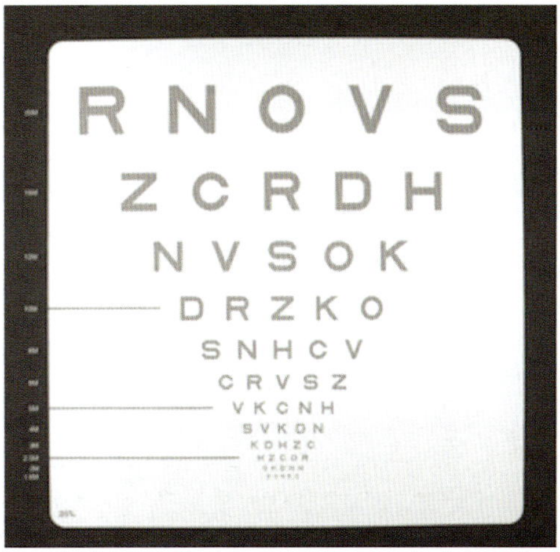

Figure 6.1 Low-contrast letter acuity chart (low-contrast Sloan letter chart, Precision Vision, LaSalle, IL). * These charts have a standardized format based on the Early Treatment Diabetic Retinopathy Study visual acuity charts, the standard used in ophthalmology clinical trials, and they have several advantages over standard Snellen charts or near vision testing cards as traditionally used in MS trials: (1) letters (Sloan letters) are designed to be equally detectable for normal observers; (2) each line has an equal number of letters (five per line); (3) spacing between letters and lines is proportional to the letter size; (4) the change in visual acuity from one line to another occurs in equal logarithmic steps (a change of three lines constitutes a doubling of the visual angle); (5) visual acuity (for high-contrast [black letters on white] chart) may be specified by Snellen notation for descriptive purposes (i.e., 20/20), by the number of letters identified correctly. This figure shows the 25% contrast level for purposes of illustrating the format; the actual contrast levels used in these trials, 2.5% and 1.25%, have substantially lighter gray letters. The charts measure 14 × 14 inches for easy use and portability in the MS clinical trial setting; charts may also be mounted on a retroilluminated cabinet, thus, eliminating the need for standardization of room lighting levels.

characteristics in clinical trial outcomes), and it can be easily understood by neurologists [43, 44]. A clinically significant change in vision has been more recently defined as a seven-letter change for the low-contrast charts and a five-letter change for the high-contrast charts, which are equivalent to two standard deviations of inter-rater difference [1, 44]. Chart portability (measuring 14 × 14 inches), the use of an retroilluminated cabinet (negating the need for standardizing room lighting levels) high-inter-rater reliability, test time efficiency, and the potential for administration by trained, nonphysician professionals make the LCSLC an excellent test in the clinical setting [32, 39, 43]. Potential limitations of letter charts include unevenness of illumination, fading of the print, and reflections from the surface [3].

Table 6.1 presents data from studies that have examined LCSLC using the Sloan charts, as well as

Table 6.1 Mean reference values from recent investigations of vision, QOL, and OCT in MS

	Disease-Free Controls	All MS	MS, No History of ON	MS, History of ON	References for Data *
High-contrast visual acuity (VA), ETDRS, number of letters correct	64 ± 5	59 ± 8	60 ± 6	58 ± 9	173 *
	(n=61 eyes)	(n=239 eyes)	(n=150 eyes)	(n=87 eyes)	
Binocular testing	66 ± 5	62 ± 8	63 ± 7	61 ± 10	62 *
	(n=324 pts)	(n=1,007 pts)	(n=544 pts)	(n=463 pts)	
Low-contrast letter acuity (2.5%), number of letters correct	34 ± 8	26 ± 11	28 ± 9	22 ± 12	173 *
	(n=61 eyes)	(n=239 eyes)	(n=150 eyes)	(n=87 eyes)	
Binocular testing	43 ± 6	36 ± 10	38 ± 9	35 ± 11	62 *
	(n=324 pts)	(n=1,007 pts)	(n=544 pts)	(n=463 pts)	
Low-contrast letter acuity (1.25%), number of letters correct	25 ± 7	16 ± 10	18 ± 10	11 ± 11	173 *
	(n=61 eyes)	(n=239 eyes)	(n=150 eyes)	(n=87 eyes)	
Binocular testing	34 ± 8	24 ± 11	26 ± 11	22 ± 12	62 *
	(n=324 pts)	(n=1,007 pts)	(n=544 pts)	(n=463 pts)	
NEI-VFQ-25 composite score,					
best score = 100	96 ± 4 (n=31 pts)	88 ± 13 (n=122 pts)	90 ± 12 (n=111 pts)	85 ± 14 (n=51 pts)	173 *
10-Item Neuro-Ophthalmic					
Supplement to the NEI-VFQ-25,	97 ± 3	87 ± 13	88 ± 12	83 ± 14	173 *
best score=100	(n=31 pts)	(n=122 pts)	(n=111 pts)	(n=51 pts)	

Time-domain (TD) OCT					
Peripapillary RNFL thickness, μm	104.5 ± 10.7	92.5 ± 16.7	95.6 ± 14.5	85.7 ± 19.0	174 *
	(n=219 eyes)	(n=1,058 eyes)	(n=730 eyes)	(n=328 eyes)	
Total macular volume, mm3	6.84 ± 0.36	6.54 ± 0.51	6.63 ± 0.48	6.36 ± 0.53	174 *
	(n=219 eyes)	(n=1,058 eyes)	(n=730 eyes)	(n=328 eyes)	
Spectral-domain (SD) OCT					
Peripapillary RNFL thickness, μm	92.9 ± 10.0	84.3 ± 12.8	87.6 ± 11.1	78.4 ± 13.6	173 *
	(n=61 eyes)	(n=239 eyes)	(n=150 eyes)	(n=87 eyes)	
Ganglion cell + inner plexiform layer (GCL+IPL), μm	88.9 ± 6.9 (n=61 eyes)	84.1 ± 8.4 (n=239 eyes)	87.0 ± 6.6 (n=150 eyes)	79.7 ± 9.2 (n=87 eyes)	173 *
Macular RNFL, μm	29.6 ± 6.0	23.5 ± 8.2	25.5 ± 7.1	20.0 ± 9.0	173 *
	(n=61 eyes)	(n=239 eyes)	(n=150 eyes)	(n=87 eyes)	

Abbreviations: MS = multiple sclerosis; ETDRS = Early Treatment Diabetic Retinopathy Study; QOL = quality of life; NEI-VFQ-25 = 25-Item National Eye Institute Visual Functioning Questionnaire; TD = time-domain (OCT-3 platform); SD = spectral-domain (Cirrus platform); OCT = optical coherence tomography; RNFL = retinal nerve fiber layer

* Reference with asterisk is source of data presented in table; other published studies contain similar data. Table adapted from reference [1].

high-contrast VA by ETDRS, OCT measures, and quality-of-life (QOL) scales using MS, optic neuritis (ON), and disease-free controls as an example [1]. These data may be used to provide initial reference values and should be viewed in the context of (1) the continually evolving field of vision in MS and neurologic disease, (2) the potential challenge inherent in applying group data to individual patients, and (3) the perspective that even the small observed differences in mean OCT values have been shown to correlate with clinically meaningful changes in visual function and QOL.

Low-contrast letter acuity: clinical correlates

On a standard Snellen VA chart, a 20/20 letter occupies a very small area (0.083 degree of vision), which is equivalent to 18 to 24 cycles per degree, the high-frequency end of the contrast-sensitivity function [3]. On the other hand, the peak of contrast sensitivity occurs between a spatial frequency of 3 and 6 cycles per degree (the equivalent visual frequency of the 20/200 line on the Snellen chart), a range responsible for activities like discerning a bus from a car [3]. This peak contrast sensitivity has been shown to be the most important visual factor in predicting performance on activities of daily function [3].

Far from being an academic exercise without any real-world applications, low-contrast vision has been shown to play an important role in the ability to carry out activities of daily living (e.g., pouring liquids, using tools) [46, 47], reading [31, 47–49], mobility [50], negotiating stairs [51], driving [52], and facial recognition [53–55], and influences perceived disability [56]. Further, diminished contrast sensitivity has been associated with an increased risk for falls in older adults [57, 58].

There is evidence that impaired contrast sensitivity is as disabling as visual field loss and more disabling than VA loss [59]. Decreased contrast sensitivity has been shown to negatively impact patients' quality of life. In a study of multiple sclerosis (MS) patients, a two-line difference in low-contrast acuity was associated with a deterioration of greater than four points on the NEI-VFQ-25 (25-Item National Eye Institute Visual Functioning Questionnaire) composite score, indicating an impaired quality of life [60]. The NEI-VFQ-25 domains most associated with diminished contrast acuity in this study included those for general vision, near and distance activities, role difficulties, and driving. Reduced contrast sensitivity was also associated with poorer scores on other measures of quality of life, including the Impact of Visual Impairment Scale (IVIS) and the Short Form 36 Health Survey (SF-36) [60]. Decreased binocular low-contrast vision has also been shown to correlate with the Extended Disability Status Scale (EDSS) and the MS Functional Composite (MSFC) scores, both measures of disability in MS patients [39]. In fact, deterioration of low-contrast vision can predict future EDSS decline [39].

How well a patient sees in high-spatial-frequency channels, which is captured by standard tests of high-contrast visual acuity (e.g., Snellen charts), does not necessarily predict visual function at intermediate or lower frequencies [2, 3, 61]. Contrast sensitivity testing can detect apparently occult evidence of visual dysfunction that would otherwise be absent on standard tests of visual acuity. As will be discussed later, a number of disorders can often affect contrast sensitivity and spare high-contrast visual acuity, especially early in the course of the disease. Thus, contrast sensitivity is a sensitive measure of disease progression, and it is a valuable clinical trial outcome tool in ophthalmic and neurologic disorders.

Binocular summation and binocular inhibition

VA may be measured monocularly (with either eye separately) or binocularly (with both eyes together). While measuring binocular acuity saves time and avoids patient fatigue, comparing monocular to binocular scores is important to ascertain the effects of binocular summation or inhibition [62]. Binocular summation is a phenomenon in which VA improves under binocular viewing conditions (i.e., better than the scores of either eye). In contradistinction, binocular inhibition results in worse VA than when viewing with either eye alone [62, 63]. Low-contrast acuity has been shown to be more sensitive than high-contrast VA in assessing the effect of binocular summation [62, 64].

Two hypotheses have been proposed to explain the phenomenon of binocular summation. "Probability Summation" assumes complete independence of the two eyes and predicts enhancement of binocular over monocular vision due to the statistical consideration that a binocular observer has two opportunities to detect weak signals. "Neural Summation" posits that binocular superiority exceeds that which would be expected from probability summation alone and attributes this phenomenon to cortical interactions (layer VI) [65]. The deterioration in binocular summation following acute optic neuritis (AON) may be a consequence of complex cortical reorganization and support the neural summation hypotheses [66]. Decreased binocular summation, or frank binocular inhibition, in MS patients is more common in older age groups, those with a prior history of AON, and those with a greater inter-ocular VA difference [62]. Better binocular summation was associated with higher NEI-VFQ-25 scores (which, in turn, suggests a better quality of life) [62]. Alternately, binocular summation is decreased with age [64] and in strabismus [65].

Disorders affecting low-contrast vision

Contrast sensitivity can be affected as part of the normal aging process, as well as in various ophthalmic, neurologic, and psychiatric conditions. Impaired contrast sensitivity has been observed in myopia [67], cataract [68, 69], pseudophakia [70], meridional amblyopia [71], strabismus [65], dermatochalasis [72], non-penetrating corneal foreign bodies [73], age-related macular degeneration [74–76], xerophthalmia [77], birdshot chorioretinopathy [78], retinitis pigmentosa [79–80], diabetic retinopathy [81, 82], and glaucoma [83–85].

In addition to MS, other neurologic disorders that may compromise low-contrast vision include Parkinson's disease [38, 86–89], Alzheimer's disease [20, 90–92], Duchenne muscular dystrophy [93], neurofibromatosis type 1 [94], migraine [95, 96], pseudotumor cerebri [97–100], Friedreich's ataxia [101], a left parieto-occipital infectious lesion, and a left occipital meningioma [102]. Reduced contrast sensitivity has also been observed in schizophrenia [103] and depression [104, 105]. Diminished contrast sensitivity is a common, albeit under recognized, side effect of many medications, including ethambutol [106] and tiagabine [107]. Exposure to solvents has also been implicated in decreased contrast sensitivity [108–110].

Impaired contrast sensitivity under photopic conditions with increasing spatial frequencies occurs in older adults, as part of the normal aging process, due to both optical and neural changes [111, 112]. By age 75, almost half of adults have cataracts, which impair contrast sensitivity by absorbing light, scattering light, and increasing disability glare [69, 113]. Notwithstanding the effects of pupillary miosis, higher lens density, increased optical aberrations, and increased intraocular light scattering on retinal illuminance, age-related visual pathway changes also conspire to further diminish contrast-sensitivity in older adults [64, 111]. Rod photoreceptor density is particularly affected by aging compared to cone photoreceptor density, which remains relatively stable [114]. Rod photoreceptor degeneration may result from deficits in rhodopsin regeneration [113]. Furthermore, at the cortical level, studies in senescent monkeys have demonstrated that cortical neurons exhibit lower optimal spatial and temporal frequencies, decreased contrast sensitivity, diminished spatial resolution, and reduced higher temporal frequency cut-offs when compared to younger monkeys [115, 116]. FDT perimetry has been shown to be useful in detecting age-related contrast-sensitivity impairment [112, 117, 118].

The progressive loss of dopaminergic neurons, the hallmark of Parkinson's disease (PD), also affects the retina [119]. Retinal dopaminergic deficiency is hypothesized to cause physiological dysfunction of dopaminergic amacrine, horizontal, and interplexiform cells that subsequently compromises the receptive field properties of RGCs. Pattern electroretinography (PERG) can be used to detect RGC dopaminergic dysfunction in PD patients, and, indeed, levdopa treatment improves delayed PERG latencies [89, 113, 120, 121]. Compared to the standard, high-contrast checkerboard pattern, low-contrast PERG is more sensitive in detecting RGC dysfunction in PD [88, 89]. Likewise, contrast sensitivity using chart-based testing is diminished in PD [38, 87]. Besides retinal abnormalities, pathologic changes elsewhere in the afferent visual pathway contribute to visual dysfunction in PD patients. Specifically, the lateral geniculate nuclei and visual cortices may also be affected by the neurodegenerative processes of PD [122–124]. Orientation-specific loss of contrast sensitivity in PD may provide evidence for cortical involvement [125, 126].

Several studies have reported impaired contrast sensitivity in Alzheimer's disease (AD) [90–92]. Using FDT, a more recent study [20] showed that decreased contrast sensitivity, most notably in the bilateral upper-right visual field quadrant, was associated with poorer cognitive measures in

AD and mild cognitive impairment. In AD, the outer retina (i.e., photoreceptors) is normal, as evidenced by normal full-field electroretinography [127]. However, like PD, the PERG is abnormal, signifying RGC dysfunction [127, 128], the possible consequence of retinal amyloid deposition [129]. Specifically, electroretinographic abnormalities are most pronounced for high-temporal-frequency patterns, indicating selective impairment of the large M-type RGCs [128]. Pathologically, neurodegenerative changes have been noted in the central M-pathway in the lateral geniculate nucleus and visual cortices [130–134], as well as in the retina [135–142]. Furthermore, glaucoma, cataracts, and macular degeneration (all of which also compromise contrast sensitivity) are more frequent among AD patients [143].

Structure meets function: low-contrast acuity and OCT in multiple sclerosis

MS is arguably the neurologic disorder in which low-contrast acuity, as well as OCT, have been most widely tested in recent years. MS frequently affects both the afferent and efferent visual pathways. Visual dysfunction occurs in 80% of patients and is the presenting feature in 50% [144, 145]. Acute optic neuritis (AON) is the presenting feature in 20% of cases, and 50% of MS patients develop AON during the course of their disease [146]. However, virtually all patients have evidence of optic nerve demyelination at autopsy [147, 148], indicating that occult, subclinical optic nerve demyelination occurs in the vast majority of MS patients, whether or not they develop clinical symptoms and signs of AON.

The eloquence of the afferent visual pathway and the frequency of AON in MS make it an ideal system to use as a model to understand the pathobiological underpinnings of the disease, as well as to develop sensitive biomarkers that can be applied to clinical trials of neuroprotective, and even neuro-restorative, therapies. The robust utility of optical coherence tomography (OCT) in detecting axonal damage in MS is explored at length throughout this book, but it remains possible that early pathologic changes that begin at a cellular level (particularly in the postgeniculate visual pathway) may easily escape the resolution of even the most sensitive OCT. Before any structural changes become evident, these pathologic perturbations may manifest as functional abnormalities that may be detected by means of sensitive electrophysiological assessments or tests of visual function. It is important to identify such early dysfunction, since it may represent a potentially reversible state of visual compromise; detecting these abnormalities would permit timely therapeutic interventions that would potentially stop the disease process, prevent future disability, and even reverse the damage.

Although the EDSS [149] is widely used as an outcome measure for clinical trials in MS, this scale is heavily skewed in favor of the motor system involved in ambulation and lacks any sensitivity with regard to other salient manifestations of MS-related disability, including fatigue, heat sensitivity, cognition, and, in particular, visual function. The MSFC was developed to serve as a more sensitive measure of the multidimensional manifestations of MS-related disability and included the quantitative tests of arm function (the 9-hole Peg Test), leg function (the timed 25-foot walk), and cognition (the PASAT3) [150–152], but it is devoid of any measure of visual function. For a long time, the only measure of visual function in MS patients was the hand-held Snellen chart, which measured high-contrast visual acuity (VA) [153].

While convenient and reproducible, the use of the Snellen chart in MS patients is limited by several inherent problems. First, Snellen VA is tested at the near distance, and it may potentially be difficult for presbyopic patients [32]. Second, despite normal high-contrast VA, there may be pathologic evidence of severe visual pathway demyelination [147] and RNFL thinning [154, 155]. Finally, as discussed earlier, Snellen VA only tests higher-spatial-frequency levels and is insensitive to impairment of intermediate to lower spatial frequencies. By contrast (pun intended), low-contrast vision testing has proven to be a more sensitive measure of visual function in MS. Many studies have shown that, despite recovery of standard, high-contrast VA to 20/20 or better following an attack of AON, patients continue to have persistent abnormalities of low-contrast vision [32, 34–37, 43, 44, 153–171].

Decreased contrast acuity correlates with RNFL thinning and reduced macular volume [44, 154, 155]. Poorer contrast sensitivity has been associated with a higher MS lesion load, particularly in the postgeniculate visual pathway [168, 172], suggesting that postgeniculate visual processing plays an important part in contrast sensitivity. It would be easy to assume that

RNFL thinning reflects pregeniculate damage while impaired contrast sensitivity (without OCT changes) indicates postgeniculate lesions. Reich et al. [172], however, dispelled this simple dichotomy and showed that postgeniculate MS lesions were associated with RNFL thinning as well. The precise mechanisms for retinal changes resulting from postgeniculate damage remain unclear, but they may be related to trans-synaptic degeneration.

Further, low-contrast acuity been shown to be the best measure that distinguishes MS patients from disease-free controls, accounting for age [39, 153]. As a trial outcome for natalizumab (in the AFFIRM and SENTINEL clinical trials), low-contrast acuity was sensitive enough to detect treatment effects and visual changes sustained over time, demonstrating the superiority of natalizumab as a disease-modifying agent [43]. As discussed previously, contrast sensitivity correlates well with various measures of visual dysfunction and disability in MS.

Summary

While impaired low-contrast vision is not pathognomonic for any particular disease, the presence of diminished contrast sensitivity can alert the clinician to the presence of a pathologic disorder and help explain the bases of a patient's visual complaints, particularly if other tests of visual structure and function are apparently normal. When used in conjunction with OCT, contrast sensitivity can provide useful and valuable information that will allow clinicians and researchers to follow disease progression. Contrast sensitivity testing can provide information that complements that garnered from structural (e.g., OCT) and functional measures (e.g., visual fields, color vision, electrophysiologic tests) of the afferent visual system. Contrast sensitivity can now be easily tested in busy clinical or research settings with commercially-available charts as well as established, efficient testing protocols. Evidence from MS clinical trials has demonstrated that contrast acuity is a reliable, sensitive measure of visual function that can be used to follow disease evolution and response to therapy.

References

1. Sakai RE, Feller DJ, Galetta KM, et al. Vision in multiple sclerosis: the story, structure-function correlations,and models for neuroprotection. *J Neuroophthalmol* 2011; **31**: 362–73
2. Owsley C. Contrast sensitivity. *Ophthalmol Clin N Am* 2003; **16**: 171–7
3. Richman J, Spaeth GL, Wirotsko B. Contrast sensitivity basics and a critique of currently available tests. *J Cataract Refract Surg* 2013; **39**: 1100–6
4. Pelli DG, Bex P. Measuring contrast sensitivity. *Vision Res* 2013; **90**: 10–4
5. Gouras P. Identification of cone mechanisms in monkey ganglion cells. *J Physiol* 1968; **199**: 533–47
6. Levanthal AG, Roedick RW, Dreher B. Retinal ganglion cell classes in the Old World monkey: morphology and central projections. *Science* 1981; **213**: 1139–42
7. Shapley R, Perry VH. Cat and monkey retinal ganglion cells and their visual function roles. *Trends Neurosci* 1986; **9**: 235
8. Dreher B, Fukada Y, Roedick RW. Identification, classification and anatomical segregation of cells with X-like and Y-like properties in the lateral geniculate nucleus of old-world primates. *J Neurophysiol* 1976; **258**: 433–52
9. Hubel DH, Wiesel TN. Laminar and columnar distribution of geniculo-cortical fibers in the macaque monkey. *J Comp Neurol* 1972; **146**: 421–50
10. Hendrickson AE, Wilson JR, Ogren MP. The neuroanatomical organization of pathways between the dorsal lateral geniculate nucleus and visual cortex in Old World and New World primates. *J Comp Neurol* 1978; **182**: 123–36
11. Blasdel GG, Lund JS. Termination of afferent axons in macaque striate cortex. *J Neurosci* 1983; **3**: 1389–413
12. Hubel DH, Wiesel TN. Effects of varying stimulus size and color on single lateral geniculate cells in Rhesus monkeys. *Proc Natl Acad Sci U S A* 1966; **55**: 1345–6
13. Kaplan E, Shapley RM. X and Y cells in the lateral geniculate nucleus of macaque monkeys. *J Physiol* 1982; **330**: 125–43
14. Derrington AM, Lennie P. Spatial and temporal contrast sensitivities of neurons in lateral geniculate nucleus of macaque. *J Physiol* 1984; **357**: 219–40
15. Livingstone MS, Hubel DH. Psychophysical evidence for separate channels for the perception of form, color, movement, and depth. *J Neurosci* 1987; **7**: 3416–68
16. Lee BB, Martin PR, Valberg A. Sensitivity of macaque retinal ganglion cells to chromatic and luminance flicker. *J Physiol* 1989; **414**: 223–43
17. Lee BB, Pokorny J, Smith VC, et al. Luminance and chromatic modulation sensitivity of macaque ganglion cells and human observers. *J Opt Soc Am A* 1990; **7**: 2223–36
18. Laycock R, Crewther SG, Crewther DP. A role for the 'magnocellular advantage' in visual impairments in neurodevelopmental and psychiatric disorders. *Neurosci Biobehav Rev* 2007; **31**: 363–76

19. McKendrick AM, Sampson GP, Walland MJ, Badcock DR. Contrast sensitivity changes due to glaucoma and normal aging: low-spatial frequency losses in both magnocellular and parvocellular pathways. *Invest Ophthalmol Vis Sci* 2007; **48**: 2115–22
20. Risacher SL, Wudunn D, Pepin SM, et al. Visual contrast sensitivity in Alzheimer's disease, mild cognitive impairment, and older adults with cognitive complaints. *Neurobiol Aging* 2013; **34**: 1133–44
21. Anderson AJ, Johnson CA. Frequency-doubling technology perimetry. *Opthalmol Clin North Am* 2003; **16**: 213–25
22. De Monasterio FM, Gouras P. Functional properties of ganglion cells of the rhesus monkey retina. *J Physiol* 1975; **251**: 167–95
23. Wiesel TN, Hubel DH. Spatial and chromatic interactions in the lateral geniculate body of the rhesus monkey. *J Neurophysiol* 1966; **29**: 1115–56
24. Hicks TP, Lee BB, Vidyasagar TR. The responses of cells in macaque lateral geniculate nucleus to sinusoidal gratings. *J Physiol* 1983; **337**: 183–200
25. Hendry SH, Yoshioka T. A neurochemically distinct third channel in the macaque dorsal lateral geniculate nucleus. *Science* 1994; **264**: 575–7
26. Johnson JK, Casagrande VA. Distribution of calcium-binding proteins within the parallel visual pathways of a primate (Galago crassicaudatus). *J Comp Neurol* 1995; **356**: 238–60
27. Hendry SH, Casagrande VA. A common pattern for a third visual channel in the primate LGN. *Soc Neurosci Abstr* 1996; **22**: 1605
28. Goodchild AK, Martin PR. The distribution of calcium-binding proteins in the lateral geniculate nucleus and visual cortex of a New World monkey, the marmoset, *Callithrix jacchus. Vis Neurosci* 1998; **15**: 625–42
29. Xu X, Ichida JM, Allison JD, et al. A comparison of koniocellular, magnocellular, and parvocellular receptive field properties in the lateral geniculate nucleus of the owl monkey (Aotus trivirgatus). *J Physiol* 2001; **531**: 203–18
30. Pelli DG, Robson JG, Wilkins AJ. Designing a new letter chart for measuring contrast sensitivity. *Clin Vision Sci* 1988; **2**: 187–99
31. Leat SJ, Woo GC. The validity of current clinical tests of contrast sensitivity and their ability to predict reading speed in low vision. *Eye* 1997; **11**: 893–9
32. Balcer LJ, Baier ML, Pelak VA, et al. New low-contrast vision charts: reliability and test characteristics in patients with multiple sclerosis. *Mult Scler* 2000; **6**: 163–71
33. Bodis-Wollner I, Diamond SP. The measurement of spatial contrast sensitivity in cases of blurred vision associated with cerebral lesions. *Brain* 1976; **99**: 695–710
34. Regan D, Silver R, Murray TJ. Visual acuity and contrast sensitivity in multiple sclerosis – hidden visual loss: an auxiliary diagnostic test. *Brain* 1977; **100**: 563–79
35. Kupersmith MJ, Seiple WH, Nelson JI, Carr RE. Contrast sensitivity loss in multiple sclerosis. Selectivity by eye, orientation, and spatial frequency measured with the evoked potential. *Invest Ophthalmol Vis Sci* 1984; **25**: 632–9
36. Nordmann JP, Saraux H, Roullet E. Contrast sensitivity in multiple sclerosis: a study in 35 patients with and without optic neuritis. *Ophthalmologica* 1987; **195**: 199–204
37. Regan D, Neima D. Low-contrast letter charts as a test of visual function. *Ophthalmology* 1983; **90**: 1192–200
38. Regan D, Neima D. Low-contrast letter charts in early diabetic retinopathy, ocular hypertension, glaucoma, and Parkinson's disease. *Br J Ophthalmol* 1984; **68**: 885–9
39. Baier ML, Cutter GR, Rudick RA, et al. Low-contrast letter acuity testing captures visual dysfunction in patients with multiple sclerosis. *Neurology* 2005; **64**: 992–5
40. Bailey IL, Lovie JE. New design principles for visual acuity letter charts. *Am J Optom Physiol Opt* 1976; **53**: 740–5
41. Ferris FL, Kassoff A, Bresnick GH, et al. New visual acuity charts for clinical research. *Am J Ophthalmol* 1982; **94**: 91–6
42. Ferris FL, Bailey I. Standardizing the measurement of visual acuity for clinical research studies: guideline from the Eye Care Technology Forum. *Ophthalmology* 1996; **103**: 181–2
43. Balcer LJ, Galetta SL, Calabresi PA, et al. Natalizumab reduces visual loss in patients with relapsing multiple sclerosis. *Neurology* 2007; **68**: 1299–304
44. Talman LS, Bisker ER, Sackel DJ, et al. Longitudinal study of vision and retinal nerve fiber layer thickness in multiple sclerosis. *Ann Neurol* 2010; **67**: 749–60
45. Rubin GS, Roche KB, Prasada-Rao P, Fried LP. Visual impairment and disability in older adults. *Optom Vis Sci* 1994; **71**: 750–60
46. Szylick JS, Seiple W, Fishman GA, et al. Perceived and actual performance of daily tasks: relationship to visual function tests in individuals with retinitis pigmentosa. *Ophthalmology* 2001; **108**: 65–75
47. Rubin GS, Legge GE. Psychophysics of reading. VI – The role of contrast in low vision. *Vision Res* 1989; **29**: 79–91

48. Whittaker SG, Lovie-Kitchin J. Visual requirements for reading. *Optom Vis Sci* 1993; **70**: 54–65

49. Crossland MD, Rubin GS. Text accessibility by people with reduced contrast sensitivity. *Optom Vis Sci* 2012; **89**: 1276–81

50. Marron JA, Bailey IL. Visual factors and orientation-mobility performance. *Am J Optom Physiol Opt* 1982; **59**: 413–26

51. Startzell JK, Owens DA, Mulfinger LM, Cavanagh PR. Stair negotiation in older people: a review. *J Am Geriatr Soc*; **48**: 567–80

52. Freeman EE, Munoz B, Turano KA, West SK. Measures of visual function and their association with driving modification in older adults. *Invest Opthalmol Vis Sci* 2006; **47**: 514–20

53. Owsley C, Sekuler R, Boldt C. Aging and low-contrast vision: face perception. *Invest Ophthalmol Vis Sci* 1981; **21**: 362–5

54. Owsley C, Sloane ME. Contrast sensitivity, acuity, and the perception of "real world" targets. *Br J Ophthalmol* 1987; **71**: 791–6

55. McCulloch DL, Loffler G, Colguhoun K, et al. The effects of visual degradation on face discrimination. *Ophthalmic Physiol Opt* 2011; **31**: 240–8

56. Elliott DB, Hurst MA, Weatherhill J. Comparing clinical tests of visual function with the patient's perceived visual disability. *Eye* 1990; **4**: 712–7

57. Lord S, Dayhew J. Visual factors for falls in older people. *J Am Geriatr Soc* 2001; **49**: 508–15

58. French D, Campbell R, Spehar A, et al. Drugs and falls in community dwelling older people: a national veterans study. *Clin Therapeutics* 2006; **28**: 619–30

59. Leat SJ, Legge GE, Bullimore MA. What is low vision? A re-evaluation of definitions. *Optom Vis Sci* 1999; **76**: 198–211

60. Mowry EM, Loquidice MJ, Daniels AB, et al. Vision related quality of life in multiple scleorsis: correlation with new measures of low and high contrast letter acuity. *J Neurol Neurosurg Psychiatry* 2009; **80**: 767–72

61. Elliot DB, Whitaker D. How useful are contrast sensitivity charts in optometric practice? Case reports. *Optom Vis Sci* 1992; **69**: 378–85

62. Pineles SL, Birch EE, Talman LS, et al. One eye or two: a comparison of binocular and monocular low-contrast acuity testing in multiple sclerosis. *Am J Ophthalmol* 2011; **152**: 133–40

63. Newman NJ, Wolfe JM, Steward MI, Lessell S. Binocular visual function in patients with a history of monocular optic neuritis. *Clin Vision Sci* 1991; **6**: 95–107

64. Gillespie-Gallery H, Konstantakopoulou E, Harlow JA, Barbur JL. Capturing age-related changes in functional contrast sensitivity with decreasing light levels in monocular and binocular vision. *Invest Ophthalmol Vis Sci* 2013; **54**: 6093–103

65. Pineles SL, Velez FG, Isenberg SJ, et al. Functional burden of strabismus: decreased binocular summation and binocular inhibition. *JAMA Ophthalmol* 2013; **131**: 1413–19

66. Gallo A, Esposito F, Sacco R, et al. Visual resting-state network in relapsing-remitting MS with and without previous optic neuritis. *Neurology* 2012; **79**: 1458–65

67. Collins JW, Carney LG. Visual performance in high myopia. *Curr Eye Res* 1990; **9**: 217–23

68. Hess R, Woo G. Vision through cataracts. *Invest Ophthalmol Vis Sci* 1978; **17**: 428–35

69. Abrahamsson M, Sjostrand J. Impairment of contrast sensitivity function (CSF) as a measure of disability glare. *Invest Ophthalmol Vis Sci* 1986; **27**: 1131–6

70. Gil MA, Varon C, Rosello N, et al. Visual acuity, contrast sensitivity, subjective quality of vision, and quality of life with 4 different multifocal IOLs. *Eur J Ophthalmol* 2012; **22**: 175–87

71. Freedman RD, Thibos LN. Contrast sensitivity in humans with abnormal visual experience. *J Physiol* 1975; **247**: 687–710

72. Rogers SA, Khan-Lim D, Manners RM. Does upper lid blepharoplasty improve contrast sensitivity? *Ophthal Plast Reconstr Surg* 2012; **28**: 163–5

73. Coe CD, Bower KS, Brooks DB, et al. Effect of blast trauma and corneal foreign bodies on visual performance. *Optom Vis Sci* 2010; **87**: 604–11

74. Sjostrand J, Frisen L. Contrast sensitivity in macular disease: a preliminary report. *Acta Ophthalmol (Copenh)* 197;**55**: 507–14

75. Kleiner RC, Enger C, Alexander MF, Fine SL. Contrast sensitivity in age-related macular degeneration. *Arch Ophthalmol* 1988; **106**: 55–7

76. Owsley C, Sloane ME, Skalka HW, et al. A comparison of the Regan Low-Contrast Letter Charts and contrast sensitivity testing in older patients. *Clin Vis Sci* 1990; **5**: 325–34

77. Rolando M, Lester M, Macri A, Calabria G. Low spatial-contrast sensitivity in dry eyes. *Cornea* 1993; **17**: 376–9

78. Kappel PJ, Monnet D, Yu F, et al. Contrast sensitivity among patients with birdshot chorioretinopathy. *Am J Ophthalmol* 2009; **147**: 351–6

79. Lindberg CR, Fishman GA, Anderson RJ, Vasquez V. Contrast sensitivity in retinitis pigmentosa. *Br J Ophthalmol* 1981; **65**: 855–8

80. Yioti GC, Kalogeropoulos CD, Aspiotis MB, Stefaniotou MI. Contrast sensitivity and color vision in eyes with retinitis pigmentosa and good visual

acuity: correlations with SD-OCT findings. *Ophthalmic Surg Lasers Imaging* 2012; **43**: S44-S53

81. Midena E, Segato T, Bottin G, et al. The effect on the macular function of laser photocoagulation for diabetic macular edema. *Graefes Arch Clin Exp Ophthalmol* 1992; **230**: 162–5
82. Greenstein VC, Chen H, Hood DC, et al. Retinal function in diabetic macular edema after focal laser photocoagulation. *Invest Ophthalmol Vis Sci* 2000; **41**: 3655–64
83. Stamper RL. The effect of glaucoma on central visual function. *Trans Am Ophthalmol Soc* 1984; **82**: 792–826
84. Johnson CA. Psychophysical measurement of glaucomatous damage. *Surv Ophthalmol* 2001; **45**: S313-S318
85. Gandolfi SA. Improvement in spatial contrast sensitivity threshold after surgical reduction of intraocular pressure in unilateral high-tension glaucoma. *Invest Ophthalmol Vis Sci* 2005; **46**: 197–201
86. Skrandies W, Gottlob I. Alterations of visual contrast sensitivity in Parkinson's disease. *Hum Neurobiol* 1986; **5**: 255–9
87. Kupersmith MJ, Shakin E, Siegel IM, et al. Visual system abnormalities in patients with Parkinson's disease. *Arch Neurol* 1982; **39**: 284–6
88. Peppe A, Stanzione P, Pierelli F, et al. Low contrast stimuli enhance PERG sensitivity to the visual dysfunction in Parkinson's disease. *Electroencephalogr Clin Neurophysiol* 1992; **82**: 453–7
89. Langheinric T, Tebartz van Elst L, Lagreze WA, et al. Visual contrast response functions in Parkinson's disease: evidence from electroretinograms, visually evoked potentials and psychophysics. *Clin Neurophysiol* 2000; **111**: 66–74
90. Cronin-Golomb A, Corkin S, Rizzo JF, et al. Visual dysfunction in Alzheimer's disease: relation to normal aging. *Ann Neurol* 1991; **29**: 41–52
91. Gilmore GC, Levy JA. Spatial contrast sensitivity in Alzheimer's disease: a comparison of two methods. *Optom Vis Sci* 1991; **68**: 790–4
92. Sadun AA, Borchert M, DeVita E, et al. Assessment of visual impairments in Alzheimer's disease. *Am J Ophthalmol* 1987; **104**: 113–20
93. Barboni MT, Nagy BV, de Araujo Moura AL, et al. ON and OFF electroretinography and contrast sensitivity in Duchenne muscular dystrophy. *Invest Ophthalmol Vis Sci* 2013; **54**: 3195–204
94. Ribeiro MJ, Violante IR, Bernardino I, et al. Abnormal achromatic and chromatic contrast sensitivity in neurofibromatosis type 1. *Invest Ophthalmol Vis Sci* 2012; **53**: 287–93
95. Braunitzer G, Rokszin A, Kobor J, Benedek G. Is the development of visual contrast sensitivity impaired in children with migraine? An exploratory study. *Cephalalgia* 2010; **30**: 991–5
96. Shepherd AJ, Beaumont HM, Hine TJ. Motion processing deficits in migraine are related to contrast sensitivity. *Cephalalgia* 2012; **32**: 554–70
97. Wall M. Contrast sensitivity testing in pseudotumor cerebri. *Ophthalmology* 1986; **93**: 4–7
98. Verplanck M, Kaufman DI, Parson T, et al. Electrophysiology versus psychophysics in the detection of visual loss in pseudotumor cerebri. *Neurology* 1988; **38**: 1789–92
99. Buncie JR, Tytla ME. Contrast sensitivity in shunted hydrocephalus. *Invest Ophthalmol Vis Sci* 1989; **30**: 407
100. Wall M, Conway MD, House PH, et al. Evaluation of sensitivity and specificity of spatial resolution and Humphrey automated perimetry in pseudotumor cerebri patients and normal subjects. *Invest Ophthalmol Vis Sci* 1991; **32**: 3306–12
101. Lynch DR, Farmer JM, Rochestie D, Balcer LJ. Contrast letter acuity as a measure of visual dysfunction in patients with Friedreich ataxia. *J Neuroophthalmol* 2002; **22**: 270–4
102. Bodis-Wollner I. Visual acuity and contrast sensitivity in patients with cerebral lesions. *Science* 1972; **178**: 769–71
103. Halasz I, Levy-Gigi E, Kelemen O, et al. Neuropsychological functions and visual contrast sensitivity in schizophrenia: the potential impact of comorbid posttraumatic stress disorder (PTSD). *Front Psychol* 2013; **4**: 136
104. Bubl E, Kern E, Ebert D, et al. Seeing gray when feeling blue? Depression can be measured in the eye of the diseased. *Biol Psychiatry* 2010; **68**: 205–8
105. Bubl E, Ebert D, Kern E, et al. Effect of antidepressive therapy on retinal contrast processing in depressive disorder. *Br J Psychiatry* 2012; **201**: 151–8
106. Santaella RM, Fraunfelder FW. Ocular adverse effects associated with systemic medications: recognition and management. *Drugs* 2007; **67**: 75–93
107. Sorri I, Kalviainen R, Mantyjarvi M. Color vision and contrast sensitivity in epilepsy patients treated with initial tiagabine monotherapy. *Epilepsy Res* 2005; **67**: 101–7
108. Boeckelmann I, Pfister EA. Influence of occupational exposure to organic solvent mixtures on contrast sensitivity in printers. *J Occup Environ Med* 2003; **45**: 25–33
109. Gong Y, Kishi R, Kasai S, et al. Visual dysfunction in workers exposed to a mixture of organic solvents. *Neurotoxicology* 2003; **24**: 703–10
110. Costa TL, Barboni MT, Moura AL, et al. Long-term occupational exposure to organic solvents affects

color vision, contrast sensitivity, and visual fields. *PLoS One* 2012; **7**: e42961

111. Owsley C. Aging and vision. *Vision Res* 2011; **51**: 1610–22
112. Mateus C, Lemos R, Silva MF, et al. Aging of low and high level vision: from chromatic and achromatic contrast sensitivity to local and 3D object motion perception. *PLoS One* 2013; **8**: e55348
113. Jackson GR, Owsley C. Visual dysfunction, neurodegenerative diseases, and aging. *Neurol Clin* 2003; **21**: 709–28
114. Curcio CA, Milican CL, Allen KA, et al. Aging of the human photoreceptor mosaic: evidence for selective vulnerability of rods in central retina. *Invest Ophthalmol Vis Sci* 1993; **34**: 3278–96
115. Zhang J, Wang X, Wang Y, et al. Spatial and temporal sensitivity degradation of primary visual cortical cells in senescent rhesus monkeys. *Eur J Neurosci* 2008; **28**: 201–7
116. Yang Y, Liang Z, Liang Z, et al. Aging affects contrast response functions and adaptation of middle temporal visual area neurons in rhesus monkeys. *Neuroscience* 2008; **156**: 748–57
117. Adams CW, Bullimore MA, Wall M, et al. Normal aging effects for frequency doubling technology perimetry. *Optom Vis Sci* 1999; **76**: 582–7
118. Anderson AJ, Johnson CA, Fingeret M, et al. Characteristics of the normal database for the Humphrey Matrix Perimeter. *Invest Ophthalmol Vis Sci* 2005; **46**: 1540–8
119. Harnois C, Di Paolo T. Decreased dopamine in the retinas of patients with Parkinson's disease. *Invest Ophthalmol Vis Sci* 1990; **31**: 2473–5
120. Nightingale S, Mitchell KW, Howe JW. Visual evoked cortical potentials and pattern electroretinograms in Parkinson's disease and control subjects. *J Neurol Neurosurg Psychiatry* 1986; **49**: 1280–7
121. Gottlob I, Scneider E, Heider W, et al. Alteration of visual evoked potentials and electroretinograms in Parkinson's disease. *Electroencephalogr Clin Neurophysiol* 1987; **66**: 349–57
122. Reader TA, Quesney LF. Dopamine in the visual cortex of the cat. *Experimentia* 1986; **42**: 1242–4
123. Parkinson D. Evidence for a dopaminergic innervations of cat primary visual cortex. *Neuroscience* 1989; **30**: 171–9
124. Papadopoulos GC, Parnavelas JG. Distribution and synaptic organization of dopaminergic axons in the lateral geniculate nucleus of the rat. *J Comp Neurol* 1990; **294**: 356–61
125. Regan D, Maxner C. Orientation-selective visual loss in patients with Parkinson's disease. *Brain* 1987; **110**: 415–32
126. Bulens C, Meerwaldt JD, Van der Wildt GJ. Effect of stimulus orientation on contrast sensitivity in Parkinson's disease. *Neurology* 1988; **38**: 76–81
127. Katz B, Rimmer S, Iragui V, et al. Abnormal pattern electroretinogram in Alzheimer's disease: evidence for retinal ganglion cell degeneration. *Ann Neurol* 1989; **26**: 221–5
128. Trick GL, Barris MC, Bickler-Bluth M. Abnormal pattern electroretinogram in patients with senile dementia of the Alzheimer's type. *Ann Neurol* 1989; **26**: 226–31
129. Koronyo Y, Salumbides BC, Black KL, Koronyo-Hamaoui M. Alzeheimer's disease in the retina: imaging retinal Aβ plaques for early diagnosis and therapy assessment. *Neurodegener Dis* 2012; **10**: 1–9
130. Armstrong RA. Visual field defects in Alzheimer's disease patients may reflect differential pathology in the primary visual cortex. *Optom Vis Sci* 1996; **73**: 677–82
131. Hof PR, Morrison JH. Quantitative analysis of a vulnerable subset of pyramidal neurons in Alzheimer's disease: II. Primary and secondary visual cortex. *J Comp Neurol* 1990; **301**: 55–64
132. Leudba G, Saini K. Pathology of subcortical visual centres in relation to cortical degeneration in Alzheimer's disease. *Neuropathol Appl Neurobiol* 1995; **21**: 410–22
133. McKee AC, Au R, Cabral HJ, et al. Visual association pathology in preclinical Alzheimer disease. *J Neuropathol Exp Neurol* 2006; **65**: 621–30
134. Mielke R, Kessler J, Fink G, et al. Dysfunction of visual cortex contributes to disturbed processing of visual information in Alzheimer's disease. *Int J Neurosci* 1995; **82**: 1–9
135. Blanks JC, Hinton DR, Sadun AA, Miller CA. Retinal ganglion cell degeneration in Alzheimer's disease. *Brain Res* 1989; **501**: 364–72
136. Curcio CA, Drucker DN. Retinal ganglion cells in Alzheimer's disease and aging. *Ann Neurol* 1993; **33**: 248–57
137. Hinton DR, Sadun AA, Blanks HC, Miller CA. Optic-nerve degeneration in Alzheimer's disease. *N Engl J Med* 1986; **315**: 485–7
138. Paquet C, Boissonnot M, Roger F, et al. Abnormal retinal thickness in patients with mild cognitive impairment and Alzheimer's disease. *Neurosci Lett* 2007; **420**: 97–9
139. Parisi V, Restuccia R, Fattapposta F, et al. Morphological and functional retinal impairment in Alzheimer's disease patients. *Clin Neurophysiol* 2001; **112**: 1860–7
140. Sadun AA, Bassi CJ. Optic nerve damage in Alzheimer's disease. *Ophthalmology* 1990; **97**: 9–17

141. Tsai CS, Ritch R, Schwartz B, et al. Optic nerve head and nerve fiber layer in Alzheimer's disease. *Arch Ophthalmol* 1991; **109**: 199–204
142. Valenti DA. Neuroimaging of retinal nerve fiber layer in AD using optical coherence tomography. *Neurology* 2007; **69**: 1060
143. Valenti DA. Alzheimer's disease: visual system review. *Optometry* 2010; **81**: 12–21
144. McDonald WI, Barnes. The ocular manifestations of multiple sclerosis. 1. Abnormalities of the afferent visual system. *J Neurol Neurosurg Psychiatry* 1992; **55**: 747–52
145. Leibowitz U, Alter M. Optic nerve involvement and diplopia as initial manifestations of multiple sclerosis. *Clin Neurosci* 1994; **2**: 180–8
146. Balcer LJ. Optic Neuritis. *N Engl J Med* 2006; **354**: 1273–80
147. Ulrich J, Groebke-Lorenz W. The optic nerve in multiple sclerosis. A morphological study with retrospective clinic-pathological correlations. *Neuro-ophthalmology* 1983; **3**: 149–59
148. Lumsden CE. The neuropathology of multiple sclerosis. In: Vinken PJ, Bruyn GW, editors. *Handbook of Clinical Neurology* New York: Elsevier 1970. p. 161–216
149. Kurtzke JF. Rating neurologic impairment in multiple sclerosis: an Expanded Disability Status Scale (EDSS). *Neurology* 1983; **33**: 1444–52
150. Rudick R, Antel J, Confavreux C, et al. Recommendations from the National Multiple Sclerosis Society Clinical Outcomes Assessment Task Force. *Ann Neurol* 1997; **42**: 379–82
151. Miller DM, Rudick RA, Cutter G, et al. Clinical significance of the multiple sclerosis functional composite: relationship to patient-reported quality of life. *Arch Neurol* 2000; **57**: 1319–24
152. Rudick RA, Cutter G, Reingold S. The multiple sclerosis functional composite: a new clinical outcome measure for multiple sclerosis trials. *Mult Scler* 2002; **8**: 359–65
153. Balcer LJ, Baier ML, Cohen JA, et al. Contrast letter acuity as a visual component for the Multiple Sclerosis Functional Composite. *Neurology* 2003; **61**: 1367–73
154. Fisher JB, Jacobs DA, Markowitz CE, et al. Relation of visual function to retinal nerve fiber layer thickness in multiple sclerosis. *Ophthalmology* 2006; **113**: 324–32
155. Bock M, Brandt AU, Kuchenbecker J, et al. Impairment of contrast visual acuity as a functional correlate of retinal nerve fibre layer thinning and total macular volume reduction in multiple sclerosis. *Br J Ophthalmol* 2012; **96**: 62–7
156. Zimmern RL, Campbell FW, Wilkinson IMS. Subtle disturbances of vision after optic neuritis elicited by studying contrast sensitivity. *J Neurol Neurosurg Psychiatry* 1979; **42**: 407–12
157. Regan D, Raymond J, Ginsburg AP, Murray TJ. Contrast sensitivity, visual acuity and the discrimination of Snellen letters in multiple sclerosis. *Brain* 1981; **104**: 333–50
158. Patterson VH, Foster DH, Heron J, Mason RJ. Multiple sclerosis. Luminance threshold and measurements of temporal characteristics of vision. *Arch Neurol* 1981; **38**: 687–9
159. Kupersmith MJ, Nelson JI, Seiple WH, Carr RE, Weiss PA. The 20/20 eye in multiple sclerosis. *Neurology* 1983; **33**: 1015–20
160. Pace R, Woo GC. Contrasta sensitivity function for vision testing in suspected demyelinating disease. *Lancet* 1984; **8373**: 405–6
161. Ashworth B, Aspinall PA, Mitchell JD. Visual function in multiple sclerosis. *Doc Ophthalmology* 1989; **73**: 209–24
162. Honan WP, Heron JR, Foster DH, et al. Visual loss in multiple sclerosis and its relation to previous optic neuritis, disease duration and clinical classification. *Brain* 1990; **113**: 975–87
163. Russell MHA, Murray IJ, Metcalfe RA, Kulikowski JJ. The visual defect in multiple sclerosis and optic neuritis. *Brain* 1991; **114**: 2419–35
164. Leys MJ, Candaele CM, De Rouck AF, Odom JV. Detection of hidden visual loss in multiple sclerosis. A comparison of pattern-reversal visual evoked potentials and contrast sensitivity. *Doc Opthalmol* 1991; **77**: 255–64
165. Trobe JD, Beck RW, Moke PS, Cleary PA. Contrast sensitivity and other vision tests in the Optic Neuritis Treatment Trial. *Am J Ophthalmol* 1996; **121**: 547–53
166. Beck RW, Gal RL, Bhatti MT, et al. Optic Neuritis Study Group. Visual function more than 10 years after optic neuritis: experience of the Optic Neuritis Treatment Trial. *Am J Ophthalmol* 2004; **137**: 77–83
167. Wender M. Value of Pelli-Robson contrast sensitivity chart for evaluation of visual system in multiple sclerosis patients. *Neurol Neurochir Pol* 2007; **41**: 141–3
168. Wu GF, Schwartz ED, Lei T, et al. Relation of vision to global and regional brain MRI in multiple sclerosis. *Neurology* 2007; **69**: 2128–35
169. Optic Neuritis Study Group. Visual function 15 years after optic neuritis: a final follow-up report from the Optic Neuritis Treatment Trial. *Ophthalmology* 2008; **115**: 1079–82

170. Keltner JL, Johnson CA, Cello KE, et al. Optic Neuritis Study Group. Visual field profile of optic neuritis: a final follow-up report from the Optic Neuritis Treatment Trial from baseline through 15 years. *Arch Ophthalmol* 2010; **128**: 330–7

171. Graves J, Galetta SL, Palmer J, et al. Alemtuzumab improves contrast sensitivity in patients with relapsing-remitting multiple sclerosis. *Mult Scler* 2013; **19**: 1302–9

172. Reich DS, Smith SA, Gordon-Lipkin EM, et al. Damage to the optic radiation in multiple sclerosis is associated with retinal injury and visual disability. *Arch Neurol* 2009; **66**: 998–1006

173. Walter SD, Ishikawa H, Galetta KM, Sakai RE, Feller DJ, Wilson JA, Maguire MG, Galetta SL, Frohman E, Calabresi PA, Schuman JS, Balcer LJ. Ganglion cell loss in relation to visual disability in multiple sclerosis. *Ophthalmology* **119**: 1250–57

174. Burkholder BM, Osborne B, Loguidice MJ, Bisker E, Frohman TC, Conger A, Ratchford JN, Warner C, Markowitz CE, Jacobs DA, Galetta SL, Cutter GR, Maguire MG, Calabresi PA, Balcer LJ, Frohman EM. Macular volume determined by optical coherence tomography as a measure of neuronal loss in multiple sclerosis. *Arch Neurol* 2009; **66**: 1366–72

Chapter 7

Optical coherence tomography and electrophysiology of the visual pathway

A. Klistorner, C. L. Fraser, C. Yiannikas, and S. L. Graham

While modern spectral-domain OCT technology can deliver visualization of individual retinal layers, allowing for a substantial shift in our knowledge of both ophthalmic and neurological conditions, it provides only structural information about the retina. To fully understand the visual system, structure and function should be examined together.

Visual electrophysiology tests represent an objective way to assess the function of the visual pathway. The visual system can be interrogated using a variety of testing paradigms, which have been standardized by the International Society for Clinical Electrophysiology of Vision (ISCEV). The most commonly performed tests include the full-field electroretinogram (ERG), pattern ERG (PERG), and visual evoked potentials (VEP), which provide a summed response from the retinal elements being tested. Additional topographical information can be assessed through the use of multifocal technologies, such as a multifocal ERG (mfERG) and multifocal VEP (mfVEP). The series of tests allow clinical assessment of conditions including suspected retinal dystrophy, neurological disease or unexplained visual loss.

By coupling the information from OCT and electrophysiology, it is possible to perform structural and functional assessment of the various cell populations within the retina, as well as the optic nerve fibers. This combination of tests is most commonly used in the diagnosis and management of retinal disease, which is beyond the scope of this chapter. Instead we will concentrate on the use of these techniques in neurological conditions, predominantly multiple sclerosis.

Anatomical substrate of clinical electrophysiology recordings

An understanding of the anatomical origins of the measured electrophysiological signals allows better correlation between the responses measured and the anatomical appearance on OCT.

Anatomical origin of the full-field electroretinogram

The electroretinogram (ERG) represents the electrical response of different cellular elements of the retina to light. The ERG is a simple clinical test that can be performed with the use of corneal electrodes. ISCEV full-field ERG stimuli are presented using the ganzfeld dome, which results in even illumination across the entire retina in patients with dilated pupils. The electrical responses recorded during the ERG are generated by the retinal neurons directly or by changes in the retinal glia secondary to the activity of the retinal neurons.

The relative contributions of various retinal types are different under dark-adapted (scotopic) and light-adapted (photopic) conditions or different levels of stimulus intensity. The rod photoreceptors are involved in the generation of responses under scotopic conditions, when very dim blue light is used for stimulation. Cone photoreceptors require much brighter stimulus and are better recorded under photopic conditions. Full-field flashes stimulate the entire retina and are used to elicit the major waveform responses in the typical ERG, providing diagnostic information about rod and cone photoreceptors and inner retinal function across the entire retina, but with no localizing information.

A typical ERG protocol includes the following: after dark-adaptation, a dim scotopic stimulus is presented, resulting in a pure rod response. This is the only electrophysiology test that is rod specific. While the patient remains dark-adapted, stimuli of increasing intensity generate combined dark-adapted

Optical Coherence Tomography in Neurological Disease, ed. Peter A. Calabresi, Laura J. Balcer, and Elliot M. Frohman. Published by Cambridge University Press.

cone and rod responses. Then, after a period of light adaptation, a single flash stimulus drives a pure cone response.

ERG a-wave

ERG waveforms show an initial negative deflection (a-wave) originating from the photoreceptor layer. The photoreceptor response to light absorption in the outer segments results in hyperpolarization. The a-wave is not seen, however, in the rod specific stimulus conditions (fully dark-adapted with dimmer flash).

ERG b-wave

The first positive deflection, called the b-wave, originates primarily from optic nerve (ON) bipolar cells, with a small contribution from the Muller cells. These ON bipolar cells are driven by the stimulated photoreceptors.

Oscillatory potentials can be recognized as multiple wavelets on the up-slope of the b-wave (and isolated with appropriate high pass filters). Their exact origin and clinical significance is still debated. The ratio of b-to a-wave in bright flash conditions can be used as a marker of inner retinal pathology, with a reduction typical of such conditions as melanoma associated retinopathy (MAR) or carcinoma associated retinopathy (CAR), but also in more benign conditions such as congenital stationary night blindness.

In summary, the standard ERG assesses the photoreceptor and inner nuclear layer, and its integrity determines the function of the retina through to the ganglion cells.

Anatomical origin of the pattern electroretinogram

The overall response from the retina produced by alternating black and white checkerboard pattern stimulation without a net change in stimulus luminance (rather than diffuse flash) is called the pattern electroretinogram (PERG). It has been suggested that the retinal ganglion cells are the prime generators of this response.

As the macula comprises less than 5% of the total retinal area, maculopathy usually does not affect the full-field ERG response. The PERG stimulus, however, is projected directly to the macula. With no stray light (since there is no change in total retinal illumination), the PERG can be used diagnostically to differentiate macular damage from diffuse retinal pathology.

The PERG consists of two peaks: an initial positive deflection (P50) occurs at approximately 50 milliseconds with a following negative deflection occurring at approximately 95 milliseconds (N95). It is believed that the second component largely arises from retinal ganglion cells spiking output activity.

Reduction in the P50 amplitude, or an increase in the P50 latency, suggests macular dysfunction anterior to the ganglion cells [1]. A reduction in P50 usually leads to a consecutive reduction of the N95 component. The ratio between the P50 and N95 is, therefore, not reduced in these cases.

Abnormalities confined to the N95 component, leaving P50 unaffected, are seen in diseases of the optic nerve. Reported examples include optic nerve demyelination, Leber's Hereditary Optic Neuropathy, and autosomal dominant optic atrophy [2].

In summary, the PERG is driven by macular photoreceptors but its second component arises predominantly from the retinal ganglion cells.

Anatomical origin of the multifocal electroretinogram

The multifocal electroretinogram (mfERG) allows simultaneous but independent stimulation of multiple retinal areas. The stimulus is presented on a computer monitor and change in illumination of individual areas is driven by pseudo-random sequences. Responses are derived from a single continuous ERG recording using cross-correlation mathematical techniques. The stimulus pattern is designed to produce local responses of approximately equal amplitudes (i.e., the stimulus area is scaled to be slightly larger with eccentricity).

The typical mfERG is a cone-driven response from a radius of 20–30 degrees around the fovea. The rods do not contribute to the mfERG. Like the standard ERG, the mfERG is formed by bipolar cell activity with smaller contributions from the photoreceptors.

mfERG responses are largely independent of refractive error, but they are critically dependent on good fixation and patient cooperation. Patients with poor vision typically have poor fixation, making test interpretation difficult.

The mfERG is used as an alternative to PERG as a test of macular function. The information is used in association with full-field ERG and VEP in order to localize the cause of visual loss to a widespread retinal abnormality, macular abnormality, or optic nerve disease. The localizing information from mfERG is helpful in diagnosing conditions with specific macular involvement such as hydroxychloroquine (Plaquenil) maculopathy.

Anatomical origin of the visual evoked potential

The visual evoked potential (VEP) represents the response of the visual cortex to optical stimulation. It was proposed as a means of assessing the integrity of the visual pathway in optic neuritis (ON) more than 30 years ago [3], and is understood to be generated at the level of striate cortex by combined activity of postsynaptic potentials [4]. The magnitude of the VEP reflects the number of functional afferent fibers reaching striate cortex and the degree of synaptic activity in V1. Therefore, its amplitude is determined by the severity of the acute inflammation along the visual pathway and subsequent axonal degeneration [5]. The timing of the response (latency) reflects the degree of demyelination along the visual pathway. Delayed VEP latency reflects a reduction of conduction speed due to a change from saltatory to continuous membrane conduction after demyelination [6]. Subsequent shortening of VEP latency is thought to represent the process of optic nerve remyelination [5, 7]. Although remyelination may not be solely responsible for the recovery of VEP latency, as other factors such as reorganization of the ion channel distribution and cortical plasticity may also play a role, it is believed to be the major factor [8]. The VEP signal is typically recorded at the scalp overlying the occiput.

Since central vision is disproportionally represented in the striate cortex, the full-field VEP is a macular-dominated response. A normal macula is necessary for normal VEP recordings, and it is prudent to prove normal macula structure and function before attributing abnormalities in VEP to optic nerve pathology.

The two most common ways to elicit a cortical response are flash and pattern stimulation. The Flash VEP (response to bright flash) has significant interindividual test variability, but it is useful in infants and patients with nystagmus. Pattern-reversal (checkerboard or gratings) VEP is less variable between subjects than flash VEP, with the P100 latency being less variable between subjects than its amplitude. There is often a difference in nomenclature between ophthalmologists and neurologists. Ophthalmologists record an initial positive deflection at approximately 100 milliseconds, referred to as P100, whereas neurologists often use reverse polarity and record the same response as N100. P100/N100 amplitude is reduced in many different optic nerve disorders. P100 latency delay has been described as typically occurring in demyelination.

Multifocal visual evoked potential

The multifocal VEP (mfVEP) is a cortical response to simultaneous but independent stimulation of multiple areas of the visual field. As mentioned earlier, the conventional full-field VEP is greatly dominated by the macular response due to its cortical overrepresentation [9]. Being the vector sum of numerous differently oriented dipoles, which are often opposite due to the cortical anatomy of the striate cortex around the calcarine sulcus, the waveform of the full-field VEP is also prone to cancellation and distortion. This can result in under- or overestimation of amplitude and detection of apparent rather than real latency delay [10]. In contrast, the mfVEP enables simultaneous recording from multiple regions of the visual field, allowing more detailed topographical assessment of small groups of axons within the optic nerve. Due to the small size of the stimulated cortical area, mfVEP also eliminates cancellation effects, providing real representation of amplitude and latency [11–15].

The size of individual segments is cortically scaled to stimulate approximately equal cortical areas (similar to the mfERG, but with more substantial change in size with eccentricity) (Figure 7.1). Therefore, the mfVEP is ideal to study spatial and temporal evolution of optic nerve demyelinated lesions with high precision.

Similarly to full-field VEP recordings, mfVEP responses are dependent on the integrity of the entire visual pathway.

Applications in optic neuritis and multiple sclerosis

The advent of VEPs in the 1970s first allowed clinicians to assess neural conduction in the optic nerve. Halliday demonstrated that diagnostic confirmation of optic neuritis can be made using latency

Table 7.1 Summary of electrophysiological tests

Test	Stimulus	Signal generation	Visual region
Full-field ERG	Diffuse flash using Ganzfeld dome	Photoreceptors (rods,cones), bipolar cells	Pan-retinal
Pattern ERG	Reversing black/white checkerboard; 15 ° and 30 ° field size	Macular photoreceptors, retinal ganglion cells	Macula
Pattern VEP	Reversing black/white checkerboard; ≥15 °	Cortical neurons within primary visual cortex	Large field, macular dominated
Multifocal ERG	Flickering black/white hexagons; 40°-50° diameter	Cone photoreceptors and bipolar cells	Topographical responses within macula
Multifocal VEP	Reversing black/white dartboard; 60° diameter	Cortical neurons within primary visual cortex	Topographical responses within visual field

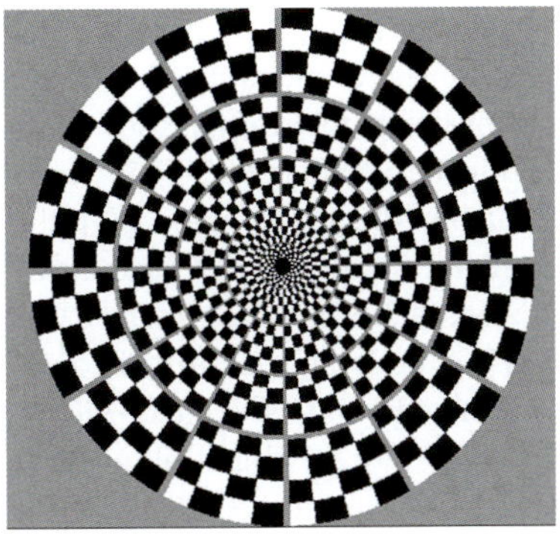

Figure 7.1 Multifocal stimulus employed in mfVEP recording. Each sector (area 4 × 4 checks) reverses polarity according to a pseudo-random sequence. Temporal sector (T) corresponds to central visual field, superior sector (S)-to inferior visual field, and inferior sector (I)-to superior visual field.

Reprinted with permission from Klistorner et al., Multifocal VEP And OCT in optic neuritis: a topographical study of the structure-function relationship, *Doc Ophthalmol*, 2009; 118: 129–37.

delays of full-field VEP [3, 16]. Due to advances in neuroimaging techniques, such as magnetic resonance imaging (MRI), the VEP was neglected for many years. However, recently the focus in multiple sclerosis (MS) research is shifting back to structural and functional correlation based on OCT and electrophysiology of the optic nerve and retina.

Studies of optic neuritis evolution

Optic neuritis (ON) is an inflammatory optic neuropathy which is strongly associated with MS. Up to 75% of ON patients have been reported to eventually develop MS, with the presence of typical MRI lesions in the brain at the time of ON onset being a strong risk factor [17]. The natural history of acute ON mirrors that of acute MS relapses elsewhere in the central nervous system [18]. However, in contrast to most brain lesions, the effects of disease on the optic nerve are readily clinically apparent and potentially measurable [19]. By obtaining mfVEPs as a measure of inflammation and conduction speed, in parallel with detailed clinical measures of visual function and OCT measurements of retinal layers as a more direct assessment of axonal damage, it is possible to develop a picture of pathophysiological events produced by individual lesions as they progress. [20] Therefore, ON represents an ideal in vivo model for studying the relationship between inflammation, axonal loss, and de/remyelination following single inflammatory attack [21].

It is understood that transection of optic nerve axons during acute inflammatory demyelination leads to retrograde degeneration, which ultimately reaches the RNFL and can be accurately measured by OCT providing a structural measure of axonal loss. The amplitude of the mfVEP, on the other hand, provides a functional estimation of preserved optic nerve fibers. Therefore, application of both techniques allows comprehensive assessment of the effect of inflammatory demyelination on visual pathway [5].

Early work exploring the links between optic nerve structure and function after acute ON in MS (MSON) produced inconclusive results.

The first study comparing OCT and conventional VEP was performed by Parisi et al. in 2001 [22], who reported significantly delayed P100 latencies and reduced N75 to P100 amplitudes in the eyes of MS patients with documented ON (MSON) when compared with control and fellow eyes. There was also a significant reduction of total and temporal RNFL thickness in MSON eyes compared with the values observed in control eyes. The authors, however, did not find a significant correlation between VEP (both amplitude and latency) and RNFL thickness. The study only included 14 patients and an early model of OCT with lower resolution was used.

A study published by Trip et al. [23] in 2005 using higher-resolution OCT demonstrated a significant correlation of RNFL thickness with amplitude of the full-field VEP. Time since onset of optic neuritis in this group was three years, and patients with a previous optic neuritis episode with or without MS were included.

Pueyo et al. [24] in 2008 confirmed a correlation between RNFL thickness (temporal sector in particular) and full-field VEP amplitude in a group of 50 MS patients. This study also demonstrated a significant correlation of RNFL with VEP latency, which was explained by the fact that, contrary to Trip et al., all study patients had clinically definite multiple sclerosis (CDMS), which is more often associated with demyelinating processes. Data from the same group published two years later (2010) and based on a smaller number of patients [25] also demonstrated significant latency increase and significant amplitude decrease of VEP P100 in MS patients. However, while good correlation was reported between P100 latency and OCT mean RNFL thickness, no correlation was shown between RNFL and VEP amplitude.

This discrepancy of structure–function relationships may be attributed to several factors: first, sensitivity of time-domain OCT devices used in earlier studies was low; second, there was significant difference in the cohorts of patients studied, some studies including CIS, while others only included CDMS. Additionally, and maybe most importantly, full-field VEP recording has intrinsic problems described in the section above.

Therefore, to clarify the structure-function relationship in the visual system of MS patients with and without ON, we have undertaken several studies comparing structural changes in the optic nerve using OCT RNFL thickness compared with latency and amplitude of mfVEP [26, 27, 30]. An initial cross-sectional investigation of patients with post-acute optic neuritis demonstrated a strong correlation between RNFL thickness and mfVEP amplitude [26, 27]. To minimize the effect of inter-subject variability, between-eye asymmetry of RNFL thickness and amplitude of the mfVEPs were analyzed. There was also good topographical association between two measures (Figure 7.2) [28].

Reduction of mfVEP amplitude, however, was considerably greater compared to RNFL thinning, indicating that the functional deficit may be greater than structural loss. Some possible explanations were suggested, including:

a. larger functional loss from channel failure on the denuded, but structurally preserved axons [28];
b. ongoing inflammation in the visual pathway, possibly as part of a more diffuse, slow inflammation in the white matter [29], which may reduce mfVEP amplitude due to axonal dysfunction or conduction block in some fibers.

A longitudinal study performed within the first year of acute ON, however, demonstrated a more complex relationship between functional and structural measures of optic nerve integrity. This study showed that while during the acute stage of optic neuritis both RNFL thickness and mfVEP amplitude are influenced by the severity of inflammation, its effect on structural and functional measures is quite different. Acute loss of myelin and associated inflammation cause conduction block, which reduces or completely abolishes mfVEP amplitude. At the same time, inflammatory edema often results in thicker swollen RNFL [30–34]. This leads to a complete structure–function dissociation (Figure 7.3a).

Conduction block normally recovers within a few weeks, during which inflammation subsides, ion channels are reconstructed and conduction partially resumes, although often in a slower, continuous mode [28]. This usually leads to recovery of amplitude up to the level supported by surviving fibers. Therefore, after conduction block is over, the magnitude of the mfVEP signal becomes mainly dependent on the degree of axonal transection.

After resolution of edema, axonal degeneration becomes the predominant pathological feature affecting RNFL thickness. However, it takes time for axons transected during acute inflammation to degenerate back to the retina. Therefore, a mild degree of correlation seen at three months is mainly due to time lag between axonal transection and retrograde degeneration reaching the retina (Figure 7.3b). By six months, however, this process is completed and the direct

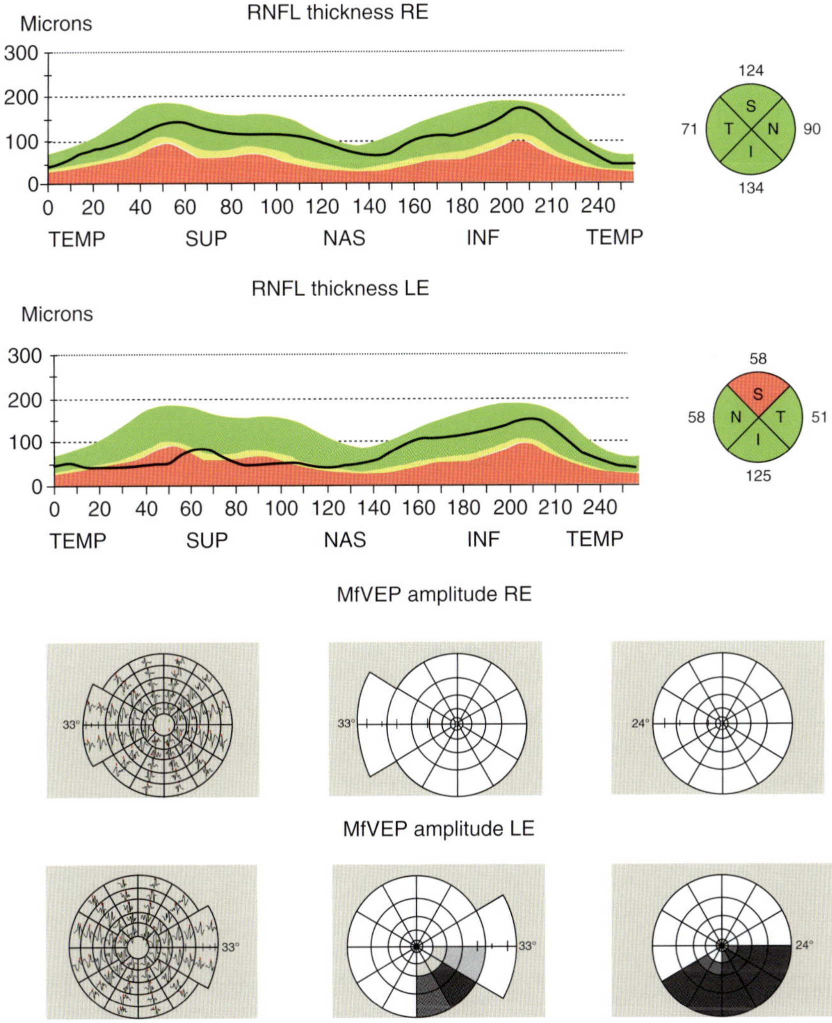

Figure 7.2 Example of topographic correspondence between RNFL thickness and mfVEP amplitude. Significant thinning of RNFL in upper sector and reduction of mfVEP amplitude in the lower area of the visual field is detected in left eye. For mfVEP, the first column represents VEP trace arrays; the second column, the Amplitude Deviation plot; and the third column, the Amplitude Asymmetry Deviation plot.

Reprinted with permission from Klistorner et al., Multifocal VEP and OCT in optic neuritis: a topographical study of the structure–function relationship, *Doc Ophthalmol*, 2009; 118: 129–37.

relationship between thinner RNFL and lower mfVEP amplitudes becomes apparent (Figure 7.3c).

Studies of the fellow eye in MS patients

An increasing number of studies have demonstrated significant axonal and neuronal loss of retinal ganglion cells (RGC) in MS patients with no previous ON (MS-NON). A recently published meta-analysis showed an average RNFL thinning of 7 μm (about 7%) in those eyes [35]. Talman et al. [36] presented evidence that this loss may even be progressive. However, the pathological basis of the RGC axonal and neuronal loss in the MS-NON eyes is not clear. Therefore, a combination of functional assessment of the visual pathway with structural OCT measurement may help to better understand the nature of this loss. Latency of mfVEP can be used as a marker of subclinical inflammatory demyelination along the visual pathway.

Using this approach, we assessed the relationship between loss of RNFL and mfVEP in NON-eyes of MS patients in early disease. Figure 7.4, which is based on a compilation of results from several studies, shows the percentage of patients with abnormally thin RNFL

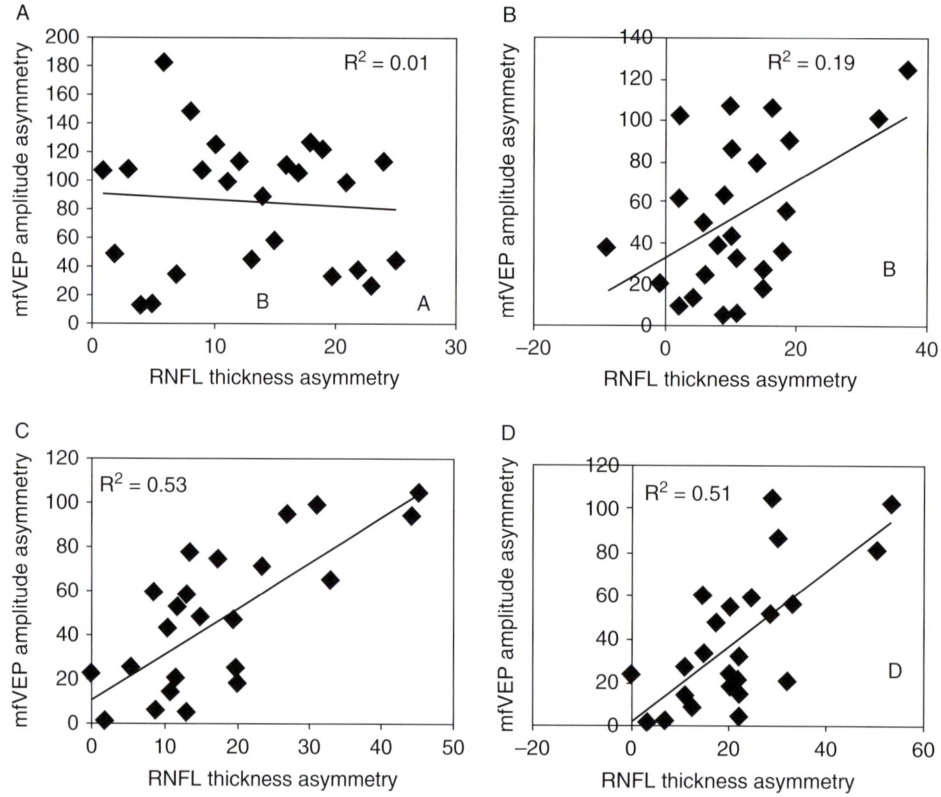

Figure 7.3 Correlation between inter-eye asymmetry of RNFL thickness and mfVEP amplitude at (A) 1 month, (B) 3 months, (C) 6 months, and (D)12 months.

Reprinted with permission from A. Klistorner et al., Interrelationship of optical coherence tomography and multifocal visual-evoked potentials after optic neuritis. *Invest Ophthalmol Vis Sci* 2010; 51: 2770–7

and delayed mfVEP latency compared to age- and gender-matched normal controls.

Only CIS patients (acute unilateral ON) were examined at one month after the onset of symptoms. All patients, however, had brain or spinal cord demyelinating lesions detected by magnetic resonance imaging (MRI) and were classified as high risk for development of MS [37]. A mixed group of CIS and CDMS patients were investigated at 12 and 36 months after the first demyelinating episode [26, 38], while only CDMS patients were included in the last group (54 months) [39].

Taken together, these results demonstrate early change of conduction along the visual pathway (which is already obvious in CIS patients) possibly caused by subclinical inflammation with loss of RGC axons to follow.

The last study is of particular interest since it demonstrated not only significant latency delay of mfVEP, but also significant reduction of total and

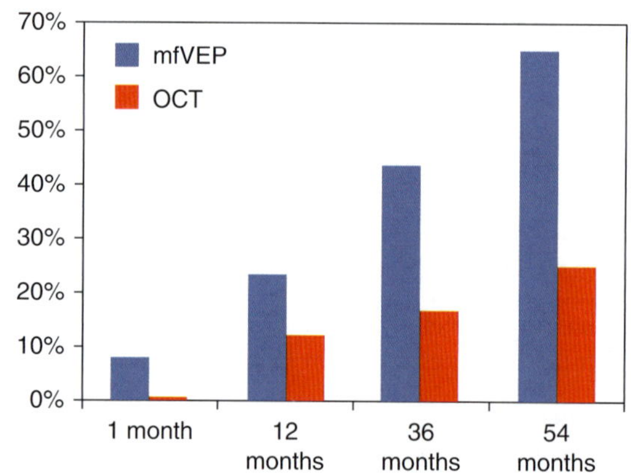

Figure 7.4 Percentage of non-optic neuritis eyes with delayed mfVEP latency (blue) and reduced RNFL thickness (red).

temporal RNFL thickness in NON eyes (including fellow eyes of ON patients). Even more interestingly, both total and temporal RNFL thickness was associated with latency of the mfVEP (Figure 7.5a, b).

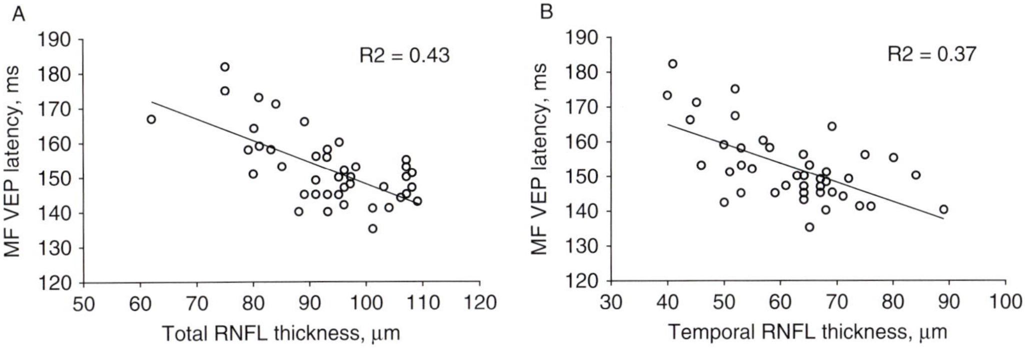

Figure 7.5 Correlation between mfVEP latency and (A) total RNFL thickness and (B) temporal RNFL thickness.
Reprinted with permission from A. Klistorner et al., Axonal loss in non-optic neuritis eyes of MS patients linked to delayed visual evoked potential. *Neurology* 2013; 80: 245.

When grouped according to latency delay, NON eyes with normal latency showed no reduction of RNFL thickness compared to controls, while eyes with delayed latency demonstrated significantly thinner RNFL. MS-NON eyes with delayed latency also had significantly thinner RNFL compared to those with normal latencies. In patients with no previous ON in either eye, delayed latency and reduced RNFL were bilateral whenever present. The binocular nature of latency delay suggests a retro-chiasmal location of demyelinating lesions. However, whether or not axonal loss is the result of retrograde degeneration triggered by optic tract lesions or caused by trans-neuronal spread of neurodegeneration from LGN neurons to RGC axons following optic radiation or cortical lesions, remains to be seen.

Chronic demyelination and neurodegeneration

While demyelination is still considered the most characteristic histopathological feature of MS, a significant association has been found between permanent functional deficit in MS and loss of axons, and it is now believed that axonal degeneration constitutes the basis for neurological disability.

It was suggested that permanent demyelination in the absence of active inflammation may contribute to axonal degeneration [40] by making axons more vulnerable to physiological stress. One of the potential mechanisms of axonal damage due to chronic demyelination may be related to ischemic insult of white matter and involves an imbalance between axonal energy demand and limited energy supply. Lack of trophic support from myelin or myelin-forming cells and disruption of normal axon–myelin interaction may also contribute to degeneration of chronically demyelinated axons [33]

While remyelination is now accepted as an early and frequent phenomenon in MS [41, 42], it is often incomplete [43] and probably limited in its duration [44]. It has previously been demonstrated that speed of VEP latency recovery significantly slows down within the first year after ON and practically does not change after that [8, 45]. Therefore, latency remains considerably prolonged in a significant proportion of patients even a few years after the demyelinating episode, indicating existence of extensive chronic demyelination.

Using mfVEP to characterize the level of optic nerve demyelination [46, 47] and optical coherence tomography to quantify RNFL thickness, it is possible to investigate the association between the degree of permanent demyelination and progressive axonal loss in a visual system of MS patients. We followed a group of 25 patients with clinically isolated acute unilateral ON for three years after onset of ON using both techniques. All patients had demyelinating MRI lesions of the brain or spine on initial MRI scans and were classified at enrollment as "possible MS." During the follow-up period, nine patients converted to CDMS.

This study demonstrated significant latency delay of mfVEP at 12 months in ON eyes as compared to normal controls. Latency delay ranged from 4 to 39 ms, indicating a high degree of demyelination for some patients. There was a small, but statistically significant, latency recovery over the follow-up period, but it remained extensively delayed even at 36 months. Fellow eyes also demonstrated significant latency prolongation at 12 months, although on a much lesser scale. Latency of the fellow eye then remained stable during entire follow-up period. RNFL thickness was significantly reduced in ON eyes at study entry point (12 months) indicating substantial axonal loss caused by axonal transection during acute inflammatory demyelination and subsequent retrograde degeneration. RNFL thickness of the fellow eye, however, was not affected.

There was a small, but significant, reduction of RNFL thickness between 12 and 36 months for both ON and fellow eyes. During the follow-up period RNFL thickness decreased on average by 1.2 μ in ON and 1.3 μ in the fellow. However, this change in RNFL thickness was not related to the degree of latency delay at 12 months for both ON and fellow eyes, indicating no association between the degree of permanent optic nerve demyelination and progressive axonal loss and raising a question about any potential role of chronic demyelination in axonal neurodegeneration, at least in the early stages of the disease. The fact that fellow eyes demonstrated a similar degree of RNFL thinning, while only showing marginal demyelination, supports this conclusion [48].

Pattern ERG studies in MS

Parisi et al. [22] reported significant reduction of PERG P50 and N95 amplitudes, as well as a delay of the P50 latency, in MSON eyes when using 15-min arc checks stimulation. In addition, the OCT temporal RNFL thickness was significantly correlated with the PERG P50 latency and N95 amplitude. The study was small (14 patients) and employed an early model of OCT. Correlation of N95 amplitude with RNFL and macular thickness, but not with P50 latency was also reported by Almarcegui et al [25].

In contrast, the study of patients with optic neuritis by Trip et al. [23] produced quite different results. The authors demonstrated no association of RNFL thickness with any of the PERG measures.

Cortical plasticity in MS

Following optic neuritis, RGC axons show retrograde degeneration back to the retina, which results in RNFL thinning. This process is believed to be completed by six months [49]. It was, however, demonstrated that in MS patients the RNFL continues to deteriorate after that (and even regardless of a history of ON). A progressive loss of optic nerve fibers even one year after the attack was also detected in longitudinal MRI studies of the optic nerve mean area [18, 50].

The mechanism of RNFL loss is uncertain, but may be related to ongoing primary axonal degeneration, subclinical inflammation or retro-chiasmal inflammatory demyelination with retrograde changes.

After recovery of acute conduction block, which typically takes 4–8 weeks, axonal degeneration becomes the predominant pathological process determining amplitude of the VEP, since loss of optic nerve fibers limits the transmission of the afferent stimulus to the visual cortex [51]. It is expected, therefore, that in the post-acute period changes in amplitude of mfVEP should fall in parallel with changes in the optic nerve structural integrity measure (RNFL thickness). In other words, that progressive axonal degeneration should lead to progressive decline of the mfVEP amplitude.

A recent study, however, presented a different picture – contrary to expectation and despite the loss of RNFL fibers, significant improvement of the mfVEP amplitude was observed between six and 12 months after an episode of acute ON. It was suggested that the findings of increased post-synaptic activity in the striate cortex (as measured by improvement of the mfVEP amplitude) coupled with simultaneous reduction of cortical input (RNFL thinning) supports the concept of continuous cortical reorganization in post-acute optic neuritis [52].

Neural reorganization has been described after acute optic neuritis and is considered to be one of the mechanisms responsible for recovery of function from the acute attack. Various mechanisms including increased expression of sodium channels, neuronal or synaptic changes, increased recruitment of parallel pathways, and cortical reorganization, including functional expansion of surviving neurons are thought to be involved in this process. While the exact site of neuroplasticity in the hierarchy of the visual system still remains a matter of controversy [51, 53, 54], continuous recovery of mfVEP amplitude suggests that it may (at least partially) occur below or at the level of primary visual cortex.

Applications in generalized neurological disease

Increasingly, ophthalmic examination is allowing for greater understanding of the disease processes in neurological conditions that were not classically associated with direct ocular pathology.

Parkinson's disease

Parkinson's disease (PD) is generally considered a "movement disorder"; it is now understood that alterations in dopaminergic cells affects the entire visual system from the retina to areas of the central nervous system that subserve vision. In the retina dopamine is found within amacrine and interplexiform cells [55]. The PERG specifically records a response consequent on the pre-ganglionic retinal circuitry that is controlled by these amacrine and interplexiform cells. Both PERG and VEP abnormalities can be detected in PD patients with specific foveal stimulus parameters. Interestingly, patients treated with L-dopa show higher PERG amplitudes compared to untreated patients, but never reach the amplitudes seen in normal controls [56]. The loss of macular PERG correlates with studies showing that on OCT there is loss of the temporal retinal nerve fiber layer thickness at the optic disc [57] and a thinning of the inner plexiform layer at the fovea [58].Other studies have shown alterations in EOG [59] and mfERG in correlation with loss of the inferior and temporal RNFL thickness [60].

Alzheimer's disease

Alzheimer's disease (AD) is a progressive neurodegenerative condition resulting in dementia. As in PD, there is increasing evidence that the retina is also affected in the pathophysiological process. Studies have documented that the mean RNFL thickness at the optic disc is reduced in AD compared to controls, with particular loss of the fibers from the superior quadrant [61, 62]. In addition, these OCT changes were shown to correlate with reduced P1 amplitudes of mfERG in both the foveal and peri-foveal regions [62].

Monitoring medication side effects

The retina and central nervous system are particularly sensitive to the effects of toxic insults. Many medications in common use have known effects on the electrophysiology and structural OCT changes. Some examples are presented below.

Hydroxychloroquine (Plaquenil)

In the retinal pigment epithelium, chloroquine phosphate remains at higher concentration than in the liver [63]. Hydroxychloroquine retinopathy typically results in reduced b-wave amplitudes on ERG with prolonged latency in advanced cases and a bull's eye pattern of reduced function on mfERG, with localized reduction in response amplitudes in ring 2, best detected by analyzing ring ratios [64]. In late cases, a corresponding bull's eye retinal appearance is seen clinically [65]. The OCT shows a loss of RPE cells, initially as a ring around the macula, and autofluorescence patterns are disrupted relatively early.

Vigabatrin (Sabril)

Vigabatrin is used as an anti-epileptic medication, particularly for the management of infantile spasms. It works by increasing the concentration of gamma-amino butyric acid (GABA) in the brain. However, it also increases GABA in the retina and is associated with visual field constriction.

A study of Vigabatrin patients with visual field constriction [66] shows reduced b-wave amplitude for the rod responses and the combined rod-cone response. Lesser, but significant reduction of a-wave was also detected. Significant positive correlations were found between the total averaged RNFL thickness, superior and inferior RNFL thickness, and reduced standard ERG parameters. The authors concluded that Vigabatrin is retino-toxic on several levels, from photoreceptors to ganglion cells.

Using OCT and mfVEP to characterize the nature of nonconventional MRI techniques

While MRI has proven to be a very sensitive tool in confirming diagnosis of MS and monitoring of treatment trials, it is pathologically nonspecific. It has been suggested that nonconventional MRI techniques such as the magnetization transfer ratio (MTR) may provide more specific characterization of underlying pathological processes [67–69].

MTR imaging is a measure of the exchange of protons between free water and macromolecules in membranes. It is believed MTR is affected by either dilution of protons caused by edema or loss of tissue structure, in particular the structure of myelin. While animal research has demonstrated a strong relationship between the level of myelination and MTR [70, 71], human studies are inconclusive.

Our group performed analysis of optic nerve MTR, RNFL thickness and latency of mfVEP in 23 patients with a single unilateral episode of ON and ten healthy controls [72]. We found a significant reduction of MTR value in ON eyes. A strong correlation of MTR was demonstrated with RNFL thickness and mfVEP amplitude, but not with the level of latency delay, suggesting that MTR reduction is related to axonal loss, rather than demyelination.

Limitations of electrophysiology testing

The standards of electrophysiological tests published by ISCEV allow for comparison of results between laboratories. As yet there is no ISCEV standard for the mfVEP. Our recommendation is that at least two orthogonal channels are needed in mfVEP recording to ensure a satisfactory detection without cancellation of the variously oriented dipoles that combine to form the conventional VEP. By measuring the responses that are most reproducible between patients, alterations in these results can provide diagnostic information. However, it is important to note that patient compliance influences responses recorded. Frequent blinking, loss of fixation, and intentional defocusing can result in reduced-quality responses, particularly for PERG, mfERG, and mfVEP, which have small amplitude signals, requiring considerable signal averaging. Patients who have poor vision and/or amblyopia may have abnormal responses due to inability to fixate further complicating test interpretation. The PERG and the mfVEP are acuity dependent, with a reduction in signals seen in the central rings of the mfVEP when acuity falls below 6/12. Lack of concentration can affect the mfVEP via the intrusion of alpha rhythm, and we have found that a changing fixation target is helpful to engage the patient and reduce alpha-rhythm contamination.

In summary, the use of both electrophysiology as a functional measure and OCT as a structural measure provides better insight into mechanisms of neurodegenerative diseases when the visual system is used as a model. In clinical trials of potentially neuroprotective and remyelinating drugs an assessment of structural and functional changes will be valuable to determine beneficial effects of therapy.

References

1. Holder GE. Pattern electroretinography (PERG) and an integrated approach to visual pathway diagnosis. *Prog Ret Eye Res* 2001; **20**: 531–61.
2. Holder GE, Gale RP, Acheson JF, Robson AG. Electrodiagnostic assessment in optic nerve disease. *Curr Opin Neurol* 2009; **22**: 3–10.
3. Halliday AM, McDonald WI, Mushin J. Delayed visual evoked response in optic neuritis. *Lancet* 1972; **i**: 982–5.
4. Fahle M, Bach M. Origin of the visual evoked potentials. In: Heckenlively JR, Arden GB, editors. *Principles and practice of clinical electrophysiology of vision.* Cambridge: The Mit Press 2006. p. 207–234.
5. Jones SJ, Brusa A. Neurophysiological evidence for long-term repair of MS lesions: implications for axon protection. *J Neurolog Sci* 2003; **206**: 193–8.
6. Waxman SG. Altered distributions and functions of multiple sodium channel subtypes in multiple sclerosis and its models. In: Waxman SG, editor. *Multiple sclerosis as a neuronal disease.* Amsterdam: Elsevier, 2005.
7. Klistorner A, Graham SL, Fraser C, Garrick R, Nguyen T, Paine M, et al. Electrophysiological evidence for heterogeneity of lesions in optic neuritis. *Invest Ophthalmol Vis Sci.* 2007; **48**: 4549–56.
8. Brusa A, Jones SJ, Plant GT. Long-term remyelination after optic neuritis. *Brain.* 2001; **124**: 468–79.
9. Yiannikas C, Walsh JC. The variation of the pattern shift visual evoked response with the size of the stimulus field. *Electroencephalography & Clinical Neurophysiology* 1983; **55**: 427–435.
10. Halliday AM, Darbett G, Blumhardt LD, Kriss A. The macular and submacular subcomponents of the pattern evoked response. In: B LDaG, editor. *Human evoked potentials.* New York: Plenum Publishing; 1979. p. 135–451.
11. Klistorner AI, Graham SL, Grigg JR, Billson FA. Multifocal topographic visual evoked potential: improving objective detection of local visual field defects. *Invest Ophthalmol Vis Sci.* 1998; **39**(6): 937–50.
12. Klistorner A, Fraser C, Garrick R, Graham SL, Arvind H. Correlation between full-field and multifocal VEPs in optic neuritis. *Doc Ophthal.* 2008; **116**: 19–27.
13. Hood DC, Odel JG, Zhang X. Tracking the recovery of local optic nerve function after optic neuritis: a multifocal VEP study. *Invest Ophthalmol Vis Sci* 2000; **41**: 4032–8.
14. Graham SL, Klistorner A, Goldberg I. Clinical Application of objective perimetry using multifocal VEP in Glaucoma Practice. *Arch Ophthalmol* 2005; **123**: 729–39.
15. Laron M, Cheng H, Xhang B, Schiffman JS, Tang RA, Frishman LJ. Assessing visual pathway function in multiple sclerosis patients with multifocal visual evoked potentials. *Mult Scler* 2009; **15**: 1431–41.
16. Fredericksen JL, Petrera J. Serial visual evoked potentials in 90 untreated patients with acute optic neuritis. *Surv Ophthalmol* 1999; **44**: S54–62.
17. Ghezzi A, Martinelli V, Torri V et al. Long-term follow-up of isolated optic neuritis: the risk of developing multiple sclerosis, its outcome, and the prognostic role of paraclinical tests. *J Neurol* 1999; **246**: 770–5.
18. Hickman SJ, Toosy AT, SJJ, Altman DR, Mizszkiel KA, MacManus DG, et al. A serial MRI study following optic nerve mean area in acute optic neuritis. *Brain* 2004; **127**: 2498–505.
19. Youl BD, Turano G, Miller DH, Towell AD, MacManus DG, Moore SG, et al. The pathophysiology

of acute optic neuritis. An association of gadolinium leakage with clinical and electrophysiological deficits. *Brain* 1991; **114**: 2437–50.

20. Miller DH. Natural history of multiple sclerosis: when do axons degenerate? In: Waxman SG, editor. *Multiple sclerosis as a neuronal disease.* Amsterdam: Elsevier 2005. p. 185–200.
21. Frohman EM, Fujimoto JG, Frohman TC, Calabresi PA, Cutter GR, Balcer LJ. Optical coherence tomography: a window into the mechanisms of multiple sclerosis. *Nature Neurol* 2008; **4**: 664–775.
22. Parisi V, Manni G, Centofanti M, Gandolfi SA, Olzi D, Bucci MG. Correlation between optical coherence tomography, pattern electroretinogram, and visual 7evoked potentials in open-angle glaucoma patients. *Ophthalmology* 2001; **108**(5): 905–12.
23. Trip A, Schlottmann PG, Jones SJ, Altman DR, Garway-Heath DF, Thompson AJ, et al. Retinal nerve fiber layer loss and visual disfunction in optic neuritis. *Ann Neurol* 2005; **58**: 383–91.
24. Pueyo V, Martin J, Fernandez J, Almarcegui C, Ara J, Egea C, et al. Axonal loss in the retinal fiber layer in patients with multiple sclerosis. *Mult Scer* 2008; **14**: 609–14.
25. Almarcegui C, Dolz I, Pueyo V, Garcia E, Fernandez FJ, Martin J, et al. Correlation between functional and structural assessments of the optic nerve and retina in multiple sclerosis patients. *Clin Neurophysiol* 2010; **40**: 129–35.
26. Klistorner A, Arvind H, Nguyen T, Garrick R, Paine M, Graham S, et al. Inflammation, demyelination and axonal loss in post-acute optic neuritis. *Ann Neurol* 2008; **61**: 325–31.
27. Klistorner A, Arvind H, Nguyen T, Garrick R, Paine M, Graham S, et al. Multifocal VEP and OCT in optic neuritis: a topographical study of the structure–function relationship. *Doc Ophthal* 2009; **118**: 129–37.
28. Smith KJ, Waxman SG. The conduction properties of demyelinated and remyelinated axons. In: Waxman SG, editor. *Multiple sclerosis as neuronal disease.* Amsterdam: Elsevier Academic Press; 2005, p. 85–100.
29. Lassmann H. New Concepts on progressive multiple sclerosis. *Cur Neurol Neurosci Reports* 2007; **7**: 239–44.
30. Foster RE, Whalen CC, Waxman SG. Reorganisation of the axonal membrane of demyelinated nerve fibres: morphological evidence. *Science* 1980; **210**: 661–3.
31. Bostock H, Sears TA. The internodal axon membrane: electrical excitability and continious conduction in segmental demyelination. *J Physiol (London)* 1978; **280**: 273–301.
32. Shrager P, Simon W, Kazarinova-Noyes K. Na+ channel reorganisation in demyelinated axons. In: SG W, editor. *Multiple sclerosis as a neuronal disease.* Amsterdam: Elsevier; 2005.
33. Peterson J, Kidd D, Trapp BD. Axonal degeneration in multiple sclerosis: the histopathological evidence. In: Waxman SG, editor. *Multiple sclerosis as a neuronal disease.* Amsterdam: Elsevier; 2005. p. 165–184.
34. Pro MJ, Pons ME, Liebmann JM, Ritch R, Zafar S, Lefton D, et al. Imaging of the optic disk and retinal nerve fiber layer in acute optic neuritis. *J Neurolog Sci.* 2006; **250**: 114–9.
35. Petzold A, de Boer JF, Schippling S, Vermersch P, Kardon R, Green A, et al. Optical coherence tomography in multiple sclerosis: a systematic review and meta-analysis. *The Lancet (Neurol)* 2010; **9**: 921–32.
36. Talman LS, Bisker ER, Sackel BS, Long DA, Galetta KM, Ratchford JN, et al. Longitudinal study of vision and retinal nerve fiber layer thickness in multiple sclerosis. *Ann Neurol* 2010; **67**: 749–60.
37. Klistorner A, Arvind H, Garrick R, Graham SL, Paine M, Yiannikas C. Interrelationship of optical coherence tomography and multifocal visual-evoked potentials after optic neuritis. *Invest Ophthalmol Vis Sci* 2010; **51**(5): 2770–7.
38. Klistorner A, Garrick R, Paine M, Graham SL, Arvind H, Van Der Walt A, et al. Relationship between chronic demyelination of the optic nerve and short term axonal loss. J Neurol Neurosurg Psychiatry. 2011; Epub ahead of print.
39. Klistorner A, Garrick R, Barnett MH, Graham SL, Arvind H, Sriram P, et al. Axonal loss in non-optic neuritis eyes of patients with multiple sclerosis linked to delayed visual evoked potential. *Neurol* 2013; **15**: 242–5.
40. Bruck W. Inflammatory demyelination is not central to the pathogenesis of multiple sclerosis. *J Neurol.* 2005; **252**(Suppl 5): V/10-V/5.
41. Patrikios P, Stadelmann C, Kutzelnigg A, Rauschka H, Schmidbauer M, Laursen H, et al. Remyelination is extensive in a subset of multiple sclerosis patients. *Brain* 2006; **129**: 3165–72.
42. Prineas JW, Barnard RO, Kwon EE, Sharer LR, Cho ES. Multiple sclerosis: remyelination of nascent lesions. *Ann Neurol* 1993; **33**: 137–51.
43. Prineas JW, Kwon EE, Goldenberg PZ, Ilyas AA, Quarles RH, Benjamins JA, et al. Multiple sclerosis. Oligodendrocyte proliferation and differentiation in fresh lesions. *Lab Invest* 1989; **61**: 489–503.
44. Blakemore WF, Chari DM, Gilson JM, Crang AJ. Modelling large areas of demyelination in the rat reveals the potential and possible limitations of transplanted glial cells for remyelination in the CNS. *Glia* 2002; **38**: 155–68.
45. Klistorner A, Arvind H, Garrick R, Yiannikas C, Graham SL. Remyelination of optic nerve lesions: spatial and temporal factors. *Mult Scler* 2010; **16**: 786–95.
46. Klistorner A, Arvind H, Nguyen T, Garrick R, Paine M, Graham S, et al. Axonal loss and myelin in early ON loss in postacute optic neuritis. *Ann Neurol* 2008; **64**(3): 325–31.
47. You Y, Klistorner A, Thie J, Graham SL. Latency delay of visual evoked potential is a real measurement of

demyelination ina rat model of optic neuritis. *Invest Ophthalmol Vis Sci* 2011; **52**: 6911–8.

48. Raz N, Chokron S, Ben-Hur T, Levin N. Temporal reorganization to overcome monocular demyelination. *Neurology*. August 20, 2013; **81**(8): 702–9. doi: 10.1212/WNL.0b013e3182a1aa3e. Epub July 19, 2013. PubMed PMID: 23873970.
49. Costello F, Hodge W, Pan YI, Eggenberger E, Coupland S, Kardon R. Tracking retinal nerve fiber layer loss after optic neuritis: a prospective study using optical coherence tomography. *Mult Scler* 2008; **14**: 893–905.
50. Hickman SJ, Brierley CMH, Brex PA, MacManus DG, Scolding NJ, Compston DAS, et al. Continuing optic nerve atrophy following optic neuritis: a serial MRI study. *Multiple sclerosis* 2002; **8**: 339–42.
51. Toosy AT, Hickman SJ, Mizszkiel KA, Jones SJ, Plant GT, Altman DR, et al. Adaptive cortical plasticity in higher visual areas after optic neuritis. *Ann Neurol* 2005; **57**: 622–33.
52. Raz N, Dotan S, Benoliel T, Chokron S, Ben-Hur T, Levin N. Sustained motion perception deficit following optic neuritis: Behavioral and cortical evidence. *Neurology*. June 14, 2011; **76**(24): 2103–11. doi: 10.1212/WNL.0b013e31821f4602. PubMed PMID: 21670440.
53. Korsholm K, Madsen KH, Fredericksen JL, Skimmingr A, Lund TE. Recovery from optic neuritis: anROI-based analysis of LGN and visual cortical areas. *Brain* 2007; **130**: 1244–53.
54. Werring DJ, Bullmore ET, Toosy AT, Miller DH, Barker GJ, MacManus DG, et al. Recovery from optic neuritis is associated with a change in the distribution of cerebral response to visual stimulation: a functional magnetic resonance imaging study. *Journal of Neurology, Neurosurgery & Psychiatry* 2000; **68**(4): 441–9.
55. Archibald NK, Clarke MP, Mosimann UP, Burn DJ. The retina in Parkinson's disease. *Brain* 2009; **132**: 1128–45.
56. Tagliati M, Bodis-Wollner I, Yahr MD. The pattern electroretinogram in Parkinson's disease reveals lack of retinal spatial tuning. *Electroencephalogr Clin Neurophysiol* 1996; **100**: 1–11.
57. Kirbas S, Turkyilmaz K, Tufekci A, Durmus M. Retinal nerve fiber layer thickness in Parkinson disease. *J Neuroophthalmol* 2013; **33**: 62–t5.
58. Adam CR, Shrier E, Ding Y, Glazman S, Bodis-Wollner I. Correlation of inner retinal thickness evaluated by spectral-domain optical coherence tomography and contrast sensitivity in Parkinson disease. *J Neuroophthalmol* 2013.
59. Nowacka B, Lubinski W, Karczewicz D. Ophthalmological and electrophysiological features of Parkinson's disease. *Klin Oczna* 2010; **112**: 247–52.
60. Moschos MM, Tagaris G, Markopoulos I, Margetis I, Tsapakis S, Kanakis M, et al. Morphologic changes and functional retinal impairment in patients with Parkinson disease without visual loss. 2011; **21**: 2429.
61. Kirbas S, Turkyilmaz K, Anlar O, Tufekci A, Durmus M. Retinal nerve fiber layer thickness in patients with Alzheimer disease. *J Neuroophthalmol* 2013; **33**: 58–61.
62. Moschos MM, Markopoulos I, Chatziralli I, Rouvas A, Papageorgiou SG, Ladas I, et al. Structural and functional impairment of the retina and optic nerve in Alzheimer's disease. *Curr Alzheimer Res* 2012; **9**: 782–8.
63. Meier-Ruge W. Drug induced retinopathy. *CRC Toxicol* 1972; **1**: 325–60.
64. Lyons JS, Severns ML. Using multifocal ERG ring ratios to detect and follow Plaquenil retinal toxicity: a review. *Doc Ophthalmol* 2009; **118**: 29–36.
65. Marmor MF, Kellner U, Lai TY, Lyons JS, Mieler WF. Revised recommendations on screening for chloroquine and hydroxychloroquine retinopathy. *Ophthalmology* 2011; **118**: 415–22.
66. Kjellstrom U, Andreasson S, Ponjavic V. Attenuation of the retinal nerve fibre layer and reduced retinal function assessed by optical coherence tomography and full-field electroretinography in patients exposed to vigabatrin medication. *Acta Ophthalmol* 2013.
67. Tjoa CW, Benedict RH, Dwyer MG, Carone DA, Zivadinov R. Regional specificity of magnetization transfer imaging in multiple sclerosis. *J Neuroimaging* April 2008; **18**(2): 130–6. doi: 10.1111/j.1552-6569.2007.00198.x.
68. Gallo A, Rovaris M, Benedetti B, Sormani MP, Riva R, Ghezzi A, et al. A brain magnetization transfer MRI study with a clinical follow up of about four years in patients with clinically isolated syndromes suggestive of multiple sclerosis. *J Neurol*. January 2007; **254**(1): 78–83. Epub February 14, 2007. PubMed PMID: 17508141.
69. Tortorella P, Rocca MA, Mezzapesa DM, Ghezzi A, Lamantia L, Comi G, et al. MRI quantification of gray and white matter damage in patients with early-onset multiple sclerosis. *J Neurol*. July 2006; **253**(7): 903–7. Epub March 6, 2006. PubMed PMID: 16511645.
70. Deloire-Grassin MS, Brochet B, Quesson B, Delalande C, Dousset V, Canioni P, et al. In vivo evaluation of remyelination in rat brain by magnetisation transfer imaging. *J Neurol Sci* 2000; **178**: 10–16.
71. Zaaraoui W, Deloire M, Merie M, Girard C, Raffard G, Biran M, et al. Monitoring demyelination and remyelination by magnetization transfer imaging in the mouse brain at 9.4 T. *Magn Res Mat Phys*. 2008; **21**: 357–62.
72. Klistorner A, Chaganti J, Garrick R, Moffat K, Yiannikas C. Magnetisation transfer ratio in optic neuritis is associated with axonal loss, but not with demyelination. *Neuroimage* 2011; **56**(1): 21–6.

Chapter 8

Optical coherence tomography and electrophysiology of the optic nerve head

Shin C. Beh, Zane Schnurman, Darrel Conger, Amy Conger, Benjamin M. Greenberg, Elliot M. Frohman, and Teresa C. Frohman

Introduction

It is reasonable to predict that functional disruptions precede any measurable structural changes in the nervous system and retina. Early pathologic changes that begin at a cellular level may easily evade the resolution of highly sensitive structural metrics but may be detected by electrophysiologic means. It is possible that early dysfunction represents a potentially reversible state of visual compromise, and, therefore, timely detection of such dysfunction would allow therapeutic interventions that would halt the pathological process, prevent future disability, and potentially even reverse the accrued damage, even before structural changes of retinal nerve fiber layer or ganglion cell layer thinning are evident on OCT.

Visual perimetry, visual acuity, contrast vision testing, and color testing (time-tested neuro-ophthalmic methods of investigating visual function) are contingent upon the active participation of a cooperative patient and are, therefore, prone to variability. However, these assessments themselves are considered valid and of adequate utility to have rendered them the gold standards for clinical evaluation. Alternately, each of these tests are lacking in sufficient sensitivity such that a more than insignificant burden of disease activity could have been sustained within the visual system before such changes translate into corresponding functional consequences. For instance, evidence confirms the hypothesis that, in glaucoma, significant damage to the retinal ganglion cells (RGC) may occur before visual field deficits are detectable [1, 2]. An analogue of this observation reflects a similar discordance between changes in the burden of radiographic measures of disease activity in multiple sclerosis (MS) and the surprising lack of commensurate clinical concomitants, the so-called clinic-radiologic paradox [3]. In contradistinction, extremely modest alterations in tissue architecture (e.g., very few brain hyperintensities on T2 or FLAIR-weighted MR imaging sequences, or subtle to no identifiable changes in the thickness of retinal layers), can nonetheless be associated with disabling physiologic changes within the central nervous system (CNS).

In the elegant study by Naismith and colleagues, the authors demonstrated discrete changes in visual evoked potential (VEP) response metrics in patients with acute optic neuritis (ON) at a time when corresponding abnormalities of the retinal nerve fiber layer thickness (RNFL) had not yet been sufficiently manifested to document the changes, even with the application of high-definition spectral-domain OCT imaging techniques [4]. This important observation confirms the principle that pathophysiologic mechanisms, such as changes in axonal transmission properties (due to demyelination, ion channel perturbations, intra-axonal neurofilamentous, and microtubular deconstruction; changes in the thresholds for membrane depolarization; and the commensurate requirements for meeting an escalated requirement for intra-axonal ATP) may antedate the detection of changes in retinal architecture. The compromise in signal fidelity fails to provide the brain with critical visual information and actually serves to predict the localization and magnitude of tissue injury. Both the localization and magnitude of tissue injury are germane to influencing the integrity of normal visual system circuit capabilities (i.e., vision, adjustment of the pupillary aperture across various lighting conditions to optimize foveation while reducing chromatic aberration associated with peripheral lens distortions, and for the

Optical Coherence Tomography in Neurological Disease, ed. Peter A. Calabresi, Laura J. Balcer, and Elliot M. Frohman. Published by Cambridge University Press.

transmission of light information into the hypothalamus, which relates to a myriad of important physiologic processes). Given the evidence-based observations underscored earlier, we are at a crossroads with respect to the need for objective, convenient, tolerated, and time-efficient electrophysiologic techniques that provide for the capability to precisely define both stimulus and response characteristics in conjunction with a highly stringent low test–retest variability.

Ultimately, the principal thrust of such testing paradigms must be the ability to accurately, objectively, and reproducibly monitor the physiologic signatures associated with RGC neurobiology. A sensitive electrophysiologic technique that allows early detection of RGC or optic nerve dysfunction in neurologic diseases like MS would permit timely institution of immunomodulatory agents, or neuroprotective and even neuro-restorative therapies that might serve to arrest or at least attenuate the inflammatory cascades affiliated with MS, particularly, that culminate in progressive disability.

Electrophysiologic investigations of the afferent visual system

Visual-evoked potentials (VEPs)

A well-established technique in neuro-ophthalmology, VEPs refer to electrical potentials believed to be generated in the primary visual cortex (recorded on the scalp in close proximity to the calcarine fissure) and are elicited by a brief photic stimuli [5–7]. Visually evoked potential cortical responses reflect the functional integrity of the retino-geniculo-calcarine pathway; hence, any lesion along the afferent visual pathway (e.g., optic neuritis, chiasmitis, tract, geniculate, optic radiation, or occipital lesions) may produce abnormalities in magnitude or timing responses associated with VEP responses.

Visual evoked potentials: limitations

There are several limitations to the application of conventional VEP studies in clinical practice and in clinical investigation. First, the full-field illumination used in VEP elicits a compound waveform that represents a consolidated global-field response, which is a derivative of both abnormal and normal cortical generators and thereby lacks the spatial resolution necessary in order to identify geographically discrete areas of dysfunction [7]. Second, approximately 65% of the cortical response network is generated by the central 2° of the visual field [8]. Further, since the macular response (particularly driven by the lower field) dominates the VEP, spatially prominent dysfunctional areas confined to the upper field distribution may still evade capture by conventional VEP techniques [7, 9]. Third, inter-individual heterogeneity of striate cortical anatomy, as well as the contribution of extra-striate regions to the VEP response, combine to intensify the broad variation in what constitutes "normal" response metrics [10–18]. Finally, VEP abnormalities may arise from lesions anywhere along the retino-cortical pathway, rendering the technique lacking in the all important localization aspect of systems analysis in neurology and neurobiology.

Multifocal visual evoked potentials (mfVEP)

The application of multifocal VEP (mfVEP) overcomes the poor spatial resolution, as well as the dominance of the central and lower fields inherent to conventional VEPs. Instead mfVEP parcellates the central 24°– 32° of vision into 60 segments (each of which has a 4 × 4 black-and-white checked grid that contrast-reverses according to a pseudo-random m-sequence) and allows evoked responses to be generated simultaneously from multiple areas of the visual field. This permits topographical analysis of the afferent visual system (thus improving the detection of small, localized lesions) without a significant increase in recording time. Additionally, the contribution from extra-striate regions is smaller to that in VEP [7, 19–23].

The utilization of mfVEP has its most powerful application for the purpose of characterizing the intra-individual interocular mfVEP comparison technique, with evidence demonstrating clear superiority over the monocular mfVEP technique [7; 24–27]. This interocular technique is suitable for monocular/unilateral pathologies (e.g., non-arteritic ischemic anterior optic neuropathy). Notwithstanding the inherent advantages of mfVEP technology, this advanced method of visual system physiology is not without important limitations. First, a major drawback of mfVEPs is the lack of normative values [7], a significant obstacle to the wide employment of this technique in clinical investigation and principally related to the wide inter-individual variability in cortical anatomy. Further, diseases like MS often affect both retinas and optic nerves, and this may confound accurate interocular comparisons. Second, while the mfVEP is sensitive for detection of central defects, areas of dysfunction outside the central 10° may be missed due to sparser sampling [25]. Lastly, like conventional VEPs, mfVEP abnormalities may occur from lesions anywhere along the retino-cortical pathway.

Electroretinography (ERG)

Conventional ERG

Conventional full-field ERG (cERG) generates a single compound waveform (recorded over the cornea) in response to a brief flash delivered via a Ganzfeld bowl to represent the activity of the entire retina [28, 29]. It is useful for evaluating retinal disorders, in particular those that affect the health of the rods and cones (e.g., retinitis pigmentosa, toxic retinopathies).

The cone response may be isolated by recording the cERG under light-adapted (photopic) conditions, by using a stimulus wavelength above 680 nm or with a 30 Hz flicker. Alternately, the rod response may be isolated by scotopic conditions, that is, dark-adaptation for 45 minutes, followed by a short-wavelength stimulus as a single flash, or a 10 Hz flicker [30,31].

Photopic responses generate small b-wave amplitudes with short latencies (~30 ms). Scotopic conditions result in larger b-wave amplitudes and longer latencies (~60 ms) [30]. There is little contribution from the RGC population to the cERG [32, 33], limiting its utility in assessing pathologies of the inner retinal layers (those layers closest to the vitreous) and optic nerve. Additionally, since the cERG represents a global summed retinal response, small areas of dysfunction are subordinated by the principal retinal response. Unlike the VEP (where the central 2° of vision dominates the response), the foveal response represents less than 2% of the ERG response [34]; therefore, central scotomas may easily be missed.

Pattern ERG (PERG)

PERG is a biphasic response of smaller amplitude than the cERG and is a useful method of assessing inner retinal function. Utilizing an achromatic, 0.5–1 s phase reversing checkerboard pattern (similar to VEP) that maintains constant luminance, the PERG isolates nonlinear (i.e., inner retinal) responses [30, 35]. PERG generation is hypothetically contingent upon the functional integrity of the RGCs and is disrupted in diseases affecting the inner retina and optic nerve (as a consequence of retrograde RGC degeneration) [30; 36–42]. However, there is evidence that the PERG response may not be purely contingent upon nonlinear (i.e., RGC) components [43]. Additionally, PERG responses are dominated by macular RGC contributions [44, 45]; hence, peripheral areas of dysfunction may escape detection. Finally, the PERG is also limited by poor spatial resolution; like the cERG, the massed response may easily miss localized areas of dysfunction.

Photopic negative response (PhNR)

The PhNR is a component of the photopic ERG that represents the activity of the RGCs and their axons, as well as the integrity of K^+ currents in retinal glial cells [40, 46–47]. In primates, the PhNR is eliminated by intravitreal tetrodotoxin (which abolishes RGC activity) and in glaucoma models [46]. In human beings, it is diminished in diseases that affect the RGCs and their axons, including MS, glaucoma, non-arteritic acute ischemic optic neuropathy (NAION), compressive optic neuropathy, traumatic optic neuropathy, autosomal dominant optic atrophy, and central retinal artery occlusion [40; 48–53]. Interestingly, epilepsy ataxia sensorineural deafness (EAST) syndrome, an autosomal recessive mutation affecting the inward-rectifying potassium channel, is also associated with PhNR abnormalities [47]. Retrobulbar optic nerve disruption without RGC perturbation (i.e., before retrograde degeneration occurs) does not appear to affect the PhNR, implicating an intraocular RGC source for this waveform [50]. Therefore, it is possible that early optic nerve disease may not be detected until intraocular RGC dysfunction begins. Further, since the PhNR utilizes a full-field stimulus like the cERG, it may fail to capture small yet discretely localized definitive defects.

Multifocal ERG (mfERG)

The application of mfERG helps overcome the limited spatial resolution of the cERG. In mfERG, the retina is stimulated (under photopic conditions) by a hexagonal array subtending the central 20°–25° of vision. The stimulus array is scaled in size to elicit responses that are equal in amplitude across the retina, with the central hexagons being smaller than the peripheral ones [30]. The mfERG takes a single, continuous electrical signal from the eye and mathematically extracts and isolates a response profile (i.e., a "mini ERG") for each element of the display, thereby operationally executing a topographical interrogation of the retina, in conjunction with a corresponding nonlinear analysis of retinal responses [20, 29, 54–55]. The first-order kernel responses of the mfERG (the most commonly measured parameter), consists of an initial negative deflection (N1), a positive component (P1), and a second negative deflection (N2). It has been shown that N1 and P1 are analogous to the a- and b-waves of the cERG, respectively [29]. While the first-order kernel responses are devoid of significant contributions from the RGC pool, higher-order kernels (the largest of which is the second-order kernel first slice, K2.1) are generated by flash interactions (i.e., modification of responses induced by a preceding photic stimulus) and are purely nonlinear, representing predominantly inner retinal (in particular, RGC) function [56–57, 61].

The optic nerve head component (ONHC)

When retinal responses are derived by means of the standard (fast) multifocal flicker protocol, analysis of the K2.1 revealed several induced components, including a unique, and long-latency, electrophysiologic signature waveform (with respect to the retinal component (RC), the so-called optic nerve head component (ONHC) response [56]. The origination of the ONHC responses have been hypothesized to be generated in the vicinity of the optic nerve head (ONH). The stereotyped geometric configuration of the RGC axons within the RNFL traverse the neural retinal rim (at which point they sharply bend out of the plane of the inner retina and into the optic cup), concomitant with their physiologic transformation from unmyelinated axonal membrane conduction to saltatory conduction properties, as they penetrate the lamina cribrosa and obtain oligodendrocyte-derived myelin internodes (Figure 8.1) [56].

Subsequent modifications in the mfERG stimulus paradigm (specifically, by appending one or more global flashes after the m-frame to emphasize the fast adaptive mechanisms that give rise to the induced components) have improved the ability to elucidate RGC activity in the first-order kernel mfERG responses [57]. As stated previously, it was with the second-order first slice K2.1 that enabled us to elucidate the ONHC. Response waveforms obtained by these global flash paradigms consist of a direct component and several induced components (which are dominated by the RC and ONHC) [57–58]. The RC represents the contributions of diversified elements across different layers of the retina. Alternately, the normal ONHC response is derived from the inner retinal, with an onset latency that is related to the distance from the retinal patch of stimulation to the optic nerve head.

While the RC response is directly derived from the patch of retinal stimulation and recorded by the corneal electrode, the ONHC response is contingent on the integrity of the RGC, its axon, and the associated propagation of the action potential from the patch of retinal stimulation, beyond which it travels to the optic nerve head, and subsequently across the lamina cribrosa. With these principles in mind, we can understand how those patches of retinal stimulation that are closest to the optic nerve head will reveal ONHC responses of shortest latency, while those patches stimulated furthest away will generate the longest latency responses (resembling a chevron-like pattern; Figure 8.2).

The ONHC in animal studies

Pig eyes are morphometrically quite similar to human eyes, and also demonstrate a late positive mfERG waveform (referred to as the P3 peak) [59] that bears a striking resemblance to the ONHC response in human beings. As in the human ONHC response, the P3 peak is predominantly related to RGC activity, a hypothesis that has been corroborated by studies that demonstrated abolishment of these late responses following the administration of tetrodotoxin, isoflurane, and NMDA, and by its time-related deterioration following optic nerve section [59–60]. While the P3 did not demonstrate the expected changes in latency with distance from the optic nerve head (as in human beings and primates), this may be due to interspecies morphometric differences [59].

Macaques also demonstrate a very prominent ONHC (due to the high number of RGCs) [61]. Its elimination by intravitreal TTX [62–64] and disruption in advanced glaucoma [33] indicates the prominent contribution of RGC activity to this waveform.

The normal human ONHC

Our group sought to study the characteristics of the optic nerve head component response (ONHC) responses in a cohort of normal human subjects. We demonstrated two principal response waveforms: the retinal component (RC) and ONHC (Figure 8.2). The RC is a conspicuous, large-amplitude waveform consisting of an initial negative trough, a positive deflection, followed by a second

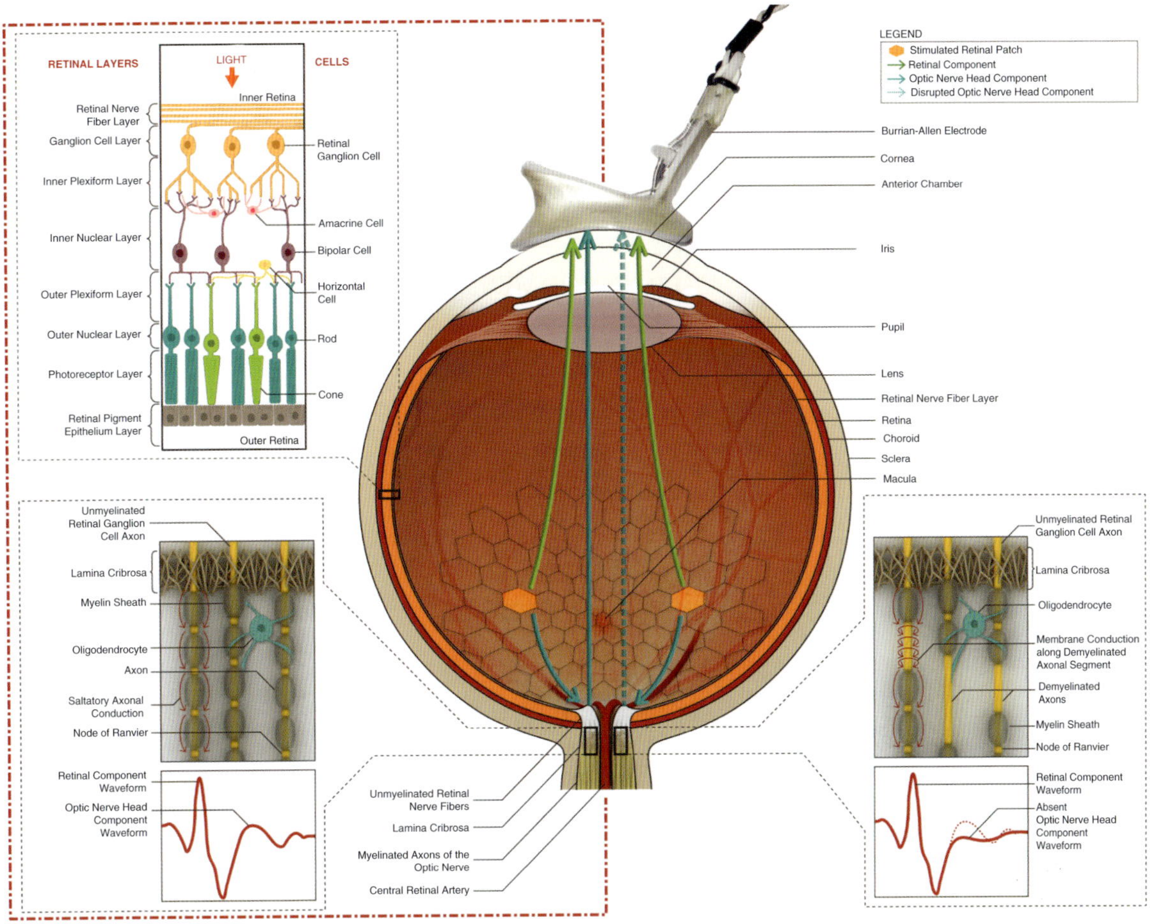

Figure 8.1 Generation of the optic nerve head component response

This illustration details how the retinal component (RC) and optic nerve head component (ONHC) responses are generated within the retina and subsequently detected and characterized by multifocal electroretinographic (mfERG) techniques. The patient is exposed to stimuli consisting of 103 hexagons, the map of which we illustrate within the posterior part of the globe of the eye. Each stimulus consists of five frames – the first contains focal flashes (controlled by the VERIS pseudo-random m-sequence), the second and fourth contain global flashes, and the third and fifth frames are dark.

The photic stimulus generates response first in the photoreceptors and then in the retinal ganglion cells. In this illustration, the retinal patches of stimulation (orange hexagons) will yield electrical responses that are detected at the corneal surface with a Burian-Allen electrode. The large-amplitude RC (teal arrow) is directly derived from the stimulated retinal patch, representing the response of multiple cell types within the retina, with only a modest contribution made by the retinal ganglion cells. However, a smaller, later waveform following the RC is designated as the ONHC waveform. The action potential that is generated at the stimulated retinal patch is propagated (membrane conduction) via the retinal ganglion cell axons in the retinal nerve fiber layer to the optic nerve head.

The ONHC response (solid green arrow) is generated as this action potential traverses the lamina cribrosa and its conduction transforms from membrane to saltatory conduction (as the optic nerve axons obtain oligodendrocyte myelination). As the ONHC is generated at the optic nerve head region, its latency is contingent upon the distance of the stimulated retinal patch from this region (i.e., the farther the patch, the longer the latency) and the thickness of the axons transmitting the action potential (i.e., the thicker the axons, the shorter the latency). In the context of ocular or neurologic disease that affects the RGC, RGC axons, or optic nerve myelin, the ONHC would appear abnormal or be completely lost (broken green arrow).

negative trough. The RC response demonstrated constant peak latency, irrespective of distance or eccentricity from the optic nerve head. This finding supports the hypothesis that the RC is composed of various cellular responses (and not purely RGC activity) and is directly derived from each stimulated retinal patch [56, 65].

The ONHC is the positive waveform occurring immediately following the second negative trough of the RC. Its peak latency varied with distance and eccentricity from the ONH. Within rings of equal eccentricity, the ONHC peak latency was directly proportional to the distance of the stimulated retinal patch from the optic

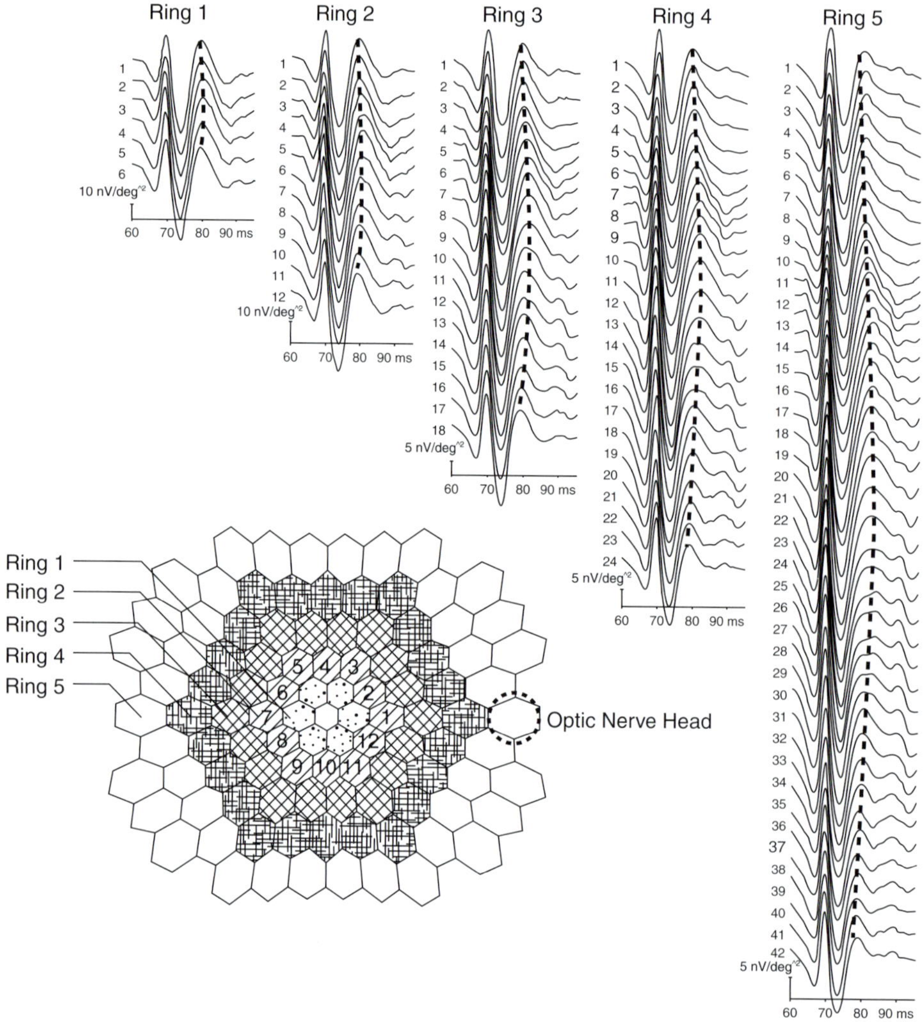

Figure 8.2 The appearance of the normal optic nerve head component response.

The stimulus array consists of hexagonal patches arranged in a series of concentric rings, each progressively more eccentric from the fovea centralis. Ring 1 is the closest to the fovea, and Ring 4 the farthest away. By convention, the stimulation pattern begins at the peripapillary zone, then proceeds superiorly, temporally, and inferiorly, and ultimately returns to the peripapillary zone. This results in the progressive increase and subsequent decrease in the ONHC latency (for patches of equal eccentricity from the fovea centralis) and gives rise to the chevron-like pattern (marked by the dashed lines) of the ONHC response when displayed in the trace array. This chevron-like pattern is an important feature seen in normal ONHC responses.

nerve head. This observation supports the hypothesis that the ONHC is ultimately generated in the region of the optic nerve head and is, therefore, dependent on the time needed for an action potential to travel via membrane conduction from the RGC to the optic nerve head, at which point the axons bend into the optic cup, penetrate the lamina cribrosa, and become myelinated.

Within rings of equal eccentricity (meaning a circular pattern of retinal patch stimulation, with each patch equidistant to the center point of the ring), the ONHC latency is contingent upon the length of the axons transmitting the stimulus to the optic nerve head. The shortest latency responses were those closest to the ONH, while those further away were delayed commensurate with their distance from the optic nerve head.

Of interest, we also found that ONHC peak latency was inversely related to eccentricity away from the central macula across successive rings (i.e., the ONHC peak latency decreased with increasing eccentricity from the central macula, in the vertical meridian). While this may seem counterintuitive (since the distance of the stimulation patch is farther away from the ONH), this finding is corroborated by changes that occur in retinal anatomy and physiology with eccentricity, and it is in keeping with principles of cable theory.

Sutter et al. showed that the calculated propagation velocities derived from concentric rings, characterized by increasing eccentricity from about 40 cm/s in Ring 1 (smallest diameter ring of retinal patch stimulation) to 120 cm/s in Ring 4 [56]; these propagation velocities are comparable to those found by means of antidromic stimulation in feline [66] and primate [67–68] optic nerves. Axonal propagation velocities in unmyelinated fibers are linearly correlated to the square root of their axon diameters ($v = k \sqrt{D}$; where $1.4 < k < 1.8$) [56, 67]; the faster conduction speed in the outer rings would imply that the axonal fibers of these rings have a greater diameter than those situated within the inner rings (consistent with axonal cable theory). Primate and human studies have shown that the mean RGC axon diameter is smallest in the immediate vicinity of the central fovea (in particular, within the papillomacular bundle; PMB) and increases as one travels eccentrically towards the superior and inferior arcuate bundles [67–72]. Even within the proximal 20° of angular distance from the fovea (i.e., the area of the retina stimulated by the hexagonal array), there is a gradual increase in axonal diameter with growing eccentricity [70]. Notably, the mean axon diameter of the inferior arcuate bundle is larger than the superior bundle [67–72], in keeping with our ONHC latency profiles, with a significantly lower latency associated with the inferior outer ring responses when compared with positionally analogous (along the vertical extent of the concentric rings) patches in the superior retinal field (data in preparation).

While the peak latencies of both the RC and ONHC demonstrated consistent characteristics between subjects, the amplitude of both waveforms were more variable, leading us to instead analyze the ONHC:RC peak amplitude ratio. The wide variation we found in the absolute values of the RC and ONHC peak amplitudes is not surprising since there is a twofold range in total RGC number in normal eyes, reflected by the number of axons in the optic nerve (between 846,000 and 1.7 million) [73]. Further, ERG amplitudes vary between healthy subjects and are influenced by factors such as fundus pigmentation [74] and globe axial length, as in high myopes [75]. This broad range makes it more difficult to establish normal parameters for both the RC and ONHC peak amplitudes, which is reflected by the wide amplitude variability.

That variability was reduced when we examined the ONHC:RC peak amplitude ratio, given that both components are affected similarly by a number of confounding factors. Pathological processes extending beyond the inner retina would be expected to affect both the RC and ONHC (while minimally impacting the ONHC:RC ratio), while a purely inner retinal disorder would predominantly affect the ONHC (decreasing the ONHC:RC ratio). In this circumstance, the ONHC:RC ratio may have utility for the identification of patients with dysfunction restricted to the inner retina.

Another characteristic we observed was that both the RC and ONHC peak amplitudes decreased with growing eccentricity from the optic nerve head, as a result of a decrease in retinal cell densities (both RGC and cones) with increasing eccentricity [56, 65, 73]. The ONHC:RC peak amplitude ratio diminished with eccentricity as a consequence of greater ONHC peak amplitude diminution [65]; this is corroborated by the declining RGC:cone density ratio with eccentricity [73].

The ONHC in neurologic and ophthalmic disease

Our investigative team has proceeded to evaluate ONHC abnormalities in a small group ($n = 7$) of MS patients with and without prior ON, and to compare the ONHC changes with those of structural (OCT, fundus photography) and functional (visual perimetry, infrared pupillometry, contrast acuity, mfVEP, and mfERG) metrics [65]. We demonstrated correspondence between abnormal visual field loss, reduced contrast acuity, reduced RNFL thickness, mfVEP cortical response asymmetry, the presence of an objective RAPD, and abnormalities of the ONHC [65]. Using a larger cohort of MS patients with prior unilateral ON (n=18), we demonstrated a robust relationship between ONHC abnormalities and low contrast visual acuity and RNFL thinning as measured by spectral-domain OCT. An example of abnormal ONHC responses in an MS patient with prior optic neuritis is provided in Figures 8.3 and 8.4.

There is evidence that abnormalities of the ONHC are present in early glaucoma in human beings [76] and in nonhuman primates (as discussed earlier).

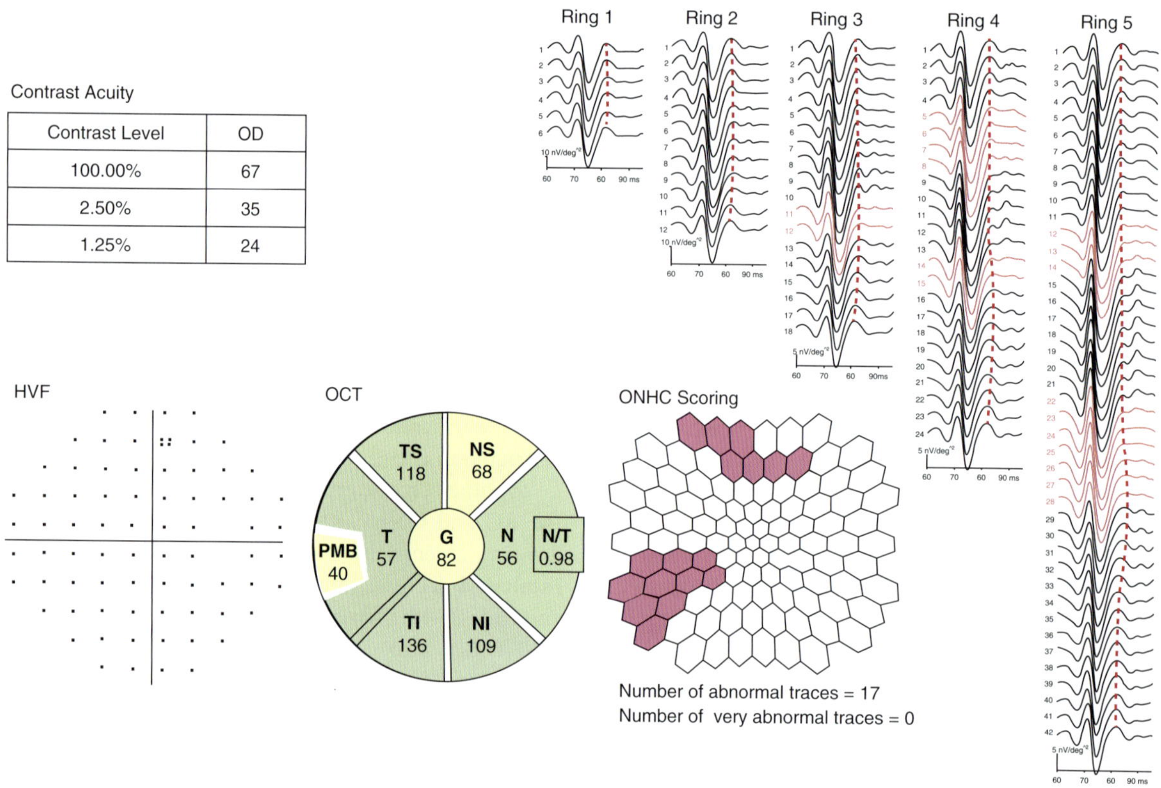

Figure 8.3 The optic nerve head component response in the eye of an MS patient without a history of optic neuritis.

Here we present data from the unaffected (historically) right eye from a patient with multiple sclerosis who had prior *left* acute optic neuritis. The upper-left text box indicates the number of correct letters identified on contrast acuity charts (at 100%, 2.5%, and 1.25% levels). Below, we show the normal pattern-deviation plot from Humphrey automated perimetry, using the 30–2 test. In the lower-left aspect of the figure, we present the retinal nerve fiber layer (RNFL) thickness analysis by spectral-domain optical coherence tomography (OCT; Spectralis, Heidelberg, Germany). The average RNFL thickness is mildly reduced (at 82 microns for the "unaffected" right eye), suggesting the presence of occult disease activity. On the right aspect of the figure, we present the concentric rings of retinal patch stimulation, with the ONHC responses aligned vertically. The waveforms traced in red are those where the ONHC is either abnormal or absent. The retinal patch topography map (bottom middle part of the figure) indicates the location of the abnormal or absent responses.

Additionally, there is anecdotal evidence that ONHC perturbation occurs in Leber's hereditary optic neuropathy (LHON) [77].

Limitations

A major drawback to the application of ONHC responses is the lack of an objective method for accurately quantifying abnormalities of this RGC-specific response. With existing technology, we are already able to quantify the amplitude and peak latency of the waveform. However, in disease states, the magnitude of response disorganization may preclude the accurate identification of latency or amplitude measures. Given this, there is a need to develop techniques that permit accurate quantitative methods for the assessment of the ONHC response.

Given the constellation of complex and time-intensive investigations, we cannot underscore enough the importance of working with highly trained and experienced neuro-ophthalmic technicians. The technician is responsible for ensuring proper scientific protocol is observed to ensure data integrity as well as safeguarding patient safety and dignity.

Finally, since the subject is required to fixate on a target during recording, uncooperative patients and those with pendular nystagmus or severely impaired visual acuity are typically excluded from participating in studies examining the ONHC.

Future directions

Any objective assessment strategy to characterize the ONHC response is likely to be contingent upon the

Contrast Acuity

Contrast Level	OD
100.00%	9
2.50%	0
1.25%	0

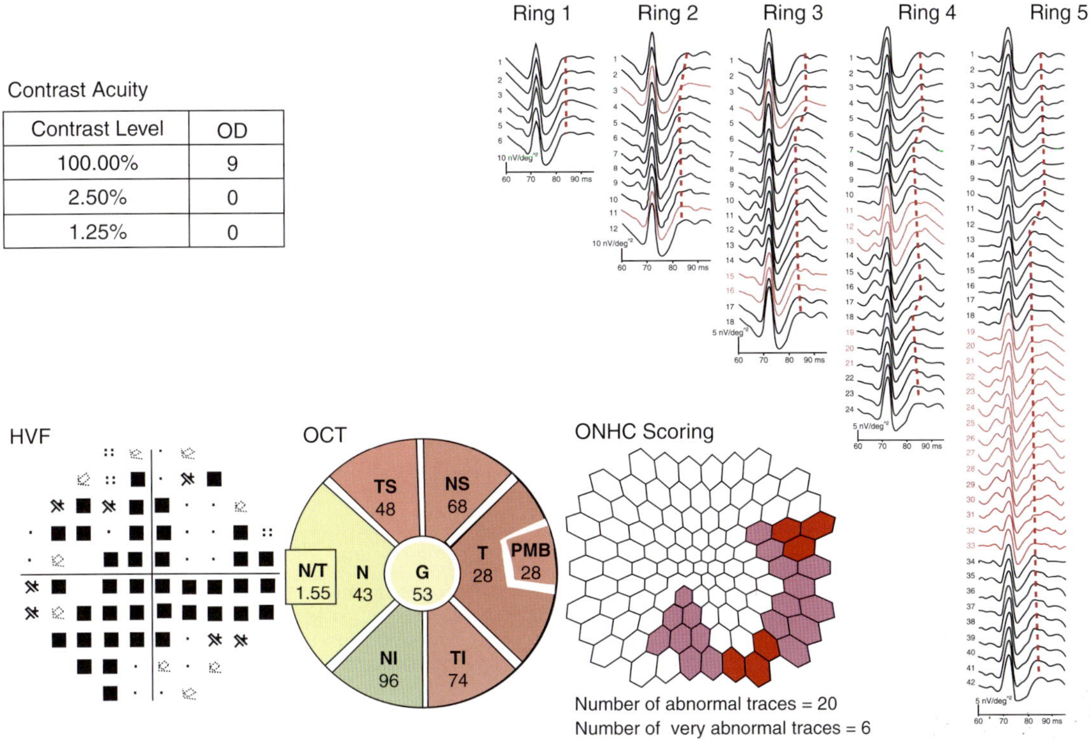

Figure 8.4 The optic nerve head component response in the eye of an MS patient previously affected by optic neuritis.
Here we present data from the same patient in Figure 8.3, but derived from the left eye that was previously affected by optic neuritis. Bedside examination revealed a severe left relative afferent pupillary defect. On ophthalmoscopic examination, there was diffuse optic disc pallor (signifying chronic changes, compositionally most consistent with astrogliosis, a cardinal histopathologic feature of chronic MS-related optic neuropathies). Note the severe loss of acuity (in both high- and low-contrast acuity levels), the broad suppression of the corresponding Humphrey visual field, and the optical coherence tomography (OCT) retinal nerve fiber layer (RNFL) topography map demonstrating diffuse thinning of the RNFL (both average and several sectors; red indicates RNFL thickness levels below 1% of predicted for a matched population). On the right aspect of the figure, note the more diffuse nature of the abnormal or absent optic nerve head component (ONHC) responses. Compared to the right eye, the waveforms are more poorly defined or absent.

high precision, valid, and reproducible methods for dissecting the mechanisms that impact the RGC from the cell body, the anatomic course of the RGC axons as they "sweep" through the RNFL and into the optic nerve head (at the neural retinal rim), and ultimately exit the eye through the lamina cribrosa en route via the retino-geniculo-calcarine pathways for vision to the rostral midbrain for eliciting the pupillary light reflexes, with the smallest number of projections navigating their way from the eye to the hypothalamus, and thereby contributing to a number of important bodily processes including mood regulation, cognitive vigilance, hunger, thirst, and satiety, thermoregulation, the neuroendocrine reflex arcs, sleep–wake cycle transitions. In this analysis scheme, we will need to precisely identify the response latency (and timing responses) in conjunction with the magnitude of ONHC responses.

The ultimate goal is to explore the relationship between structural architecture and corresponding measures of neurophysiology in the visual system, with an eye toward elucidating a surrogate biomarker (s) for the CNS in degenerative disorders in general, and for MS in particular. We propose that the ONHC response is a viable, sensitive, and objective method for assessing and monitoring RGC structure and function, as well as anterior optic nerve myelin integrity. Diseases that may be expected to result in ONHC response abnormalities include glaucoma, ischemic optic neuropathies, hereditary optic neuropathies (e.g., LHON), and demyelinating disorders (in particular, MS and neuromyelitis optica, NMO).

Early detection and treatment of glaucoma, one of the leading causes of blindness in the world, helps arrest subsequent progression to irreversible visual loss [76]. The ONHC response may, therefore, help

Table 8.1 How lesions along the afferent visual pathway may affect electrophysiologic tests of visual function

	CVEP	MfVEP	ERG	PERG	MfERG	ONHC
Outer Retina (widespread defect)	Abnormal	Abnormal	Abnormal	Normal	Abnormal	Normal
Outer Retina (focal defect)	Likely normal	Abnormal	Possibly normal	Normal	Abnormal	Normal
Inner Retina (widespread defect)	Abnormal	Abnormal	Likely normal	Abnormal	Abnormal	Abnormal
Inner Retina (focal defect)	Likely normal	Abnormal	Normal	Possibly normal	Possibly normal	Abnormal
Macula	Abnormal	Abnormal	Likely normal	Likely normal	Abnormal	Abnormal
Optic Nerve	Abnormal	Abnormal	Normal	Normal	Normal	Abnormal
Chiasm	Abnormal	Abnormal	Normal	Normal	Normal	Normal
Retrochiasmatic	Abnormal	Abnormal	Normal	Normal	Normal	Normal

This table provides some general guidelines about how various lesions along the afferent visual pathway may affect electrophysiologic tests. CVEP: conventional pattern reversal visual evoked potential; MfVEP: multifocal visual evoked potential; ERG: electroretinography; PERG: pattern electroretinography; MfERG: multifocal electroretinography; ONHC: optic nerve head component response.

Table 8.2 Summary of salient characteristics, potential applications, and limitations of the optic nerve head component (ONHC) response

Retinal Component Characteristics	• Directly generated at the stimulated retinal patch from the responses of various cell types. • RC peak latency remains constant regardless of distance from the optic nerve head (ONH) and eccentricity.
ONHC Characteristcs	• Generated in the vicinity of the ONH from inner retinal activity from the transformation of membrane to saltatory conduction (as unmyelinated RGC axons acquire oligodendrocyte myelin at the level of the lamina cribrosa). • Within rings of equal eccentricity (and across the horizontal meridian), ONHC peak latency is contingent upon the distance of the stimulation patch from the ONH; this is responsible for the "chevron-like" pattern on the trace analysis. • Across rings of increasing eccentricity in the vertical meridian, the ONHC peak latency diminishes; this is a result of increasing RGC axonal diameter as one moves from the papillomacular bundle to the superior and inferior arcuate fibers. Of note, ONHC peak latencies for retinal areas corresponding with the inferior arcuate are lower than those of the superior arcuate since axonal caliber is greater in the inferior fibers. • ONHC peak amplitude diminishes to a greater degree than the RC with growing eccentricity since RGC density decreases more steeply than those of other retinal cell types.
Potential applications of the ONHC	• Any disorder that perturbs inner retinal, RGC axons, or anterior optic nerve myelin/axonal integrity may disrupt the ONHC. Therefore, it may be useful in monitoring disease activity and treatment responses in the following disorders: multiple sclerosis, neuromyelitis optica, Leber's hereditary optic neuropathy, glaucoma, ischemic optic neuropathies, and toxic-metabolic optic neuropathies.

Table 8.2 (cont.)

ONHC compared to other electrophysiologic tests	• Compared to conventional and multifocal ERG, the ONHC assesses inner retinal and anterior optic nerve integrity. • ONHC abnormalities indicate more localized damage (inner retinal, RGC axon, or anterior optic nerve) compared to visual evoked potentials (VEP), which assess the entire retino-geniculo-calcarine pathway. • Unlike multifocal VEP studies, ONHC responses do not require interocular comparison. • ONHC responses provide superior spatial resolution compared to conventional and pattern ERG as well as conventional VEP.
Limitations of the ONHC	• The ONHC is a novel electrophysiologic metric and as such, inter-rater, intra-rater, and test–retest variability studies, as well as reliable quantification methods, are needed. • ONHC recording requires the use of mydriatic agents. • The Burian-Allen bipolar contact lens electrode is the current standard for ONHC recording and carries a small risk of corneal abrasion. Its application requires experience as well as topical corneal anesthesia. Ideally, patients should undergo slit lamp examination prior to and after ONHC recording. • As accurate recordings requires adequate fixation for the entire duration, severe visual loss or pendular nystagmus, and an inability to cooperate (e.g., children, demented patients) precludes testing.

provide localized and early evidence of RGC dysfunction in glaucoma (particularly low-tension glaucoma) and hence permit early intervention and prevention of visual loss.

With the advent of idebenone as a treatment for LHON [78], there is a need for electrophysiologic methods that can reliably monitor RGC degeneration and recovery. Larger numbers of patients and longitudinal studies are needed to evaluate if the ONHC response characteristics may have utility as a sensitive means of assessing RGC function, neuroprotection strategies, and even to detect and monitor neurorestoration.

The afferent visual system is commonly affected in demyelinating diseases like MS; abnormalities of retinal structural metrics can be objectively quantified with techniques like OCT. ONHC metrics may provide a means of detecting early disruption of optic nerve myelin integrity in MS patients. Our studies have shown that ONHC response disruption is associated with perturbations of other visual metrics. The sensitivity of the ONHC response for detecting occult optic neuropathy would make it an ideal test for those patients with subclinical or mild disease in whom other metrics may not yet reveal any obvious abnormality. The ONHC response may potentially serve as an important electrophysiologic biomarker signifying the integrity of the RGC neuron and its processes. Further, this technique may be of sufficient utility to ascertain the health of optic nerve axons and may be used to monitor the longitudinal evolution of optic neuritis, thereby representing a useful marker of visual recovery (or lack thereof). Ultimately, preservation and/or reconstitution of the ONHC response latency and waveform morphology would confirm neuroprotective and/or neurorestorative efficacy of novel neurotherapeutic agents; a prospect that could not be seriously considered in neurodegenerative disorders just a few years ago.

References

1. Quigley HA, Kerrigan–Baumrind LA, Pease ME, Kerrigan DF, Mitchell RS. The number of retinal ganglion cells in glaucoma eyes compared to threshold visual field data in the same eyes. *Invest Ophthalmol Vis Sci* 1999;**40**:S582
2. Kerrigan-Baumrind LA, Quigley HA, Pease ME, Kerrigan DF, Mitchell RS. Number of ganglion cells in glaucoma eyes compared with threshold visual field tests in the same persons. *Invest Ophthalmol Vis Sci* 2000;**41**:741–748
3. Barkhof F. The clinico-radiological paradox in multiple sclerosis revisited. *Curr Opin Neurol* 2002;**15**:239–245
4. Naismith RT, et al. Optical coherence tomography is less sensitive than visual evoked potentials in optic neuritis. *Neurology* 2009;**73**:46–52

5. Halliday AM, McDonald WI, Mushin, J. Delayed visual evoked response in optic neuritis. *Lancet* 1972;**1**:982–985
6. Halliday AM, McDonald WI, Mushin J. Visual evoked response in diagnosis of multiple sclerosis. *Br Med J* 1973;**1**:661–664
7. Hood DC, Odel JG, Winn BJ. The multifocal visual evoked potential. *J Neuro-Ophthalmol* 2003;**23**:279–289
8. Weinstein GW, Odom JV, Cavender S. Visually evoked potentials and electroretinography in neurologic evaluation. *Rev Neurol Clin* 1991;**9**:225–242
9. Fortune B, Hood DC. Conventional pattern-reversal VEPs are not equivalent to summed multifocal VEPs. *Invest Ophthalmol Vis Sci* 2003;**44**:1364–1375
10. Halliday AM, Michael WF. Changes in pattern-evoked responses in man associated with the vertical and horizontal meridians of the visual field. *J Physiol* 1970;**208**:499–513
11. Brindley GS. The variability of the human striate cortex *J Physiol* 1972;**225**:1P-3P
12. Stensaas SS, Eddington DK, Dobelle WH. The topography and variability of the primary visual cortex in man. *J Neurosurg* 1974;**40**:747–755
13. Victor JD. Isolation of components due to intracortical processing in the visual evoked potential. *Proc Natl Acad Sci USA* 1986;**83**:7984–7988
14. Srebro R. The topography of scalp potentials evoked by pattern pulse stimuli. *Vision Res* 1987;**27**:901–914
15. Schroeder CE, Tenke CE, Givre SJ, et al. Striate cortical contribution to the surface-recorded pattern-reversal VEP in the alert monkey. *Vision Res* 1991;**31**:1143–1157
16. Rademacher J, Caviness VS Jr, Steinmetz H, Galaburda AM. Topographical variation of the human primary cortices: implications for neuroimaging, brain mapping, and neurobiology. *Cereb Cortex* 1993;**3**:313–329
17. Givre SJ, Schroeder CE, Arezzo JC. Contribution of extrastriate area v4 to the surface-recorded flash VEP in the awake macaque. *Vision Res* 1994;**34**:415–428
18. Aine CJ, Supek S, George JS, et al. Retinotopic organization of human visual cortex: departures from the classical model. *Cereb Cortex* 1996;**6**,354–361
19. Fortune B, Hood DC. Conventional pattern-reversal VEPs are not equivalent to summed multifocal VEPs. *Invest Ophthalmol Vis Sci* 2003;**44**:1364–1375
20. Sutter EE. The fast m-transform: a fast computation of cross correlations with binary m-sequences. *Soc Ind Appl Math* 1991;**20**:686–694
21. Baseler HA, Sutter EE, Klein SA, et al. The topography of visual evoked response properties across the visual field. *Electroencephalogr Clin Neurophysiol* 1994;**90**:65–81
22. Baseler HA, Sutter EE. M and P components of the VEP and their visual field distribution. *Vision Res.* 1997;**37**:675–90
23. Slotnick SD, Klein SA, Carney T, Sutter E, Dastmalchi S. Using multi-stimulus VEP source localization to obtain a retinotopic map of human primary visual cortex. *Clin Neurophysiol* 1999;**110**:1793–1800
24. Grover LK, Hood DC, Ghadiali Q, et al. A comparison of multifocal and conventional visual evoked potential techniques in patients with optic neuritis/multiple sclerosis. *Doc Ophthalmol* 2008;**117**:121–128
25. Hood DC, Greenstein VC. Multifocal VEP and ganglion cell damage: applications and limitations for the study of glaucoma. *Prog Retin Eye Res* 2003;**22**:201–251
26. Hood DC, Greenstein VC, Odel JG, et al. Visual field defects and multifocal visual evoked potentials: evidence of a linear relationship. *Arch Ophthalmol* 2002;**120**:1672–1681
27. Hood DC, Zhang X, Greenstein VC, et al. An interocular comparison of the multifocal VEP: a possible technique for detecting local damage to the optic nerve. *Invest Ophthalmol Vis Sci* 2000;**411**:580–1587
28. Frishman, LJ. Origins of the electroretinogram. In: John R. Heckenlively and Geoffrey B. Arden, editors. *Principles and practice of clinical electrophysiology of vision.* 2nd ed. Cambridge, Massachusetts and London, England: Massachusetts Institute of Technology (MIT); 2006.
29. Hood DC, Odel JG, Chen CS, Winn BJ. The multifocal electroretinogram. *J Neuroophthalmol* 2003;**23**:225–235
30. Young B, Eggenberger E, Kaufman D. Current electrophysiology in ophthalmology: a review. *Curr Opin Ophthalmol* 2012;**23**:497–505
31. Marmor M, Fulton A, Holder G, et al. ISCEV standard for full-field clinical electroretinography (2008 update). *Doc Ophthalmol* 2008;**118**:69–77
32. Hood DC, Greenstein V, Frishman L, et al. Identifying inner retinal contributions to the human multifocal ERG. *Vision Res* 1999;**39**:2285–2291
33. Hare WA, Ton H, Ruiz G, et al. Characterization of retinal injury using ERG measures obtained with both conventional and multifocal methods in chronic ocular hypertensive primates. *Invest Ophthalmol Vis Sci* 2001;**42**:127–136
34. Graham SL, Klistorner A. Electrophysiology: a review of signal origins and applications to investigating glaucoma. *Aust N Z J Ophthalmol* 1998;**26**:71–85
35. Holder GE. Electrophysiological assessment of optic nerve disease. *Eye* 2004;**18**:1133–1143

36. Maffei L, Fiorentini A. Electroretinographic responses to alternating gratings in the cat. *Exp Brain Res* 1982;**48**:327–334
37. Maffei L, Fiorentini A, Bisti S, Hollander H. Pattern ERG in the monkey after section of the optic nerve. *Exp Brain Res* 1985;**59**:423–425
38. Sieving PA, Steinberg RH. Proximal retinal contribution to the intraretinal 8-Hz pattern ERG of cats. *J Neurophysiol* 1987;**57**:104–120
39. Baker CL Jr, Hess RR, Olsen BT, Zrenner E. Current source density analysis of linear and non-linear components of the primate electroretinogram. *J Physiol* 1988;**407**:155–176
40. Wang J, Cheng H, Hu Y, et al. The photopic negative response of the flash electroretinogram in multiple sclerosis. *Invest Ophthalmol Vis Sci* 2011;**53**:1315–1323
41. Froehlich J, Kaufman DI. The pattern electroretinogram: N95 amplitudes in normal subjects and optic neuritis patients. *Electroencephalogr Clin Neurophysiol* 1993;**88**:83–91
42. Holder GE. The incidence of abnormal pattern electroretinography in optic nerve demyelination. *Electroencephalogr Clin Neurophysiol* 1991;**78**:18–26
43. Vaegan, Sutter EE. Fundamental differences between the nonlinearities of pattern and focal electroretinograms. *Doc Ophthalmol* 1990;**76**:13–25
44. Lawwill T. The bar-pattern electroretinogram for clinical evaluation of the central retina. *Am J Ophthalmol* 1974;**78**:121–126
45. Arden GB, Carter RM, Macfarlan A. Pattern and Ganzfeld electroretinograms in macular disease. *Br J Ophthalmol* 1984;**68**:878–884
46. Viswanathan S, Frishman LJ, Robson JG, Harwerth RS, Smith EL, III The photopic negative response of the macaque electroretinogram: reduction by experimental glaucoma. *Invest Ophthalmol Vis Sci* 1999;**40**:1124–1136
47. Thompson DA, Feather S, Stanescu HC, et al. Altered electroretinograms in patients with KCNJ10 mutations and EAST syndrome. *J Physiol* 2011;**589**:1681–1689
48. Viswanathan S, Frishman LJ, Robson JG, Walters JW. The photopic negative response of the flash electroretinogram in primary open angle glaucoma. *Invest Ophthalmol Vis Sci* 2001;**42**:514–522
49. Rangaswamy NV, Frishman LJ, Dorotheo EU, et al. Photopic ERGs in patients with optic neuropathies: comparison with primate ERGs after pharmacologic blockade of inner retina. *Invest Ophthalmol Vis Sci.* 2004;**45**:3827–3837
50. Gotoh Y, Machida S, Tazawa Y. Selective loss of the photopic negative response in patients with optic nerve atrophy. *Arch Ophthalmol* 2004;**122**:341–346
51. Miyata K, Nakamura M, Kondo M, et al. Reduction of oscillatory potentials and photopic negative response in patients with autosomal dominant optic atrophy with OPA1 mutations. *Invest Ophthalmol Vis Sci* 2007;**48**:820–824
52. Machida S, Gotoh Y, Tanaka M, Tazawa Y. Predominant loss of the photopic negative response in central retinal artery occlusion. *Am J Ophthalmol* 2004;**137**:938–940
53. Shinoda K, Yamada K, Matsumoto CS, Kimoto K, Nakatsuka K. Changes in retinal thickness are correlated with alterations of electroretinogram in eyes with central retinal artery occlusion. *Graefes Arch Clin Exp Ophthalmol* 2008;**246**:949–954
54. Sutter EE, Tran D. The field topography of ERG components in man – I. *The photopic luminance response. Vision Res* 1992;**32**:433–446
55. Bearse MA Jr, Sutter EE. Imaging localized retinal dysfunction with the multifocal electroretinogram. *J Opt Soc Am A Opt Image Sci Vis* 1996;**13**:634–640
56. Sutter EE, Bearse MA Jr. The optic nerve head component of the human ERG. *Vision Res* 1999;**39**:419–436
57. Shimada Y, Bearse MA Jr, Sutter EE. Multifocal electroretinograms combined with periodic flashes: direct responses and induced components. *Graefes Arch Clin Exp Ophthalmol* 2005;**243**:132–141
58. Luo X, Patel NB, Harwerth RS, Frishman LJ. Loss of the low-frequency component of the global-flash multifocal electroretinogram in primate eyes with experimental glaucoma. *Invest Ophthalmol Vis Sci* 2011;**52**:3792–3804
59. Lalonde MR, Chauhan BC, Tremblay F. Retinal ganglion cell activity from the multifocal electroretinogram in pig: optic nerve section, anesthesia and intravitreal tetrodotoxin. *J Physiol* 2006;**570**:325–338
60. Ng YF, Chan HH, Chu PH, et al. Pharmacologically defined components of the normal porcine multifocal ERG. *Doc Ophthalmol* 2008;**116**:165–176
61. Hood DC, Bearse MA Jr, Sutter EE, Viswanathan S, Frishman LJ. The optic nerve head component of the monkey's (Macaca mulatta) multifocal electroretinogram (mERG). *Vision Res* 2001;**41**:2029–2041
62. Hood DC, Frishman LJ, Viswanathan S, et al. Evidence for a ganglion cell contribution to the primate electroretinogram (ERG): effects of TTX on the multifocal ERG in macaque. *Vis Neurosci* 1999;**16**:411–416
63. Frishman LJ, Saszik S, Harwerth RS, et al. Effects of experimental glaucoma in macaques on the multifocal ERG. *Multifocal ERG in laser-induced glaucoma. Doc Ophthalmol* 2000;**100**:231–251

64. Fortune B, Cull G, Wang L, Van Buskirk EM, Cioffi GA. Factors affecting the use of multifocal electroretinography to monitor function in a primate model of glaucoma. *Doc Ophthalmol* 2002;**105**:151–178
65. Frohman TC, Beh SC, Saidha S, et al. Optic nerve head component responses of the multifocal electroretinogram in MS. *Neurology* 2013;**81**:545–551
66. Stanford LR. Conduction velocity variations minimize conduction time differences among retinal ganglion cell axons. *Science* 1987;**25**:225–231
67. Fukuda Y, Watanabe M, Wakakuwa K, Sawai H, Morigawa K. Intraretinal axons of ganglion cells in the Japanese monkey (Macaca fuscata): conduction velocity and diameter distribution. *Neuroscience Research* 1988;**6**:53–71
68. Ogden TE, Miller RF. Studies of the optic nerve of the rhesus monkey: nerve fiber spectrum and physiological properties. *Vision Res* 1966;**6**:485–506
69. Ogden TE. Nerve fiber layer of the primate retina: morphometric analysis. *Invest Ophthalmol Vis Sci* 1984;**25**:19–29
70. Hebel R, Hollander H. Size and distribution of ganglion cells in the human retina. *Anat Embryol (Berl)* 1983;**168**:125–136
71. Roedick RW, Binmoeller KF, Dineen J. Parsaol and midget ganglion cells of the human retina. *J Comp Neurol* 1985;**233**:115–132
72. Fitzgibbon T, Taylor SF. Mean retinal ganglion cell axon diameter varies with location in the human retina. *Jpn J Ophthalmol* 2012;**56**:631–637
73. Curcio CA, Allen KA. Topography of ganglion cells in human retina. *J Comp Neurol* 1990;**300**:5–25
74. Wali N, Leguire LE. Fundus pigmentation and the dark-adapted electroretinogram. *Doc Ophthalmol* 1992;**80**:1–11
75. Westall CA, Dhaliwal HS, Panton CM, et al. Values of electroretinogram responses according to axial length. *Doc Ophthalmol* 2001;**102**:115–130
76. Fortune B, Johnson CA, Cioffi GA. The topographic relationship between multifocal electroretinographic and behavioral perimetric measures of function in glaucoma. *Optom Vis Sci* 2001;**78**:206–214
77. Sadun AA, Salomao SR, Berezovsky A, et al. Subclinical carriers and conversions in Leber hereditary optic neuropathy: a prospective psychophysical study. *Trans Am Ophthalmol Soc* 2006;**104**:51–61
78. Klopstock T, Yu-Wai-Man P, Dimitriadis K, et al. A randomized placebo-controlled trial of idebenone in Leber's hereditary optic neuropathy. *Brain* 2011;**134**:2677–2686

Chapter 9

Meta-analysis of optical coherence tomography in multiple sclerosis

Axel Petzold

Introduction

This chapter aims to help with a holistic interpretation of optical coherence tomography (OCT) data in multiple sclerosis (MS) research [34]. A meta-analysis will be used to combine some of the data also presented in other chapters of this book. The pooled data will give you an overview on the level of evidence on two related hypotheses:

1. Retinal axonal loss follows MS optic neuritis (MSON) and can be quantified by OCT
2. Retinal axonal loss in MS occurs independently from MSON and is less severe than MSON

These two hypotheses will be further developed using the meta-analysis to show important limitations and highlight pitfalls of OCT methodology. The chapter will conclude with a model of the development of retinal axonal loss in MS and MSON based on the present meta-analysis.

Method

Definitions

In this chapter MSON is defined by having at least one episode of optic neuritis as typically seen in MS [35]. In order to distinguish, within a given patient with MS, which eye had MSON and which one did not, the first will be called MSON-eye and the latter MS-eye.

Literature search

The literature review was conducted on all studies using OCT in MS patients between the first description of the method by Huang [20] and May 2010. Four databases were searched: Pubmed, EMBASE, Medline, Web of Science, and the Cochrane Register of Diagnostic Test Accuracy Studies. The search terms were: multiple sclerosis, MS, optic neuritis, ON, optical coherence tomography, OCT, retinal nerve fiber layer, and RNFL. All references were reviewed in order to identify those investigations where Stratus OCT was utilized (Zeiss, software version 3.0 & 4.0), given that it was the most broadly used system at time of this review. Sixty-two of ninety-nine studies were excluded because the data were not detailed enough, were based on single cases, or used different OCT technology, all precluding any further meta-analysis. Others were excluded because they were double publications of data with a change of emphasis in the interpretation, reviews, or comments. Thirty-five studies were included in the meta-analysis [1, 3, 5, 7–13, 15–18, 21, 23, 25–28, 30, 31, 36–44, 46–49].

Meta-analysis

The Cochrane Collaboration's Review Manager software package (RevMan5) was used for performing the meta-analysis. Data on RNFL thickness was used as a continuous variable. Random effects and inverse variance were used in the model. The selected effect measure was the mean difference of RNFL thickness in the eyes between: (1) MSON patients and control subjects, (2) MS patients who did not have MSON and control subjects and (3) from the same MS patients, a comparison of the MSON-eye with the MS-eye. Next, pooled regression analyses on cross-sectional data were performed using SAS software (version 9.1.3). A p-value of ≤ 0.05 was regarded as significant.

Evidence for the use of OCT in MS

OCT in MSON-eyes

There were 14 studies with data on patients with MSON-eyes and normal control eyes [1, 3, 11, 12,

Optical Coherence Tomography in Neurological Disease, ed. Peter A. Calabresi, Laura J. Balcer, and Elliot M. Frohman. Published by Cambridge University Press.

Study or Subgroup	MSON Mean	MSON SD	MSON Total	Control Mean	Control SD	Control Total	Weight	Mean Difference IV, Random, 95% CI
Albrecht 2007	74.47	22.15	21	103.4	10.96	11	3.6%	−28.93 [−40.41, −17.45]
Bock 2010	86.2	16.2	73	105.2	9.4	406	11.6%	−19.00 [−22.83, −15.17]
Burkholder 2009	85.7	19	328	104.5	10.7	219	13.8%	−18.80 [−21.30, −16.30]
Fisher 2006a	85	17	63	105	12	72	9.7%	−20.00 [−25.03, −14.97]
Frohman 2009	70.3	13.4	12	101.9	8.9	8	4.6%	−31.60 [−41.37, −21.83]
Klistorner 2008	84.5	15.1	32	104	9.2	25	7.8%	−19.50 [−25.85, −13.15]
Merle 2008	83.85	24.12	30	106.24	12.46	46	4.9%	−22.39 [−31.74, −13.04]
Pueyo 2008 (1)	84.46	0	25	104.97	0	25		Not estimable
Pulicken 2007	84.2	14.7	82	102.7	11.5	94	11.4%	−18.50 [−22.44, −14.56]
Ratchford 2009	88.3	16.5	157	102.4	11	77	12.1%	−14.10 [−17.66, −10.54]
Sepulcre 2007 (2)	0	0	24	92.3	16.7	58		Not estimable
Siger 2008	83.92	17.63	40	100.3	12.1	24	6.7%	−16.38 [−23.68, −9.08]
Trip 2005	68.7	18.8	25	102.9	14.6	15	4.2%	−34.20 [−44.64, −23.76]
Zaveri 2008	81.8	19.3	68	104.6	10.3	85	9.6%	−22.80 [−27.88, −17.72]
Total (95% CI)			**956**			**1107**	**100.0%**	**−20.38 [−22.86, −17.91]**

Heterogeneity: $Tau^2 = 9.91$; $Chi^2 = 28.03$, df = 11 (P = 0.003); $I^2 = 61\%$
Test for overall effect: Z = 16.14 (P < 0.00001)

Mean Difference IV, Random, 95% CI

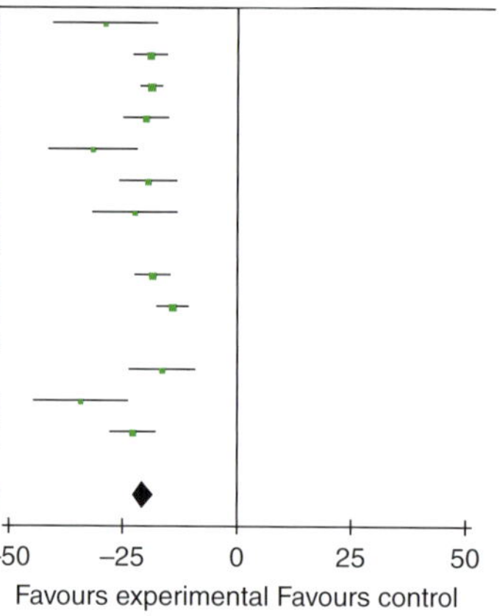

(1) Standard deviation not available from author
(2) Data (mean +/−SD) of ON eyes not published and not available from author.

Figure 9.1 Meta-analysis of OCT studies in MS patients who did suffer from MSON. The overall averaged RNFL data (mean ±SD) and number of MSON-eyes investigated are shown for patients and normal subjects. To the right are the data expressed as micron difference in RNFL thickness of eyes that had optic neuritis compared to normal eyes; the length of the horizontal bar is the 95% confidence interval for each study. Figure reprinted with permission from [34]

23, 28, 38–40, 44, 48, 49], of which 12 could be included in the meta-analysis [1, 3, 11, 12, 23, 28, 38–40, 44, 48, 49]. In total, data from 2,063 eyes were included [34].

Figure 9.1 clearly demonstrates a highly significant loss of RNFL in MSON-eyes. The estimated average RNFL loss was −20.38 μm [−22.86, −17.91]. This is about a fifth of all axons leaving the eye.

Importantly, as discussed by Andrew Henderson in Chapter 4 and Fiona Costello in Chapter 5, there are a number of other pathologies to be considered which can mimic MSON (see Table 5.2). Particularly severe RNFL loss, frequently combined with microcystic macular edema (MMO), is seen following neuromyelitis optica (NMO) and chronic relapsing inflammatory optic neuropathy (CRION) [6, 15, 33, 46]. Therefore, an important limitation of these studies is that information on previous episodes of optic neuritis was frequently sought retrospectively. In the absence of an international consensus on how to investigate patients with suspected optic neuritis, it is probable that the studies pooled for this meta-analysis were rather heterogeneous.

OCT in MS-eyes, never MSON

Sixteen studies investigated the RNFL thickness in patients with MS who did not suffer from MSON [1, 3, 11, 12, 17, 18, 21, 23, 37–40, 44, 48, 49]. Data were sufficiently detailed to permit inclusion into the meta-analysis from 15 of these studies [1, 3, 11, 12, 17, 21, 23, 38–40, 44, 48, 49]. In total 3,154 eyes were investigated.

Figure 9.2 illustrates that the estimated average RNFL loss in MS-eyes was only about a third (−7.08 μm, [−8.65, −5.52]) compared to what was seen for MSON (−20.38 μm [−22.86, −17.91]). In other words, the presumed healthy eyes of patients with MS had lost approximately a tenth of their retinal axons. This still substantial amount of unexpected axonal loss will require explanation.

OCT in MS-eyes with contralateral MSON

The reader may ask at this point if the data presented in the meta-analysis adds up. Can the gap of about 13 μm RNFL thickness between MSON eyes, MS-eyes and control eyes be explained by data derived solely from MS patients? Or may an inclusion or selection bias have been introduced on a group level such that the above two meta-analyses were flawed? To address this question a third meta-analysis was conducted. This time only MS patients with unilateral MSON were included. The OCT data from the MSON-eyes were compared to the data from the presumed unaffected eye from 27 studies [1, 3, 5, 7–9, 11–13, 16, 23, 25–27, 30, 31, 38–44, 46, 47, 49]. In total, data from 4,199 eyes were included into the meta-analysis.

Study or Subgroup	Ms–non–ON Mean	Ms–non–ON SD	Ms–non–ON Total	Control Mean	Control SD	Control Total	Weight	Mean Difference IV, Random, 95% CI
Albrecht 2007	84.59	16.03	27	103.4	10.96	11	2.6%	−18.81 [−27.67, −9.95]
Bock 2010	97	13.1	189	105.2	9.4	406	12.1%	−8.20 [−10.28, −6.12]
Burkholder 2009	95.6	14.5	730	104.5	10.7	219	12.9%	−8.90 [−10.66, −7.14]
Fisher 2006a	96	14	108	105	12	72	8.0%	−9.00 [−12.83, −5.17]
Frohman 2009	101	6	12	101.9	8.9	8	3.7%	−0.90 [−7.94, 6.14]
Gundogan 2007	107.6	16.3	78	110.9	10.3	76	7.1%	−3.30 [−7.60, 1.00]
Henderson 2008a	91.12	12.6	50	98.8	10.5	20	5.0%	−7.68 [−13.46, −1.90]
Jeanjean 2008	88.58	13.39	7	102.34	7.47	15	1.9%	−13.76 [−24.38, −3.14]
Klistorner 2008	103.8	10.8	32	104	9.2	25	5.7%	−0.20 [−5.40, 5.00]
Pueyo 2008 (1)	94.2	0	75	104.97	0	25		Not estimable
Pueyo 2009	97.93	9.08	40	105.37	9.48	20	6.0%	−7.44 [−12.46, −2.42]
Pulicken 2007	95.9	14	202	102.7	11.5	94	9.8%	−6.80 [−9.82, −3.78]
Ratchford 2009	97.4	13.9	338	102.4	11	77	10.2%	−5.00 [−7.87, −2.13]
Siger 2008	94.38	15	62	100.3	12.1	24	4.6%	−5.92 [−12.03, 0.19]
Trip 2005	94.6	14.9	25	102.9	14.6	15	2.3%	−8.30 [−17.72, 1.12]
Zaveri 2008	95.6	15	87	104.6	10.3	85	8.0%	−9.00 [−12.84, −5.16]
Total (95% CI)			**1987**			**1167**	**100.0%**	**−7.08 [−8.65, −5.52]**

Heterogeneity: $Tau^2 = 4.13$; $Chi^2 = 29.66$, df = 14 (P = 0.008); $I^2 = 53\%$

Test for overall effect: Z = 8.87 (P < 0.00001)

(1) Standard deviation not available from author.

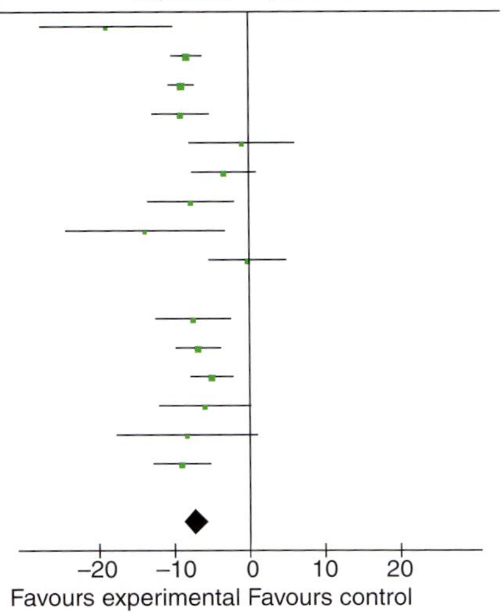

Figure 9.2 Meta-analysis of OCT studies in MS patients who did not suffer from ON, by history. The overall averaged RNFL (mean ±SD) and number of eyes investigated is shown, similarly to Figure 9.1 Note that the bar graph to the right, which summarizes the difference in RNFL in the asymptomatic eyes compared to normal eyes, shows there is loss of RNFL even in eyes supposedly not suffering from previous optic neuritis. Figure reprinted with permission from [34]

Figure 9.3 convincingly corroborates the hypothesis that a history of optic neuritis results in a greater magnitude of axonal loss when compared to MS eyes without such a history. Indeed, the estimated average RNFL loss between MSON-eyes and MS-eyes was close to 13 μm (–13.84 μm [–15.37, –11.72]; please note that, for mathematical reasons and internal consistency, the averaged amount of RNFL loss, "x", is presented as "–x").

Taken together, our findings necessarily underscore an important lingering question for the field; why and how does a substantial amount of axonal loss occur in the presumed unaffected eye of a patient suffering from MS? A possible explanation will be presented at the end of the chapter, but first, the likely time course of development of axonal loss in the MS eye is reviewed.

Time course of RNFL loss in MS

As a rule of thumb, RNFL loss becomes readily detectable to OCT about three months after an episode of acute MSON. Earlier detection of the reduction in RNFL thickness from axonal atrophy is difficult to distinguish from a reduction resulting from resolution of axonal swelling, which is common in acute MSON, as discussed by Andrew Henderson and colleagues in Chapter 4 by Fiona Costello in Chapter 5 and Robert Bermel et al in Chapter 17 of this book. Their combined data demonstrates that about 99% of axonal loss will occur within four to six following MSON.

A correlation between disease duration and the averaged overall RNFL was found by some [11, 37, 44] but not by others [18, 23] included in the meta-analysis (Figure 9.2). The divergent results may in part be explained by the variation in average disease duration and a bias in the population of MS patients studied. A meta-analysis of the published cross-sectional data remains statistically questionable, but may help to shed light on the presumed association between RNFL loss and disease duration. Clearly, accurate information will need to come from carefully conducted longitudinal studies that are executed by multiple collaborative Center teams.

Time in MS-eyes with contralateral MSON

A graph of cross-sectional data analysis illustrates that the average RNFL thickness in the unaffected eye (MS-eye) approaches ≈80 μm (which is about what is seen within one year following MSON) after about 20 years (Figure 9.4). Taking away the effect of normal ageing (about 2 μm per decade [4]), leaves a considerable amount of axonal loss of an estimated 7–9 μm per decade of MS disease duration.

Time in MS-eye, never MSON

With the advent of high-speed, high-definition, spectral-domain OCT, we are finally in a position to address one of the remaining and formidably challenging facets of retinal neurodegeneration in MS; to dichotomize MS eyes with a history of MS ON, and MS eyes with no history of MS ON (at least according to the patient and their family). The principal objective of our most recent work has been to delineate the longitudinal impact upon RNFL thickness in patients without a history of MSON. From the three studies we were able to identify [17, 18, 44], a similar picture emerged (Figure 9.5). Conspicuously, when the data is analyzed cross-sectionally, we found that, within about 12 years, thinning of the RNFL is approaching 80 μm. Of course, it is not surprising that there are outliers that collectively, upon analysis, exhibit considerable heterogeneity, with individual MS eyes distributed to either fast, slow, or average axonal degeneration. Pragmatically, the identification of novel protective and/or restorative neurotherapeutic properties would have potentially important treatment implications for the MS retina and optic nerve in particular, and for neurodegenerative disorders in general.

Time in MSON-eyes

Using a similar cross-sectional meta-analysis it can be demonstrated that following the acute axonal loss associated with MSON [7, 8, 10], little progression seems to be detectable thereafter (Figure 9.6). In fact, the RNFL thickness appears to settle around ≈80 μm within the first year. This is consistent with the clinical experience that vision remains relatively stable even many years after MSON and that the disability outcome is relatively good in patients with optic neuritis. The relevant clinical point here is that progressive visual loss following presumed MSON is hardly ever observed and alternative diagnoses need to be considered [35].

Study or Subgroup	MSON eye Mean	MSON eye SD	MSON eye Total	MS non–OM eye Mean	MS non–OM eye SD	MS non–OM eye Total	Weight	Mean Difference IV, Random, 95% CI
Albrecht 2007	74.47	22.15	21	84.59	16.03	27	2.2%	−10.12 [−21.36, 1.12]
Bock 2010	86.2	16.2	73	97	13.1	189	4.6%	−10.80 [−14.96, −6.64]
Burkholder 2009	85.7	19	328	95.6	14.5	730	5.2%	−9.90 [−12.21, −7.59]
Cheng 2007	76.12	14.92	28	96.45	11.73	33	3.5%	−20.33 [−27.15, −13.51]
Costello 2006	77.5	29.9	54	99.8	32.5	54	3.0%	−22.30 [−34.08, −10.52]
Costello 2008 (1)	89	7.2	21	105.1	3.6	21	4.8%	−16.10 [−19.54, −12.66]
Costello 2008a (2)	78.3	15.74	27	104.4	11.29	27	3.3%	−26.10 [−33.41, −18.79]
Costello 2009 (3)	82.3	19.7	33	103.7	15.5	45	3.1%	−21.40 [−29.50, −13.30]
Fisher 2006a	85	17	63	96	14	108	4.2%	−11.00 [−15.96, −6.04]
Frohman 2009	70.3	13.4	12	101.8	6	12	3.0%	−31.50 [−39.81, −23.19]
Garcia–Martin 2010	83.27	9.5	20	92.86	4.01	61	4.5%	−9.59 [−13.87, −5.31]
Grazioli 2008	81.7	19.2	29	93.6	15.3	31	2.8%	−11.90 [−20.72, −3.08]
Klistorner 2008	104	9.2	32	103.8	10.8	32	4.3%	0.20 [−4.72, −5.12]
Kochkorov 2009	89	18	16	95	14	24	2.4%	−6.00 [−16.45, −4.45]
Laron 2010	79.1	2.5	47	96.3	1.4	65	5.5%	−17.20 [−17.99, −16.41]
Merle 2010	80.81	18.4	31	96.7	15.8	29	2.9%	−15.89 [−24.55, −7.23]
Nakamura 2010	84.28	14.18	19	109.45	12.78	9	2.4%	−25.17 [−35.68, −14.66]
Oreja–Guevara 2010	76.42	16.87	18	85.52	18.62	18	2.1%	−9.10 [−20.71, 2.51]
Pulicken 2007	84.2	14.7	82	93.9	13.1	42	4.2%	−9.70 [−14.78, −4.62]
Quelli 2010	78.01	17.43	51	95.24	11.64	65	4.0%	−17.23 [−22.79, −11.67]
Ratchford 2009	88.3	16.5	157	97.4	13.9	338	5.0%	−9.10 [−12.08, −6.12]
Sepulcre 2007 (4)	85.8	13.9	122	92.3	16.7	58	4.2%	−6.50 [−11.46, −1.54]
Siepman 2010	71.15	13.46	27	90.39	13.46	38	3.6%	−19.24 [−25.88, −12.60]
Siger 2008	83.92	17.63	20	91.08	19.3	20	2.1%	−7.16 [−18.62, 4.30]
Spain 2009	75.81	5.85	24	90.93	2.95	24	5.1%	−15.12 [−17.74, −12.50]
Talman 2010	83	18	208	96	13	381	5.0%	−13.00 [−15.77, −10.23]
Zaveri 2008	81.8	19.3	68	95.6	15	87	4.0%	−13.80 [−19.37, −8.23]
Total (95% CI)			**1631**			**2568**	**100.0%**	**−13.84 [−15.97, −11.72]**

Heterogeneity: $Tau^2 = 21.31$; $Chi^2 = 173.33$, df = 26 ($P < 0.00001$); $I^2 = 85\%$
Test for overall effect: Z = 12.76 ($P < 0.00001$)

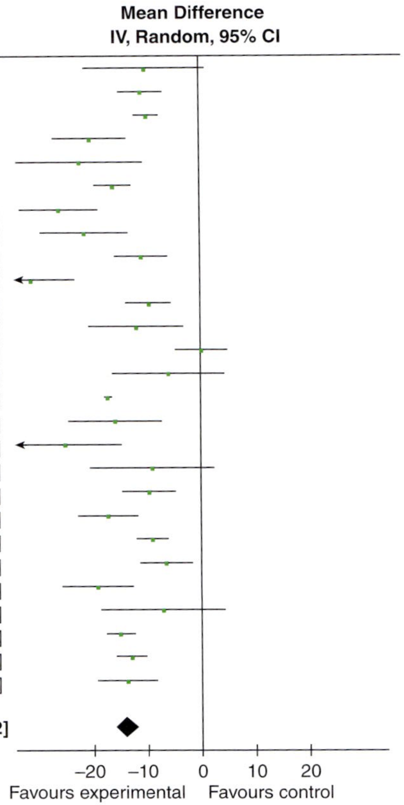

(1) Data on one year after ON. The authors also present 2-year data which is not included into this analysis.
(2) The one year after (13–18 months follow-up) data is taken. Data on standard deviation kindly provided by Dr Fiona Costello.
(3) The one year data on RRMS is presented.
(4) This study included 24 ON eyes and 98 eyes without ON. More details not available from authors.

Figure 9.3 Meta-analysis of OCT studies comparing only MS patients: MSON-eyes and MS-eyes (never affected by MSON). The overall averaged RNFL (mean ±SD) and number of eyes investigated is shown. The difference between the MSON- and MS-eyes shown in this figure is less than the difference between MSON-eyes and normal control eyes Figure 9.1 (note that the scale of the x-axis differs between the two figures). Figure reprinted with permission from [34]

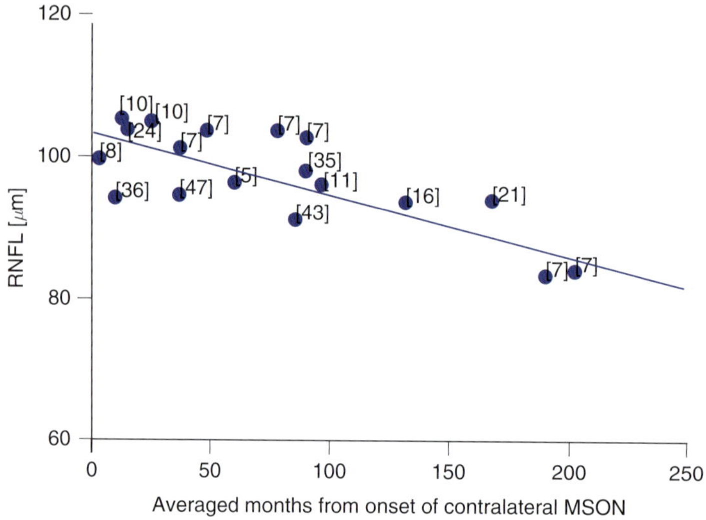

Figure 9.4 Cross-sectional, averaged longitudinal RNFL changes in the unaffected eye of MS patients who suffered from MSON (blue dots). The relatively preserved RNFL (thickness ≈ 105 μm) early in the disease may allow detection of subtle loss of retinal axons during the disease course of MS, at least on a group level. The numbers adjacent to the dots indicate the respective references.

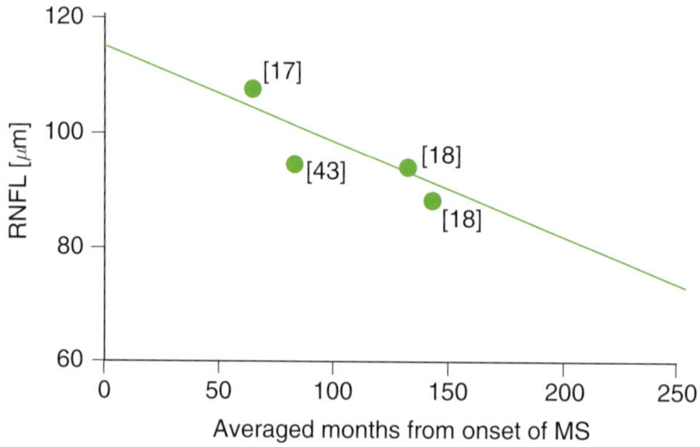

Figure 9.5 The averaged longitudinal RNFL changes in the eyes of MS patients who never suffered from MSON (green dots) suggests that subtle retinal axonal loss may be a feature of insidious axonal attrition in MS, as proposed by Hoyt et al. [19], at least on a group level. The numbers adjacent to the dots indicate the respective references.

One needs to be very careful drawing conclusions on the time course of RNFL loss in an individual eye from cross-sectional meta-analyses of averaged data. Extrapolation from this data is risky because of a possible inclusion bias of patients with early visual problems having OCT and likely exclusion of patients with severe, late progressive MS not included in an observational research study. Nevertheless, the results suggest that, in MS without MSON, there is an estimated yearly thinning of the overall RNFL in the range of ≈ 1–2 μm. Reassuringly, the data from the meta-analysis is consistent with the longitudinal data by Talman and colleagues suggesting a yearly loss of around 1 μm [47].

In this context, it should be highlighted that the current duration of phase II trials in MS is frequently around 4–6 months, thus it is not likely that OCT will provide a reliable outcome over this time scale. From the preceding data, one would expect that MS patients without MSON will require follow-up for at least two years. Again, the reader is referred to the excellent chapters by Andrew Henderson and colleagues (Chapter 4) and Robert Bermel (Chapter 17).

Limitations and pitfalls

Taken together from Evidence for the use of OCT in MS (page 103) and Time course of RNFL loss in MS

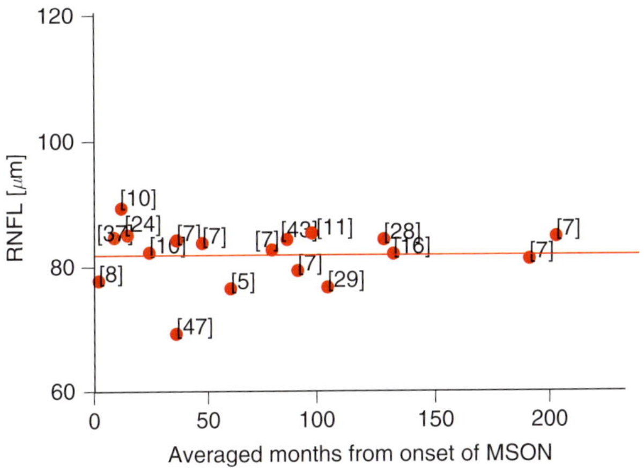

Figure 9.6 Averaged longitudinal RNFL changes in the eye affected by MSON (red dots). The degree of the damage caused to the RNFL by MSON appears cross-sectionally to be so large (RNFL thickness ≈ 80 μm) that any subtle damage that may be attributed to trans-synaptic axonal degeneration could be masked. The numbers adjacent to the dots indicate the respective references.

(page 106) in this Chapter the averaged RNFL loss is largest in MSON-eyes with −20.38 μm, followed by presumably normal MS–eyes of −7.08 μm. In addition, most damage following MSON happens rapidly within 4–12 months following the event. In contrast, in presumably normal MS-eyes, RNFL loss seems to manifest itself at a rate of around 1–2 μm per year. Taken together, these two data sets imply an accelerated rate of axonal degeneration, whereas we have another group that instead exhibits an insidiously slow and steady degeneration attributed to trans-synaptic axonal degeneration. These two presentations (rapid vs slow or retrograde axonal vs trans-synaptic retrograde axonal degeneration), on opposite ends of the injury spectrum (optic nerve vs posterior visual pathways), may be instructive with respect to the application of specific treatment modalities that may be aimed at one set of mechanisms, but not necessarily both.

Importantly, any form of optic neuritis will mask, subtle and slow axonal loss in the eye of patients with MS. Therefore, any study and analysis on a presumed relationship of RNFL loss with pathology or treatment need to carefully distinguish MS-eyes from MSON-eyes.

In the acute phase of MSON, optic disc edema and axonal swelling will mask RNFL thinning. This may considerably limit the prognostic value of OCT in the acute phase. Whether or not MMO, inner nuclear layer thickening and/or periphlebits might be of additional prognostic value remains to be seen and will be discussed in Chapter 4, 10 and 13.

The rate of RNFL loss in MS-eyes is slow. An annual decrease of around 1–2 μm is in the range of the physiological variation in humans seen with a few hours [2]. Larger changes of RNFL thickness measures can be introduced by artifacts related to the method itself. Therefore, rigorous OCT quality control criteria are required to safeguard accuracy and validity of the data. This will be discussed in chapter 18.

Putting it together: a model

At the beginning of this chapter, it was suggested that a meta-analysis may help to enable a holistic interpretation of OCT data in MS research. A possible interpretation of the data of the meta-analysis is summarized in Figure 9.7. The conceptual framework of the visual pathway model has not only inspired the present, but also other Chapters in this book. It serves as a template stimulating formulation of hypotheses which will ultimately help us to link OCT as a tool to other means of assessing structure and function with the overall aim to understand and treat neurodegeneration.

The anatomical basis is discussed in detail by Devin Mackay et al in chapter 3. In brief, retinal axons originate from ganglion cells. Retinal axons travel through the optic nerve to the chiasm, where those supplying the temporal field of vision cross to the other side. From there, axons reach the dorsal lateral geniculate nucleus (LGN), where they end and synapse. The second axon within the optic radiations project to the primary visual cortex (V1, see Figure 9.7A). In addition, to these major projections, axons from the retina also reach the tectum, V2 and V5. It is suggested that any lesion within this trajectory can cause thinning of the RNFL, as revealed by the meta-analysis. The data of the meta-analysis are further supported by histological the data presented in Chapter 3 and Chapter 14. Logically, there are three potential locations were a lesion may occur in

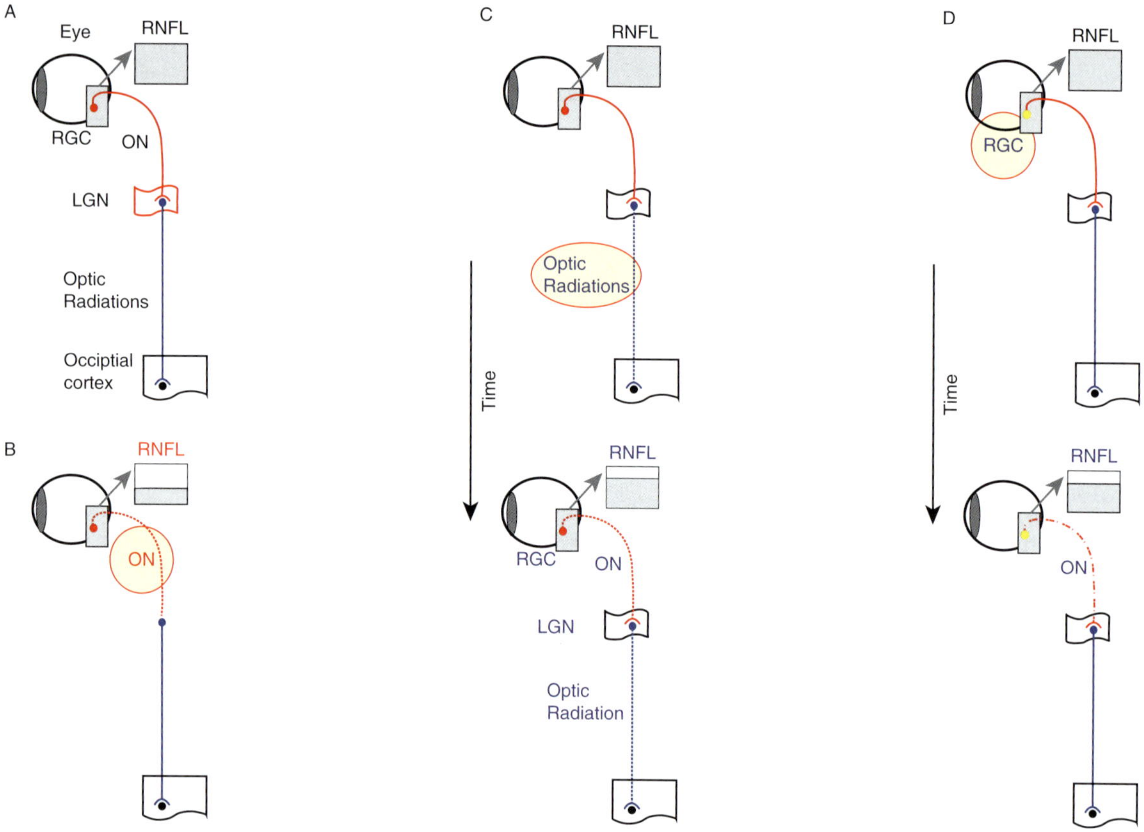

Figure 9.7 A model of the presumed relationship between RNFL thickness and MS pathology. (A) A simplified sketch of the normal human visual pathways. The retinal ganglion cells (RGC) send their unmyelinated axons into the eye, where they form the retinal nerve fiber layer (RNFL, gray inlay), travel to the optic disc, and leave the orbit. Once the axons pass the sclera, they become myelinated and form the optic nerve (ON). After passing through the chiasma, where the temporal fibers cross (not shown), they are called the optic tract. The optic tract wraps around the midbrain and enters the lateral geniculate nucleus (LGN), where all axons must synapse. After the LGN the axons fan out through the deep white matter (optic radiations) to reach the occipital cortex. (B) MSON (red) directly causes acute axonal loss in the ON (red dotted line), leading to marked thinning of the RNFL (small gray box). (C) MS lesions within the optic radiations (blue dotted line) do not immediately result in RNFL thinning. This is thought to be a chronic consequence of trans-synaptic axonal loss through the LGN. With time (black arrow) trans-synaptic axonal degeneration causes a relative smaller degree of axonal loss in the ON (red dashed-dotted line) with a quantifiable degree of RNFL loss (gray box). (D) Progressive loss of RGC (yellow dot) is a likely result of chronic changes in the anterior visual pathways themselves and causes a small degree of RNFL loss (gray box). Figure reprinted with permission from [34]

this trajectory: within the optic nerve (Figure 9.7B), at the level of the optic radiations (Figure 9.7C) or at the level of the ganglion cell (Figure 9.7D).

Possible underlying pathophysiolgoical mechanisms are:

1. Axonal transsection in the optic nerve during MSON causing retrograde axonal degeneration (that is, towards the retinal ganglion cell) and Wallerian (anterograde) axonal degeneration (towards the LGN). Because axons are densely packed in the optic nerve, a lesion is likely to affect a large number of axons, causing immediate, severe thinning of the RNFL (Figure 9.7B).
2. Axonal transsection in the optic radiations causing retrograde axonal degeneration (towards the dorsal LGN). In the dorsal LGN degeneration of a damaged axon (in the optic radiation) is passed on to a previously healthy axon (in the optic nerve) by a process called trans-synaptic axonal degeneration [22]. The likely cause for axonal transsection in the optic radiations is a MS lesion. Because axons of the optic radiations are more widespread in the brain, a single MS lesion

is likely to affect less axons, resulting in less severe RNFL thinning compared to MSON, which also takes more time to establish (Figure 9.7C).

3. Primary neurodegeneration originating from the retinal ganglion cell which subsequently leads to anterograde axonal degeneration (Figure 9.7D).

It seems conceivable that neurodegeneration of the second order neuron in the LGN and the third-order neuron in the visual cortex also may result in RNFL thinning by retrograde trans-synaptic degeneration. This will need to be tested by combining structural and functional brain imaging techniques with OCT in longitudinal studies. Likewise, a holistic model may include biomarkers able to identify axonal damage in the acute phase of inflammatory demyelinating syndromes [33, 35].

References

1 Philipp Albrecht et al. "Optical coherence tomography measures axonal loss in multiple sclerosis independently of optic neuritis." eng. In: *J Neurol* **254**.11 (Nov. 2007), pp. 1595–1596.

2 Lisanne J. Balk et al. "The physiological variation of the retinal nerve fiber layer thickness and macular volume in humans as assessed by spectral domain-optical coherence tomography." eng. In: *Invest Ophthalmol Vis Sci* **53**.3 (Mar. 2012), pp. 1251–1257.

3 Markus Bock et al. "Patterns of retinal nerve fiber layer loss in multiple sclerosis patients with or without optic neuritis and glaucoma patients." eng. In: *Clin Neurol Neurosurg* (May 2010).

4 Donald L Budenz et al. "Determinants of normal retinal nerve fiber layer thickness measured by Stratus OCT." eng. In: *Ophthalmology* **114**.6 (June 2007), pp. 1046–1052.

5 Han Cheng et al. "The relationship between visual field and retinal nerve fiber layer measurements in patients with multiple sclerosis." eng. In: *Invest Ophthalmol Vis Sci* **48**.12 (Dec. 2007), pp. 5798–5805.

6 Stacey S Choi et al. "Changes in cellular structures revealed by ultra-high resolution retinal imaging in optic neuropathies." eng. In: *Invest Ophthalmol Vis Sci* **49**.5 (May 2008), pp. 2103–2119.

7 Fiona Costello et al. "Differences in retinal nerve fiber layer atrophy between multiple sclerosis subtypes." eng. In: *J Neurol Sci* **281**.1–2 (June 2009), pp. 74–79.

8 Fiona Costello et al. "Quantifying axonal loss after optic neuritis with optical coherence tomography." eng. In: *Ann Neurol* **59**.6 (June 2006), pp. 963–969.

9 Fiona Costello et al. "Retinal nerve fiber layer and future risk of multiple sclerosis." eng. In: *Can J Neurol Sci* **35**.4 (Sept. 2008), pp. 482–487.

10 F. Costello et al. "Tracking retinal nerve fiber layer loss after optic neuritis: a prospective study using optical coherence tomography." eng. In: *Mult Scler* **14**.7 (Aug. 2008), pp. 893–905.

11 Jennifer B Fisher et al. "Relation of visual function to retinal nerve fiber layer thickness in multiple sclerosis." eng. In: *Ophthalmology* **113**.2 (Feb. 2006), pp. 324–332.

12 Elliot M Frohman et al. "Relationship of optic nerve and brain conventional and non-conventional MRI measures and retinal nerve fiber layer thickness, as assessed by OCT and GDx: a pilot study." eng. In: *J Neurol Sci* **282**.1–2 (July 2009), pp. 96–105.

13 Elena Garcia-Martin et al. "Progressive changes in the retinal nerve fiber layer in patients with multiple sclerosis." eng. In: *Eur J Ophthalmol* **20**.1 (2010), pp. 167–173.

14 Jeffrey M. Gelfand et al. "Microcystic Inner Nuclear Layer Abnormalities and Neuromyelitis Optica." eng. In: *JAMA Neurol* (Mar. 2013), pp. 1–5.

15 E. Gordon-Lipkin et al. "Retinal nerve fiber layer is associated with brain atrophy in multiple sclerosis." eng. In: *Neurology* **69**.16 (Oct. 2007), pp. 1603–1609.

16 Erica Grazioli et al. "Retinal nerve fiber layer thickness is associated with brain MRI outcomes in multiple sclerosis." eng. In: *J Neurol Sci* **268**.1–2 (May 2008), pp. 12–17.

17 Fatih C Gundogan, Seref Demirkaya, and Gungor Sobaci. "Is optical coherence tomography really a new biomarker candidate in multiple sclerosis?–A structural and functional evaluation." eng. In: *Invest Ophthalmol Vis Sci* **48**.12 (Dec. 2007), pp. 5773–5781.

18 Andrew P D Henderson et al. "An investigation of the retinal nerve fibre layer in progressive multiple sclerosis using optical coherence tomography." eng. In: *Brain* **131**.Pt 1 (Jan. 2008), pp. 277–287.

19 W. F. Hoyt, B. Schlicke, and R. J. Eckelhoff. "Fundoscopic appearance of a nerve-fibre-bundle defect." eng. In: *Br J Ophthalmol* **56**.8 (Aug. 1972), pp. 577–583.

20 D. Huang et al. "Optical coherence tomography." eng. In: *Science* **254**.5035 (Nov. 1991), pp. 1178–1181.

21 L. Jeanjean et al. "[Retinal atrophy using optical coherence tomography (OCT) in 15 patients with

multiple sclerosis and comparison with healthy subjects].” fre. In: *Rev Neurol (Paris)* **164**.11 (Nov. 2008), pp. 927–934.

22 P. Jindahra, A. Petrie, and G. T. Plant. “Retrograde trans-synaptic retinal ganglion cell loss identified by optical coherence tomography.” eng. In: *Brain* **132** (2009), pp. 628–634.

23 Alexander Klistorner et al. “Axonal loss and myelin in early ON loss in postacute optic neuritis.” eng. In: *Ann Neurol* **64**.3 (Sept. 2008), pp. 325–331.

24 Alexander Klistorner et al. “Multifocal VEP and OCT in optic neuritis: a topographical study of the structure-function relationship.” eng. In: *Doc Ophthalmol* **118**.2 (Apr. 2009), pp. 129–137.

25 A. Kochkorov et al. “Rigidity of retinal vessels in patients with multiple sclerosis.” eng. In: *Klin Monatsbl Augenheilkd* **226**.4 (Apr. 2009), pp. 276–279.

26 Michal Laron et al. “Comparison of multifocal visual evoked potential, standard automated perimetry and optical coherence tomography in assessing visual pathway in multiple sclerosis patients.” eng. In: *Mult Scler* **16**.4 (Apr. 2010), pp. 412–426.

27 Harold Merle et al. “Retinal nerve fiber layer thickness and spatial and temporal contrast sensitivity in multiple sclerosis.” eng. In: *Eur J Ophthalmol* **20**.1 (2010), pp. 158–166.

28 Harold Merle et al. “Retinal peripapillary nerve fiber layer thickness in neuromyelitis optica.” eng. In: *Invest Ophthalmol Vis Sci* **49**.10 (Oct. 2008), pp. 4412–4417.

29 R. T. Naismith et al. “Optical coherence tomography differs in neuromyelitis optica compared with multiple sclerosis.” eng. In: *Neurology* **72**.12 (Mar. 2009), pp. 1077–1082.

30 Masahiko Nakamura et al. “Early high-dose intravenous methylprednisolone is effective in preserving retinal nerve fiber layer thickness in patients with neuromyelitis optica.” eng. In: *Graefes Arch Clin Exp Ophthalmol* (Mar. 2010).

31 C. Oreja-Guevara et al. “Optic neuritis, multiple sclerosis-related or not: structural and functional study.” engspa. In: *Neurologia* **25**.2 (Mar. 2010), pp. 78–82.

32 A Petzold and GT Plant. “Chronic Relapsing Inflammatory Optic Neuropathy: a Systematic Review of 122 cases reported.” In:*J Neurol* ([Epub ahead of print]).

33 Axel Petzold. “Neurofilament phosphoforms: surrogate markers for axonal injury, degeneration and loss.” eng. In: *J Neurol Sci* **233**.1–2 (June 2005), pp. 183–198.

34 Axel Petzold et al. “Optical coherence tomography in multiple sclerosis: a systematic review and meta-analysis.” eng. In: *Lancet Neurol* **9**.9 (Sept. 2010), pp. 921–932.

35 A. Petzold et al. “The investigation of acute optic neuritis: a review and proposed protocol.” Nature Rev Neurol 2014; **10**: 447–458.

36 Victoria Pueyo et al. “Sub-clinical atrophy of the retinal nerve fibre layer in multiple sclerosis.” eng. In: *Acta Ophthalmol* (June 2009), pp. 1–5.

37 V. Pueyo et al. “Axonal loss in the retinal nerve fiber layer in patients with multiple sclerosis.” eng. In: *Mult Scler* **14**.5 (June 2008), pp. 609–614.

38 M. Pulicken et al. “Optical coherence tomography and disease subtype in multiple sclerosis.” eng. In: *Neurology* **69**.22 (Nov. 2007), pp. 2085–2092.

39 Amanda Quelly et al. “Comparison of Optical Coherence Tomography and Scanning Laser Polarimetry Measurements in Patients with Multiple Sclerosis.” eng. In: *Optom Vis Sci* (May 2010).

40 J. N. Ratchford et al. “Optical coherence tomography helps differentiate neuromyelitis optica and MS optic neuropathies.” eng. In: *Neurology* **73**.4 (July 2009), pp. 302–308.

41 A. R. Salter et al. “Retinal architecture predicts pupillary reflex metrics in MS.” eng. In: *Mult Scler* **15**.4 (Apr. 2009), pp. 479–486.

42 Jorge Sepulcre et al. “Diagnostic accuracy of retinal abnormalities in predicting disease activity in MS.” eng. In: *Neurology* **68**.18 (May 2007), pp. 1488–1494.

43 Theodora A M Siepman, Marijke Wefers Bettink-Remeijer, and Rogier Q Hintzen. “Retinal nerve fiber layer thickness in subgroups of multiple sclerosis, measured by optical coherence tomography and scanning laser polarimetry.” eng. In: *J Neurol* (May 2010).

44 Malgorzata Siger et al. “Optical coherence tomography in multiple sclerosis: thickness of the retinal nerve fiber layer as a potential measure of axonal loss and brain atrophy.” eng. In: *J Neurol* **255**.10 (Oct. 2008), pp. 1555–1560.

45 Elias S. Sotirchos et al. “In vivo identification of morphologic retinal abnormalities in neuromyelitis optica.” eng. In: *Neurology* **80**.15 (Apr. 2013), pp. 1406–1414.

46 Rebecca I Spain et al. “Thickness of retinal nerve fiber layer correlates with disease duration in parallel with corticospinal tract dysfunction in untreated multiple sclerosis.” eng. In: *J Rehabil Res Dev* **46**.5 (2009), pp. 633–642.

47 Lauren S Talman et al. “Longitudinal study of vision and retinal nerve fiber layer thickness in

multiple sclerosis." eng. In: *Ann Neurol* **67**.6 (June 2010), pp. 749–760.

48 S. Anand Trip et al. "Retinal nerve fiber layer axonal loss and visual dysfunction in optic neuritis." eng. In: *Ann Neurol* **58**.3 (Sept. 2005), pp. 383–391.

49 Maulik S Zaveri et al. "Retinal imaging by laser polarimetry and optical coherence tomography evidence of axonal degeneration in multiple sclerosis." eng. In: *Arch Neurol* **65**.7 (July 2008), pp. 924–928.

Chapter 10

Optical coherence tomography and brain magnetic resonance imaging in multiple sclerosis

Shiv Saidha and Peter A. Calabresi

Introduction

Multiple sclerosis (MS) is considered an immune-mediated disorder of the central nervous system (CNS) and is the most common nontraumatic cause of neurologic disability in early to middle adulthood throughout the developed world [1]. Although the precise etiology of MS remains to be completely elucidated, known pathologic hallmarks of MS lesions include the breakdown of the blood-brain barrier, demyelination, axonal degeneration, neuronal loss, and astrogliosis [2, 3]. Despite being conventionally designated as primarily an inflammatory demyelinating disorder of the CNS, early descriptions of MS highlight the presence of prominent axonal and neuronal pathology [4, 5]. In recent years, axonal and neuronal pathology in MS have regained considerable attention. Investigation of neurodegeneration in MS has not only led to improvements in our understanding of the biological underpinnings of the disease, but also led to a wide recognition that axonal and neuronal degeneration are the principal pathological substrates of permanent disability in MS [6–12]. Although axonal and neuronal degeneration may be the sequelae of inflammatory demyelination in MS [13–16], there may be other pathobiological processes operating as part of the disease process that contribute to their etiology.

Magnetic resonance imaging (MRI) of the brain is one of the most widely established modalities for detecting disease activity in MS. Although conventional MRI may be sensitive enough to capture inflammatory disease activity in MS by way of new or enlarging T2/FLAIR lesions or contrast-enhancing lesions, the association between MRI markers of inflammation and disability progression during the course of MS is modest at best (i.e., the clinico-radiologic paradox) [17]. Similarly, T2 lesion quantification at baseline in MS has been found to have modest predictive value for the development of disability [18]. On the other hand, MRI measures of neurodegeneration and atrophy seem to correlate better with disability progression. Numerous studies have shown that MRI measures of whole brain atrophy, such as brain parenchymal fraction (BPF), are inversely related to disability progression in MS [19, 20]. In addition to offering the capability of whole-brain volume measurement, MRI segmentation techniques enable parcellation of the brain into its component substructures, allowing the measurement of brain substructure volumes (Figure 10.1). Gray matter (GM) degeneration in particular has been shown to be extremely common in MS, beginning early in the course of MS, and may perhaps be more closely linked with disability than white matter (WM) degeneration [11, 12, 21–23]. Histopathological examination of MS brain tissue has shown that intense inflammation occurs within the cortical GM in MS, a process that appears to begin early in the course of the disease [24]. The primary antigenic target of GM inflammation in MS remains to be definitively established and may not be restricted to myelin targets.

Although cortical demyelinating lesions account for a large proportion of all brain lesions in MS (approximately 26–59%) [25, 26], the precise pathophysiologic basis underlying neuronal injury and neuronal loss in MS requires determination. While neuronal loss in MS may be caused by retrograde [13, 15] or anterograde degeneration [14], it remains unclear whether neuronal degeneration may also result from processes independent of demyelination or axonal injury in MS. Prior observations raise the possibility that

Optical Coherence Tomography in Neurological Disease, ed. Peter A. Calabresi, Laura J. Balcer, and Elliot M. Frohman. Published by Cambridge University Press.

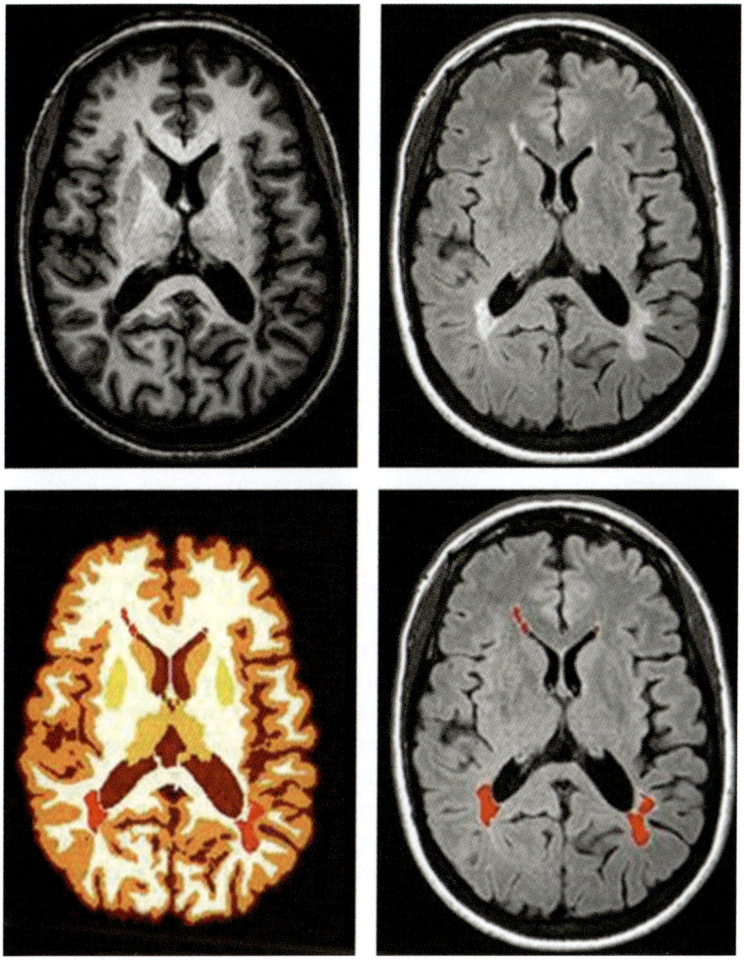

Figure 10.1 The top-left panel represents an axial MP-RAGE image in which gray–white differentiation is clear. The top-right panel represents an axial FLAIR scan in which MS lesions are obvious. The bottom-left panel represents segmentation of the brain MRI into cortical GM, cerebral WM, deep GM structures, and lesions (all of which are color-coded) by the LESION-TOADS segmentation algorithm. The bottom-right panel depicts the same axial FLAIR scan as located in the top-right panel, but with the lesions identified by the segmentation algorithm (colored red) [72].

in some instances the mechanism of GM tissue injury in MS may differ from that of WM tissue injury, and that GM injury may be the derivative of a primary neuronal pathobiology [27, 28]. This contemporary principle should emphasize the inherent potential advantages of assessing brain substructure volumes, such as cortical GM and cerebral WM volumes, rather than just whole-brain volumes in MS. For instance, measures of neurodegeneration derived from differing brain compartments could potentially reflect different pathobiological processes, which are operative in the disease process. Along this same line of reasoning, the emerging role of B-cells in the immunopathogenesis of MS has also lead to the reappraisal of MS as a primarily T-cell mediated disorder, and it is now recognized that antigen-experienced B-cell clones, which are found in lymphoid follicles in the meninges of MS patients, are also found in the brain parenchyma of MS patients [29]. Such findings serve to remind us not only of the complexity but also of the heterogeneity of MS.

Examples of nonconventional MRI techniques for dissecting mechanisms of neurodegeneration in MS include diffusion tensor imaging (DTI), magnetization transfer imaging (MTI), and magnetic resonance spectroscopy (MRS). DTI and MTI are sensitive to microstuctural tissue properties [30]. DTI utilizes information pertaining to the orientation and magnitude of water diffusion within tissue. This provides insight into the integrity of the examined tissue. DTI indices include fractional anisotropy (FA; the extent to which water diffuses along the principal eigen vector divided by the sum of diffusion in all the orthogonal plans), mean diffusivity (MD; an overall measure of water diffusion), perpendicular diffusivity ($\lambda_{\perp}$; water diffusion perpendicular to intact axon fibers), and parallel diffusivity ($\lambda_{||}$; water diffusion along or parallel to intact axon fibers). MTI relies on measuring the transfer of longitudinal magnetization between rotationally restricted hydrogen protons within macromolecules (bound to lipids or proteins) and the free water pool. The magnetization transfer ratio (MTR) is, therefore, thought to be more sensitive to myelin than conventional MRI. MRS has emerged as a technique to assess neuronal and axonal damage by measuring the concentration of brain metabolites such as N-acetyl-aspartate (NAA), which is a neuronal marker [31]. Even though nonconventional MRI techniques, such as brain substructure volumetrics, provide measures that may correlate well with disability in MS, and may therefore be informative, performing these techniques can be time-consuming, and they are generally not available in routine clinical practice. Moreover, there are a multitude of factors which may influence these measures, such as inflammation, age, disease modifying therapies, and hydration status. Consequently, there has been a drive to develop alternative techniques, including additional nonconventional MRI techniques, as well as techniques unrelated to MRI for assessing neurodegeneration in vivo in MS.

Optical coherence tomography (OCT) is a high-resolution imaging technique that conventionally enables the quantitative estimation of peripapillary-retinal nerve fiber layer (p-RNFL) thickness, as well as total or average macular thickness (a nonspecific measure of the combined thickness of all of the layers of the retina). OCT is relatively inexpensive, reproducible, easily repeatable, noninvasive, and well tolerated. Recent refinements in OCT technology have led to the powerful and highly precise capability to also automate the segmentation of the distinctive layers comprising the retina in the macular region, for the purpose of investigating the integrity of its architecture in normal subjects, and in those afflicted with disorders that target the visual system such as MS. In particular, modern, high-speed, high-definition, spectral-domain OCT is capable of rendering high-resolution images, from which the individual retinal layers can be discriminated and objectively quantified (Figure 10.2). For instance, the macular-RNFL (m-RNFL), combined ganglion cell layer and inner plexiform layer (GCIP), combined inner nuclear layer and outer plexiform layer (INL), and the outer nuclear layer, including the photoreceptor segments (ONL), can now be segmented with great facility, accuracy, and reproducibility, with highly satisfactory test–retest variability [32–35].

The innermost layer of the retina is called the RNFL and is principally composed of unmyelinated axons. In fact, under normal circumstances the retina constitutes an unmyelinated CNS structure, making it an ideal structure for investigating neurodegeneration in MS, since axonal and neuronal measures derived from the retina are not confounded by the concomitant presence of myelin. This in itself represents a major advantage of examining the process of neurodegeneration, as well as the impact of factors that may alter neurodegeneration (such as potentially neuroprotective and neurorestorative therapies), in the retina as opposed to the brain, where myelin is abundant, even in the cortical GM. The axons of the RNFL (about 1.2 million per eye) are derived from the ganglion cell neurons, which are located in the ganglion cell layer (GCL) below the RNFL (Figure 10.2). These axons coalesce at the optic discs to form the optic nerves and then exit posteriorly through the lamina cribrosa, an important zone of demarcation beyond which oligodendrocyte-derived myelin is applied to these axons retro-orbitally, thereby signifying a transition from membrane (slow) to saltatory (fast) conduction properties [36, 37].

There is a clear predilection for affliction of the optic nerves in MS, not just clinically such as from acute optic neuritis (AON), which occurs during the course of the disease in 30–70% of patients, but also subclinically, reflecting subclinical or occult optic neuropathy. Optic nerve pathology could be regarded as virtually ubiquitous in the MS disease process, since 94–99% of MS patients are found to exhibit demyelinating optic nerve lesions upon postmortem examination [38, 39]. Optic nerve demyelination (whether a derivative of acute or occult optic neuropathy) has long been recognized to result in axonal dysfunction, transection, and ultimately retrograde degeneration toward the retina (along with Wallerian degeneration distally), eventually producing atrophy of the RNFL and GCL compartments within the retina [15, 40, 41]. In keeping with evidence-based characterizations of postmortem visual system analysis in MS [40, 41], OCT has provided replete in vivo evidence of p-RNFL and GCL thinning in MS eyes, irrespective of a history of AON or not [33, 34, 42 43].

Since the RNFL represents the axonal tracts of the ganglion cell neurons, GCL reduction is believed to be

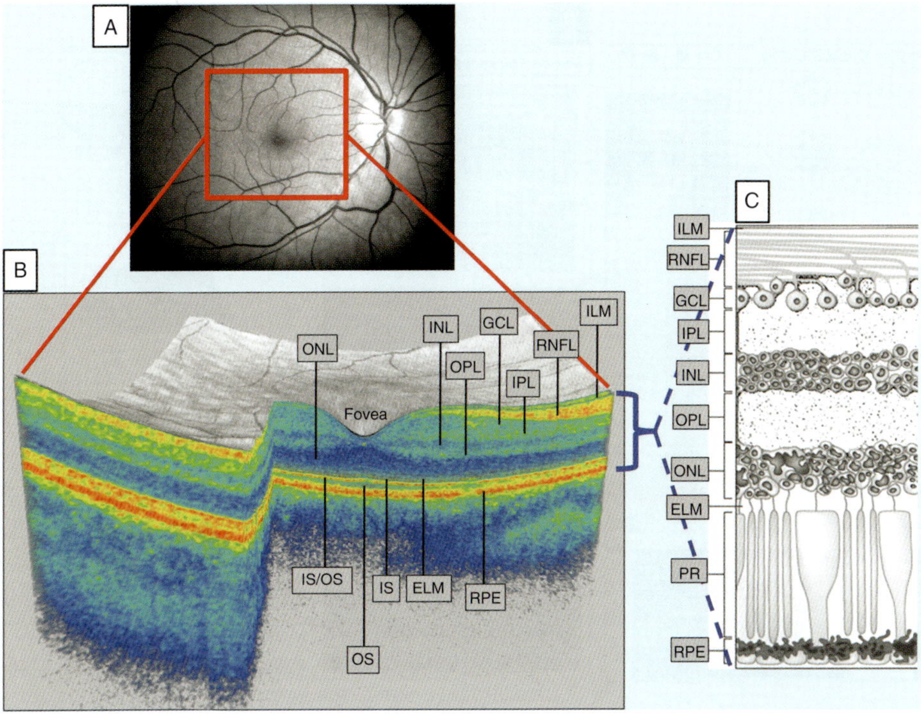

Figure 10.2 Panel A represents a fundus photograph from a healthy control. Panel B is a 3-D macular volume cube generated by Cirrus HD-OCT from the macular region denoted by the red box from the same healthy control. Note the individual layers of the retina are readily discernible, except for the ganglion cell layer (GCL) and inner plexiform layer (IPL), which are difficult to distinguish. During segmentation of the OCT image, segmentation software identifies the outer boundaries of the macular retinal nerve fiber layer (RNFL), inner plexiform layer (IPL), and outer plexiform layer (OPL), as well as the inner boundary of the retinal pigment epithelium (RPE), which is identified by the conventional Cirrus HD-OCT algorithm. The identification of these boundaries facilitates OCT segmentation, enabling the determination of the thicknesses of the macular-RNFL, GCL+IPL (GCIP), the inner nuclear layer (INL)+OPL, and the outer nuclear layer (ONL), including the inner and outer photoreceptor segments. Panel C illustrates the cellular composition of the retinal layers depicted in panel B.

Abbreviations: IS: inner photoreceptor segments; OS: outer photoreceptor segments; IS/OS: IS/OS junction; PR: photoreceptors; ILM: inner limiting membrane; ELM: external limiting membrane

Reproduced with permission from JAMA Neurology

the result of retrograde axonal degeneration of the retinal nerve fibers, i.e., reduction in both RNFL and GCL are thought to be derivative of the same pathologic processes, namely optic neuropathy (and associated tissue injury mechanisms). Despite the biologic similarity of the both the RNFL and GCL, OCT derived measures of GCIP thickness seem to have superior structure–function relationships than those of RNFL thickness [33]. This appears to be the case not only with visual measures acquired at high contrast (100%) and low contrast (2.5% and 1.25%), but also with expanded disability status scale (EDSS) estimates of global MS disability. Given the biologic similarity of both the RNFL and GCIP, and that these two retinal compartments may be regarded as mere extensions of one another, a number of potential explanations have been proposed to explain the potentially superior structure–function relationships of GCIP over p-RNFL thickness measurements. GCIP thickness measurements appear to have superior reproducibility than RNFL thickness measurements [32]. In addition, it has been proposed that the GCL may not be prone to edema, unlike the RNFL, during optic nerve inflammation [34]. Microinflammatory processes, if operative in the optic nerve(s), may therefore not confound GCIP measurements similar to RNFL measurements [32, 33].

Notwithstanding the importance of the recent and abundant evidence corroborating that both RNFL and GCL pathology are common and germane to visual system pathophysiology in MS, there is coincident evidence that deeper retinal (inner nuclear layer and outer nuclear layer) pathology also occurs in MS. Consistent with electroretinographic and

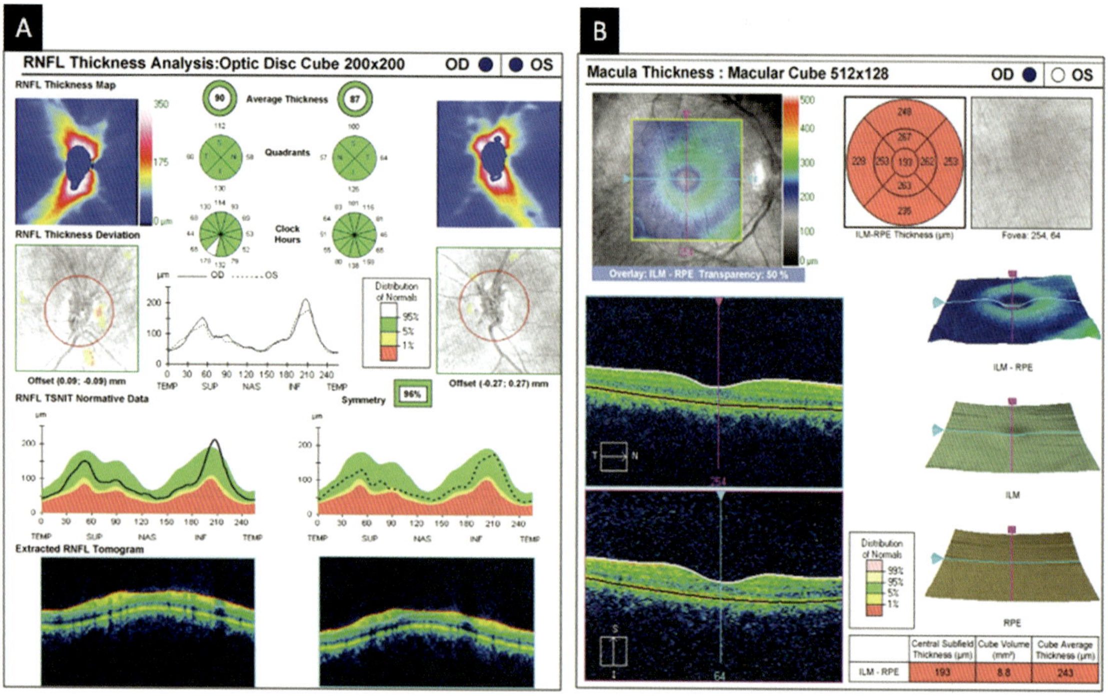

Figure 10.3 An optical coherence tomography (OCT) peripapillary retinal nerve fiber layer (p-RNFL; Panel A) and macular (Panel B) report generated by Cirrus HD-OCT (Carl Zeiss Meditec, Dublin, California) in a patient with multiple sclerosis without history of optic neuritis. The upper-middle section of Panel A displays the average p-RNFL thickness for the right eye (OD) and the left eye (OS), as well as the quadrant and clockhour measures of p-RNFL thickness for each eye. Note that the average p-RNFL thickness, as well as the quadrant and clockhour measures, is represented in colors that correspond to the normal distribution of p-RNFL thickness values. The average p-RNFL thickness (as well as quadrants and sectors) in each eye is represented in green (indicating values within normal range).

The top-right section of panel B displays quadrant measurements of retinal thickness. Again, these are represented in colors that correspond to the normal distribution of macular thickness values. The central macula represents the foveola, with the four quadrants immediately surrounding this (inner macula) representing the parafoveola. Note that the average macular thickness (cube average thickness) indicated in the bottom-right chart (as well as all of the macular quadrant thicknesses) are represented in red, indicating values less than 1% of what would be expected compared to an age-matched reference population. The macular scan of the left eye in the same patient (not shown) is similar to that of the right eye in panel B. The combination of OCT findings described in this figure fulfills our criteria for a macular-thinning-predominant (MTP) patient. Please note that this represents a patient with an average macular thickness < 1st percentile. Those with a normal average p-RNFL thickness and average macular thickness between the 1st and 5th percentile also fulfill our criteria for an MTP patient.

Reproduced with permission from *Brain*

postmortem findings [40, 44–47], OCT-segmentation demonstrates quantitative inner nuclear layer (INL) and outer nuclear layer (ONL) abnormalities in MS [32, 33, 35]. Although the definitive etiological rudiments of INL and ONL pathology in MS remains to be determined, recent observations support the possibility that a primary retinal neuronal mechanism of pathology may be operative in anterior visual system pathophysiology in a limited but not insignificant proportion of MS patients. OCT identification of INL and ONL thinning in MS eyes without a prior history of optic neuritis, in which there is relative preservation of the RNFL and GCIP, has been referred to as the macular thinning predominant (MTP) phenotype of MS [32] (Figure 10.3). The MTP phenotype may be associated with more rapid accumulation of sustained disability in MS [32], and the mechanisms of INL and ONL changes may be pathobiologically distinct from those that mediate tissue injury within the RNFL and GCL, although this remains unclear and requires further research.

Although oculohistopathological examination reveals dropout of INL neurons in up to 40% of MS eyes [40], qualitative assessment of OCT scans derived from MS patients in vivo reveal microcysts in a small proportion, which are predominantly localized to the INL [48, 49] (Figure 10.4). Again, the etiology and significance of these microcysts in MS eyes has been

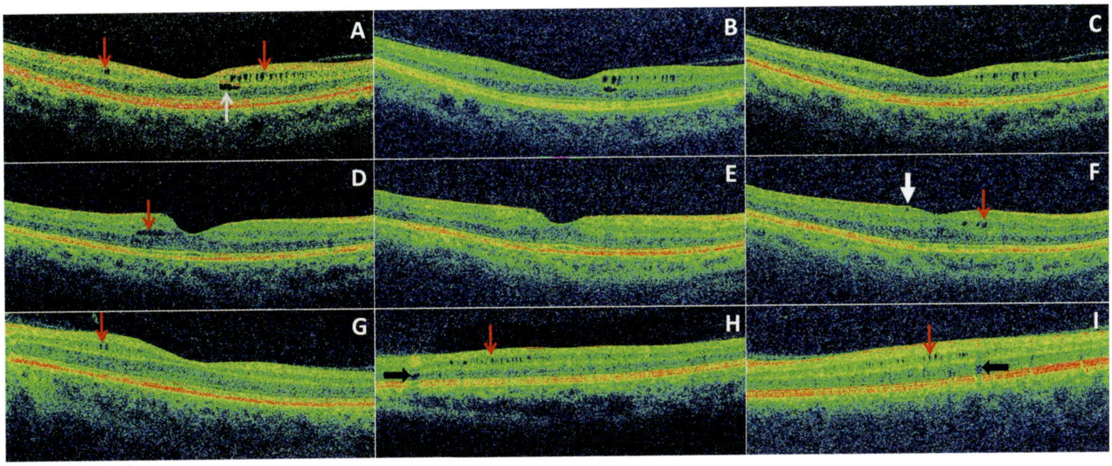

Figure 10.4 A–C: All images are from the same patient in chronological order over a three-year period. (A) Microcystic macular edema (MME) of the inner nuclear layer (INL) (red arrows) was present at baseline as well as a foveal cyst of the outer nuclear layer (ONL). (B-C) The foveal ONL cyst progressively resolved during the follow-up period.

(D-F) All images are from the same patient in chronological order over a two-year period. (D) A single INL cyst (red arrow) was present at baseline. (E) The cyst spontaneously resolved after one year. (F) Following fingolimod treatment (initiated after scan E), the patient developed new cystic changes of the INL (red arrow). An epiretinal membrane is noted (white arrow) that had been present on previous scans as well.

(G-I) Three different patients with MME of the INL (red arrows). Vessel artifacts (black arrows) are demonstrated for comparison.

Reproduced with permission from *Lancet Neurology*

the source of lively scientific debate. Some proponents have raised the possibility these microcysts may represent sites of primary retinal inflammation, on the basis that 25% of patients with macular edema demonstrating fluorescein leakage examined in an ophthalmological study exhibited similar appearing microcysts [50], microcysts in MS eyes may be dynamic in nature over time, and they may be a harbinger of more aggressive MS. Given that microcysts may be dynamic in nature, some authors have suggested that increased INL thickness in the absence of visible microcysts may enable capturing of the same process. As such, increased INL thickness at baseline has been shown to predict clinical and radiologic disease activity during follow-up [49]. On the other hand, some investigators have proposed that microcysts in MS eyes are of little significance, since they may be seen in other neuroinflammatory disorders (including neuromyelitis optica and chronic relapsing inflammatory optic neuropathy) as well as non-inflammatory disorders such as neurofibromatosis, Leber's hereditary optic neuropathy and glaucoma [51–54]. Given the array of conditions in which macular microcysts have been described, some consider them a final common pathway of retrograde degeneration, especially since there are histopathological descriptions of cavitation occurring within the INL following optic nerve transaction dating back to the 1960s [55]. Moreover, microcysts may simply represent mechanical changes resulting from vitreomacular traction, although this is not universally agreed upon [53].

Although the etiology, relevance, and significance of INL and ONL changes in MS remain to be established, there is an abundance of information highlighting the possibility of primary retinal inflammation in MS that is difficult to ignore. Despite being an unmyelinated structure, retinal periphlebitis occurs in up to 20% of MS patients [41], highlighting that myelin does not need to be present for instigating or propagating inflammation in MS. The antigenic target of this inflammation remains unknown. Interestingly, previous studies have shown that, during periods of active retinal periphlebitis, there may be concomitant breakdown of the blood-brain barrier in MS [56]. Moreover, retinal periphlebitis in MS has been shown to be a risk factor for the development of relapses, contrast enhancing lesions, as well as an increase in T1 lesion volume during follow-up [57, 58]. In addition to retinal periphlebitis, up to 16% of MS patients experience uveitis, particularly intermediate uveitis of the pars planitis subtype [59]. Activated microglia have also been demonstrated in MS retinas at postmortem examination [40]. Despite ongoing debate, all combined, these

Table 10.1 Relation between OCT-derived measures of p-RNFL thickness and MRI-derived brain volumetrics in MS

Study	n	OCT measure	MRI segmentation	Correlations: Yes	Correlations: No
		Time-domain OCT studies			
Sepulcre et al. [57]	61	Minimum p-RNFL	VBM method	WM, GM	T2 LV, T1 LV
Gordon-Lipkin et al [60]	40	Minimum p-RNFL	SIENAX	BPF, CSF	GM, WM
Grazioli et al. [61]	18/ 30	Average p-RNFL of both eyes	SIENAX	NBV, WM, T2 LV	GM, T1 LV
Siger et al.[a] [62]	51	p-RNFL in ON vs. non-ON eyes	SPM99	BPF, GM, T2 LV, T1 LV	WM
Dorr et al. [63]	104	p-RNFL of each eye[b]	SIENAX	BPF	
Pfueller et al. [65]	83	p-RNFL of each eye[b]	SIENAX	BPF	
		Spectral-domain OCT studies			
Young et al. [68]	44	p-RNFL of each eye[b] & minimum RNFL	JIM, FAST, FSL	BPF, WM	GM, BHFr, T2 LV
Zimmermann[a] et al. [69]	63	p-RNFL of ON vs. non-ON eyes[b]	SIENAX	NBV, WM, GM	
Saidha et al. [70]	84	p-RNFL of each eye & p-RNFL of ON vs. non-ON eyes[b]	LESION-TOADS	GM, caudate	NAWM, thalamus, brainstem, T2 LV

Abbreviations: OCT: optical coherence tomography; p-RNFL: peripapillary retinal nerve fiber layer; MRI: magnetic resonance imaging; VBM: voxel based morphometry; WM: white matter; GM: gray matter; LV: lesion volume; BPF: brain parenchymal fraction; CSF: cerebrospinal fluid; NBV: normalized brain volume; BHFr: black hole fraction; NAWM: normal appearing white matter

[a] Presented relationships are those from eyes without a prior history of ON.

[b] Statistical models were used to account for within-subject, inter-eye correlations in analyses from these studies.

observations may be diametrically in opposition to the long-recognized pathological polarity involving retrobulbar inflammation and its sequelae [32–35].

Time-domain OCT and the brain MRI in MS

There have been a number of studies investigating the relationships between time-domain OCT derived measures and brain MRI in MS (Table 10.1). Although several studies have consistently found that p-RNFL thickness correlates with brain parenchymal fraction (BPF) in MS [60–63], suggesting p-RNFL thickness, at least in part, reflects global CNS pathology, associations between average macular thickness (or total macular volume), a nonspecific measure of the composite thickness or volume of all of the intervening layers of the retina in the macular region, and BPF have been less consistent [60, 63]. Some studies have shown relationships between total macular volume and BPF [63], while others have not [60]. Given the lack of specificity of total macular volume or average macular thickness, however, the potential utility of this measure in MS is questionable, and thus some investigators did not examine the relationships between total macular volume and brain MRI, restricting their analyses to measures of p-RNFL thickness only [57]. More important is the lack of consistency observed in these studies between p-RNFL thickness measurements and brain-substructure volumes [57, 60–62]. Some investigators found relationships between p-RNFL thickness and BPF, but not GM or WM volumes [60], while in some studies p-RNFL thickness and both GM and WM volumes were related [57], while in others p-RNFL thickness was associated with either GM volume only [62] or WM volume only [61]. Relationships between p-RNFL thickness and T1 lesion volume, as well as T2 lesion volume, were similarly inconsistent. For example, in one study p-RNFL thickness correlated with neither T1 lesion volume nor T2 lesion volume [57], while in another it correlated with both T1 lesion volume and T2 lesion volume [62]. More specifically, on the basis of these studies, it is unclear whether p-RNFL thickness, at least as estimated with time-domain OCT technology, correlates with measures of the normal-appearing cerebral white matter (NAWM), white matter (WM) lesional morphometry, or cortical gray matter (GM) volumes. There may be several potential explanations underlying the inconsistency of the results observed in these various studies, especially with respect to the relationships of p-RNFL thickness measures with brain substructure volumes, which makes the comparability of the results derived from these different studies limited.

The patient populations included in these studies varied quite a bit with respect to sample size, MS subtype, as well as the degrees of disability and disease duration of the patients included. Treatment effects were also minimally accounted for across these various studies. There are several major methodological differences between the studies. Some studies utilized minimum p-RNFL thickness (lowest p-RNFL thickness of either eye) in analyses [57, 60], some studies utilized average p-RNFL thickness of both eyes in analyses [61], some studies utilized the p-RNFL thickness of both eyes but accounted for within-subject inter-eye correlations [63], while in some other studies comparisons were of p-RNFL thickness in eyes with and without a history of AON [62]. Interestingly, in the latter study, p-RNFL thickness in MS eyes without a history of AON correlated with BPF and GM fraction, while in MS eyes with a history of AON p-RNFL thickness correlated with neither BPF nor brain substructure volumes. In addition to these differences in the utilization of p-RNFL thickness, there were also differences in the statistical approaches and models adopted in each study. Finally, there were differences in the brain segmentation techniques employed between the studies to determine brain substructure volumes. Some studies utilized SIENAX, while others used different techniques. Moreover, not all studies investigated lesion morphometry volumes, or indeed even brain substructure volumes. For instance, in some studies only relationships between OCT measures and BPF were assessed.

The lack of consistency for relationships of p-RNFL thickness and brain substructure volumes observed in the above studies does not mitigate the consistent and encouraging observation that p-RNFL thickness and BPF appear to be related in MS, suggesting p-RNFL thickness, at least to some degree may reflect global brain atrophy and global CNS processes in MS. Investigations of relationships between time-domain OCT derived measures, principally reflecting the anterior visual pathway, and measures of the posterior visual pathways derived from nonconventional MRI techniques have also yielded interesting results in MS. In one such study, DTI indices along the optic radiation were correlated with p-RNFL thickness measures in MS, controlling for age, sex, and corresponding MRI indices along a portion of the corticospinal tract (to attempt to at least partially account for global CNS changes driving relationships) [64]. Moderate correlations of average RNFL thickness with FA and $\lambda_{\perp}$ in the OR were observed, suggesting an association between p-RNFL thickness and OR damage that may not be primarily driven by abnormalities outside of the visual system. Interestingly, p-RNFL thickness in the nasal retinal quadrant was specifically correlated with FA and $\lambda_{\perp}$ in the synaptically connected contralateral OR. Since this was a cross-sectional study, the results cannot be over-interpreted as substantiated evidence of transynaptic degeneration. Even though these results point toward a relationship between changes in the anterior visual pathway and posterior visual pathway in MS, the study does not address or help determine how the changes may be connected, that is, retrograde vs. anterograde degeneration, or coincidental concomitant pathology simultaneously afflicting both the anterior and posterior visual pathways. Another very interesting cross-sectional study utilizing time-domain OCT studied the relationships between p-RNFL thickness, global brain atrophy (as estimated by BPF), and MRS-derived NAA concentrations in the visual cortex, as well as the NAWM in MS [65]. In this study the investigators found that p-RNFL thickness measures correlated with NAA concentrations in the visual cortex, but not the NAWM, and were consistent with prior observations that RNFL thickness correlated with BPF in MS. The multivariate statistical model employed revealed that the correlation between RNFL thickness and visual cortex NAA concentration was unlikely to simply represent the consequence of global brain atrophy, as one might assume on the basis of the relationship between p-RNFL thickness and BPF, since BPF and visual cortex NAA concentrations seemed to be both independently associated with p-RNFL thickness. In fact, visual cortex NAA concentrations and BPF did not seem to be correlated with one another in this study. The investigators' findings thus highlight a potential interconnection between changes in the anterior and posterior visual pathways, beyond that which may be expected due to simple global neurodegeneration. Consistent with this observation, the study also revealed lower NAA visual cortex concentrations in subjects with a prior history of AON. Again, however, this was a cross-sectional study and, therefore, the results should not be over-interpreted to substantiate evidence of transynaptic degeneration.

Spectral-domain OCT, segmentation, and brain MRI in MS

The first analyses attempting to correlate changes in retinal architecture and global CNS pathology in MS, as described previously, utilized time-domain OCT, which has lower reproducibility and resolution than the high-speed, high-definition spectral-domain devices, which enable the rapid and near-automated acquisition of high-resolution images, in conjunction with a very low test–retest variability. [66, 67] Notwithstanding these impressive technical advancements, there has been a paucity of studies involving the utilization of spectral-domain OCT, for the purpose of studying the relationship between retinal and brain metrics in MS. While these latest studies show a similar relationship between spectral-domain derived p-RNFL thickness measurements and time-domain derived p-RNFL thickness measurements, with BPF, results of relationships with brain substructure volumes are also unfortunately conflicting (Table 10.1). In a recent study including participants with clinically isolated syndrome (CIS) or early relapsing remitting MS (RRMS), not on active treatment, in which brain volumetrics were assessed with a 1.5 T MRI, p-RNFL thickness and total macular volume independently predicted WM fraction, but not GM fraction or black hole fraction, correcting for age and history of AON [68]. However, in another recent study of just RRMS patients, in which brain volumetrics were also assessed with a 1.5 T MRI, p-RNFL thickness and TMV (albeit less so) were both significantly associated with normalized WM volume and normalized GM volume [69]. However, in this study, the authors found that the significant association of OCT measures with normalized GM volume was abolished in eyes with a history of AON (while the relationship with normalized WM volume was essentially unaffected). On the basis of this finding, which was similar to that observed by Siger et al. [62] in their study of time-domain OCT–brain MRI relationships, the authors proposed the possibility that excessive tissue damage resulting from AON may mask the underlying relationship between OCT measures and GM volume driven by global neurodegeneration in MS, as observed in eyes without a history of AON. In this study, the authors also included limited OCT segmentation data. Specifically, they assessed macular GCL thickness measures, as estimated by the composite thickness of the GCL and inner plexiform layer (GCIP). As might be expected, given the biological similarity of the GCL and RNFL (they could be regarded as extensions of one another), GCIP thickness measures exhibited relationships with brain volumetrics similar to those observed with p-RNFL thickness measures. On the basis of previous work in which GCIP thickness measures appeared to have superior structure–function relationships to p-RNFL thickness measures (33), possibly related to superior reproducibility among other potential reasons, one might have expected that GCIP thickness measures would reflect global CNS processes more strongly than p-RNFL thickness measures. However, this was not observed in this study.

A more detailed assessment of the relationships between spectral domain OCT segmentation derived retinal measures and 3 T MRI-derived brain substructure volumes has also been performed in MS [70]. Since brain substructure volumes correlate with intracranial volume (a surrogate of head size), these measures are conventionally normalized or adjusted for intracranial volume in order to account for these normal relationships. In undertaking this study, the authors also investigated whether OCT (including OCT segmentation) derived retinal measures might also correlate with head size (using intracranial volume as a surrogate) in order to potentially optimize the accuracy of their results. Indeed, the investigators of this study found that OCT measures in healthy controls and MS patients appear to correlate with intracranial volume (or head size) and, therefore, not only adjusted brain substructure volumes, but also OCT measures for intracranial volume, as part of their regression models when assessing retinal-brain relationships. In this study, p-RNFL and GCIP thickness measures exhibited relationships similar to one another with brain substructure volumes, with perhaps the relationships being interestingly slightly stronger with p-RNFL than GCIP measures. Both p-RNFL and GCIP thickness measures were associated with cortical GM volume (as well as caudate volume), but only in the eyes of MS patients without a history of AON, again raising the possibility that excessive local tissue injury following AON may mask underlying relationships that would otherwise be seen. Neither p-RNFL nor GCIP thickness measures were associated with either NAWM volume or T2 lesion volume. However, an interesting finding to emerge from this study was the unexpected and apparently strong relationship between INL thickness and T2 lesion volume, with a corresponding inverse relationship with NAWM volume in RRMS. In other words, higher INL thickness in this MS cohort appeared to be associated with higher T2 lesion volume and lower NAWM volume (Figure 10.5). The basis for this finding could not be determined as part of this cross-sectional study, although the possibility that increased INL thickness may represent part of the spectrum of macular microcysts (when the microcysts are not visible to the naked eye, for example) or even potentially retinal periphlebitis have been raised. Another interesting finding to emerge from this study was that INL and ONL changes in MS may not reflect similar global CNS processes, unlike the RNFL and GCL. For instance, ONL thickness in MS eyes only with a history of AON was associated with cerebellar WM volume and tended to towards being associated with cortical GM, caudate, thalamus, and T2 lesion volume, raising the possibility that it may be more a marker of global neurodegeneration in MS. However, the basis for these findings was not explored in this study. Overall, this represents a preliminary study, since detailed investigations of the relationships between OCT segmentation derived measures and brain MRI measures are lacking. The findings of this study need to be validated and the basis for the observed relationships need to be explored and determined.

One of the most recent studies utilizing spectral-domain OCT in MS investigated the association between damage to the anterior visual pathway (as assessed by OCT-derived measures of p-RNFL thickness and total macular volume) and posterior visual pathway (as assessed by 3 T MRI-derived volumetry and spectroscopy), both at baseline and after one year of follow-up [71]. Independent of AON history (as well as other confounders), baseline analyses revealed that visual cortex volume, visual cortex NAA, and OR lesion volumes were associated with p-RNFL thickness. Repeating the same analyses after one year of follow-up similarly revealed that visual cortex volume and OR lesion volumes were associated with p-RNFL thickness. These findings raise the possibility of retrograde transynaptic degeneration similar to prior studies. Conversely, baseline analyses revealed that patients with a prior history of severe AON had significantly lower visual cortex volumes than MS patients without a prior history of AON. Although the finding was not significant, MS patients with a prior history of mild AON also exhibited lower visual cortex volumes than MS patients without previous AON, and again although the finding was not significant, MS patients with a prior history of severe AON seemed to have reduced visual cortex volume relative to MS patients who had previously experienced mild AON. Similar to observations raised by other investigators, these findings raise the possibility of anterograde transynaptic degeneration in MS.

Summary

Although results of some investigations assessing the relationships between OCT derived measures and brain MRI in MS are conflicting, the consistently observed relationship between p-RNFL thickness and BPF is encouraging, and it provides evidence that, at least to a degree, p-RNFL thickness measures reflect global CNS processes in MS. That this cheap, easily obtainable, and repeatable, reproducible, and noninvasively acquired retinal measure may provide insight into global changes within the brains of MS

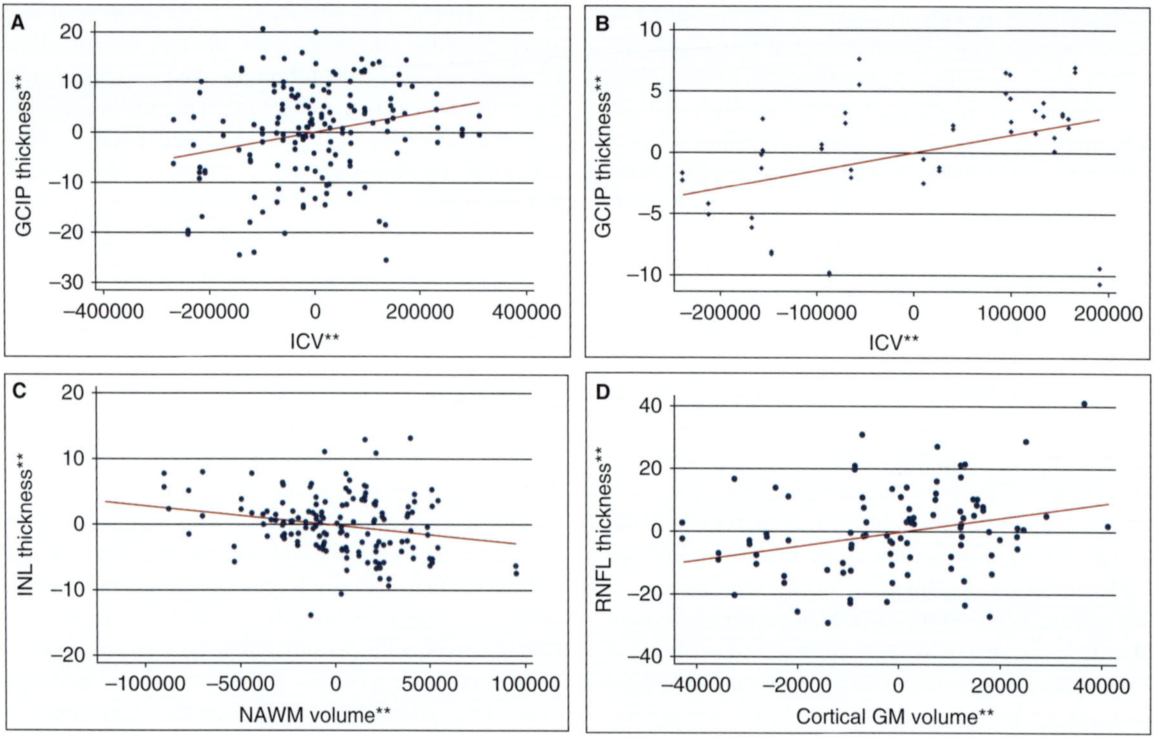

Figure 10.5 **Residual values from multivariate regression models

Panel A represents an adjusted variables plot of ganglion cell layer + inner plexiform layer (GCIP) thickness and intracranial volume (ICV) in multiple sclerosis (MS), adjusted for age, sex, and disease duration. The solid red line illustrates the independent relationship between GCIP thickness and ICV in MS. Note that, as ICV increases, GCIP thickness similarly increases, consistent with the detection of significant associations between GCIP thickness and ICV in MS ($p = 0.008$). Panel B represents an adjusted variables plot of ganglion cell layer + inner plexiform layer (GCIP) thickness and intracranial volume (ICV) in healthy controls (HCs), adjusted for age and sex. The solid red line graphically illustrates the independent relationship between GCIP thickness and ICV in HCs. As ICV increases, GCIP thickness similarly increases. Panel C represents an adjusted variables plot of inner nuclear layer (INL) thickness and normal-appearing white matter (NAWM) volume in MS, adjusted for age, sex, disease duration, and ICV. The solid red line shows the independent relationship between INL thickness and NAWM volume in MS. Note that, as INL thickness increases, NAWM volume decreases. Panel D depicts an adjusted variables plot of peripapillary retinal nerve fiber layer (p-RNFL) thickness and cortical gray matter (GM) volume in RRMS, adjusted for age, sex, disease duration, and ICV. The solid red line graphically illustrates the independent relationship between p-RNFL thickness and cortical-GM volume in RRMS.

Reproduced with permission from JAMA Neurology

patients is compelling and represents an attractive advantage of OCT relative to other emerging imaging techniques, including nonconventional MRI techniques, for assessing neurodegeneration in MS. Moreover, the possibility that one may glean information regarding different processes operative within different compartments of the brains of MS patients through the incorporation of OCT segmentation measures not only may be helpful in shedding light on the pathobiology of MS, but could turn out to be the greatest advantage of its application in MS. Nonetheless, there is need for further study of the relationships between OCT-derived measures, in particular OCT-segmentation-derived measures and brain MRI in MS, since this remains an understudied area. Specifically, there is a need for longitudinal assessments of OCT and MRI in MS, which are currently lacking. Moreover, future studies need to be more homogenous in terms of their patient inclusion, OCT and MRI devices utilized, OCT and MRI segmentation techniques employed, and their approach to analyses, in order to make the results of studies more comparable. Although much work is needed in this front, preliminary results are exciting, and if indeed they turn out to be correct, through the use of OCT, physicians may be able to gain deeper insight into ongoing processes within the brains of their MS patients at the bedside.

Disclosures: Dr. Saidha has been the recipient of a Race to Erase MS grant.

References

1. Anderson DW, Ellenberg JH, Leventhal CM, Reingold SC, Rodriguez M, Silberberg DH. Revised estimate of the prevalence of multiple sclerosis in the united states. *Ann Neurol* 1992 Mar;31(**3**):333–6.
2. Prineas J. Pathology of multiple sclerosis. in Cook S, ed. *Handbook of Multiple Sclerosis* In: New York: Marcel Dekker; 2001. p. 289–324.
3. Frohman EM, Racke MK, Raine CS. Multiple sclerosis – the plaque and its pathogenesis. *N Engl J Med* 2006 Mar 2;**354**(9):942–55.
4. Marburg O. Die sogennate akute multiple sklerose. *Jahrb Psychiatrie* 1906;**27**:211–312.
5. Putnam T. Studies in multiple sclerosis. *Arch Neurol Psych* 1936;**35**:1289–308.
6. van Waesberghe JH, Kamphorst W, De Groot CJ, van Walderveen MA, Castelijns JA, Ravid R, et al. Axonal loss in multiple sclerosis lesions: Magnetic resonance imaging insights into substrates of disability. *Ann Neurol* November 1999;**46**(5):747–54.
7. De Stefano N, Narayanan S, Francis GS, Arnaoutelis R, Tartaglia MC, Antel JP, et al. Evidence of axonal damage in the early stages of multiple sclerosis and its relevance to disability. *Arch Neurol* January 2001;**58** (1):65–70.
8. Compston A, Coles A. Multiple sclerosis. *Lancet* April 6, 2002;**359**(9313):1221–31.
9. Miller DH. Biomarkers and surrogate outcomes in neurodegenerative disease: Lessons from multiple sclerosis. *NeuroRx* April 2004;**1**(2):284–94.
10. Minneboo A, Uitdehaag BM, Jongen P, Vrenken H, Knol D, van Walderveen MA, et al. Association between MRI parameters and the MS severity scale: A 12 year follow-up study. *Multiple Sclerosis* May 2009; **15**(5):632–7.
11. Calabrese M, Atzori M, Bernardi V, Morra A, Romualdi C, Rinaldi L, et al. Cortical atrophy is relevant in multiple sclerosis at clinical onset. *J Neurol* September 2007;**254**(9):1212–20.
12. Calabrese M, Agosta F, Rinaldi F, Mattisi I, Grossi P, Favaretto A, et al. Cortical lesions and atrophy associated with cognitive impairment in relapsing-remitting multiple sclerosis. *Arch Neurol* September 2009; **66**(9):1144–50.
13. Rawes JA, Calabrese VP, Khan OA, DeVries GH. Antibodies to the axolemma-enriched fraction in the cerebrospinal fluid and serum of patients with multiple sclerosis and other neurological diseases. *Multiple Sclerosis* December 1997;**3**(6): 363–9.
14. Madigan MC, Rao NS, Tenhula WN, Sadun AA. Preliminary morphometric study of tumor necrosis factor-alpha (TNF alpha)-induced rabbit optic neuropathy. *Neurol Res* June 1996;**18**(3):233–6.
15. Shindler KS, Ventura E, Dutt M, Rostami A. Inflammatory demyelination induces axonal injury and retinal ganglion cell apoptosis in experimental optic neuritis. *Exp Eye Res* September 2008;**87**(3):208–13.
16. Frischer JM, Bramow S, Dal-Bianco A, Lucchinetti CF, Rauschka H, Schmidbauer M, et al. The relation between inflammation and neurodegeneration in multiple sclerosis brains. *Brain* May 2009;**132**(Pt 5):1175–89.
17. Kappos L, Moeri D, Radue EW, Schoetzau A, Schweikert K, Barkhof F, et al. Predictive value of gadolinium-enhanced magnetic resonance imaging for relapse rate and changes in disability or impairment in multiple sclerosis: A meta-analysis. gadolinium MRI meta-analysis group. *Lancet* March 20, 1999;**353** (9157):964–9.
18. Fisniku LK, Brex PA, Altmann DR, Miszkiel KA, Benton CE, Lanyon R, et al. Disability and T2 MRI lesions: A 20-year follow-up of patients with relapse onset of multiple sclerosis. *Brain* March 2008;**131**(Pt 3):808–17.
19. De Stefano N, Matthews PM, Fu L, Narayanan S, Stanley J, Francis GS, et al. Axonal damage correlates with disability in patients with relapsing-remitting multiple sclerosis. results of a longitudinal magnetic resonance spectroscopy study. *Brain* August 1998;**121** (Pt 8)(Pt 8):1469–77.
20. Fisher E, Rudick RA, Simon JH, Cutter G, Baier M, Lee JC, et al. Eight-year follow-up study of brain atrophy in patients with MS. *Neurology* November 12, 2002;**59** (9):1412–20.
21. Calabrese M, De Stefano N, Atzori M, Bernardi V, Mattisi I, Barachino L, et al. Detection of cortical inflammatory lesions by double inversion recovery magnetic resonance imaging in patients with multiple sclerosis. *Arch Neurol* October 2007;**64**(10):1416–22.
22. Inglese M, Oesingmann N, Casaccia P, Fleysher L. Progressive multiple sclerosis and gray matter pathology: An MRI perspective. *Mt Sinai J Med* March–April 2011;**78**(2):258–67.
23. Simon JH. Brain atrophy in multiple sclerosis: What we know and would like to know. *Multiple Sclerosis* December 2006;**12**(6):679–87.
24. Lucchinetti CF, Popescu BF, Bunyan RF, Moll NM, Roemer SF, Lassmann H, et al. Inflammatory cortical demyelination in early multiple sclerosis. *N Engl J Med* December 8, 2011;**365**(23):2188–97.
25. Brownell B, Hughes JT. The distribution of plaques in the cerebrum in multiple sclerosis. *J Neurol Neurosurg Psychiatry* November 1962;**25**:315–20.

26. Lumsden C. The neuropathology of multiple sclerosis. In: Vinken PJ, bruyn GW, eds. *Handbook of Clinical Neurology*. Amsterdam: Elsevier; 1970. pp. 217–309.
27. Bo L, Vedeler CA, Nyland HI, Trapp BD, Mork SJ. Subpial demyelination in the cerebral cortex of multiple sclerosis patients. *J Neuropathol Exp Neurol* July 2003;**62**(7):723–32.
28. Moll NM, Rietsch AM, Ransohoff AJ, Cossoy MB, Huang D, Eichler FS, et al. Cortical demyelination in PML and MS: Similarities and differences. *Neurology* January 29, 2008;**70**(5):336–43.
29. Lovato L, Willis SN, Rodig SJ, Caron T, Almendinger SE, Howell OW, et al. Related B cell clones populate the meninges and parenchyma of patients with multiple sclerosis. *Brain*. February 2011;**134**(Pt 2):534–41.
30. Oh J, Zackowski K, Chen M, Newsome S, Saidha S, Smith SA, et al. Multiparametric MRI correlates of sensorimotor function in the spinal cord in multiple sclerosis. *Multiple Sclerosis*. April 2013;**19**(4):427–35.
31. Filippi M, Rocca MA, De Stefano N, Enzinger C, Fisher E, Horsfield MA, et al. Magnetic resonance techniques in multiple sclerosis: The present and the future. *Arch Neurol* December 2011;**68**(12):1514–20.
32. Saidha S, Syc SB, Ibrahim MA, Eckstein C, Warner CV, Farrell SK, et al. Primary retinal pathology in multiple sclerosis as detected by optical coherence tomography. *Brain* February 2011;**134**(Pt 2):518–33.
33. Saidha S, Syc SB, Durbin MK, Eckstein C, Oakley JD, Meyer SA, et al. Visual dysfunction in multiple sclerosis correlates better with optical coherence tomography derived estimates of macular ganglion cell layer thickness than peripapillary retinal nerve fiber layer thickness. *Multiple Sclerosis*. August 24, 2011;
34. Syc SB, Saidha S, Newsome SD, Ratchford JN, Levy M, Ford E, et al. Optical coherence tomography segmentation reveals ganglion cell layer pathology after optic neuritis. *Brain* October 17, 2011;
35. Seigo MA, Sotirchos ES, Newsome S, Babiarz A, Eckstein C, Ford E, et al. In vivo assessment of retinal neuronal layers in multiple sclerosis with manual and automated optical coherence tomography segmentation techniques. *J Neurol* March 15, 2012;
36. Frohman EM, Fujimoto JG, Frohman TC, Calabresi PA, Cutter G, Balcer LJ. Optical coherence tomography: A window into the mechanisms of multiple sclerosis. *Nat Clin Pract Neurol* December 2008;**4**(12):664–75.
37. Saidha S, Eckstein C, Ratchford JN. Optical coherence tomography as a marker of axonal damage in multiple sclerosis. *CML – Multiple Sclerosis* 2010;**2**(2):33–43.
38. Toussaint D, Perier O, Verstappen A, Bervoets S. Clinicopathological study of the visual pathways, eyes, and cerebral hemispheres in 32 cases of disseminated sclerosis. *J Clin Neuroophthalmol* September 1983;**3** (3):211–20.
39. Ikuta F, Zimmerman HM. Distribution of plaques in seventy autopsy cases of multiple sclerosis in the united states. *Neurology* June 1976; **26**(6 PT 2): 26–8.
40. Green AJ, McQuaid S, Hauser SL, Allen IV, Lyness R. Ocular pathology in multiple sclerosis: Retinal atrophy and inflammation irrespective of disease duration. *Brain* April 21, 2010;**133**(6):1591–601.
41. Kerrison JB, Flynn T, Green WR. Retinal pathologic changes in multiple sclerosis. *Retina* 1994;**14**(5): 445–51.
42. Naismith RT, Xu J, Tutlam NT, Trinkaus K, Cross AH, Song SK. Radial diffusivity in remote optic neuritis discriminates visual outcomes. *Neurology* May 25, 2010;**74**(21):1702–10.
43. Talman LS, Bisker ER, Sackel DJ, Long DA,Jr, Galetta KM, Ratchford JN, et al. Longitudinal study of vision and retinal nerve fiber layer thickness in multiple sclerosis. *Ann Neurol* June 2010;**67**(6):749–60.
44. Papakostopoulos D, Fotiou F, Hart JC, Banerji NK. The electroretinogram in multiple sclerosis and demyelinating optic neuritis. *Electroencephalogr Clin Neurophysiol* January–February 1989;**74**(1):1–10.
45. Forooghian F, Sproule M, Westall C, Gordon L, Jirawuthiworavong G, Shimazaki K, et al. Electroretinographic abnormalities in multiple sclerosis: Possible role for retinal autoantibodies. *Doc Ophthalmol* September 2006;**113**(2):123–32.
46. Gundogan FC, Demirkaya S, Sobaci G. Is optical coherence tomography really a new biomarker candidate in multiple sclerosis? – A structural and functional evaluation. *Invest Ophthalmol Vis Sci* December 2007;**48**(12):5773–81.
47. Gills JP,Jr. Electroretinographic abnormalities and advanced multiple sclerosis. *Invest Ophthalmol* December 1966;**5**(6):555–9.
48. Gelfand JM, Nolan R, Schwartz DM, Graves J, Green AJ. Microcystic macular edema in multiple sclerosis is associated with disease severity. *Brain* June 2012;**135** (Pt 6):1786–93.
49. Saidha S, Sotirchos ES, Ibrahim MA, Crainiceanu CM, Gelfand JM, Sepah YJ, et al. Microcystic macular edema, thickness of the inner nuclear layer of the retina, and disease characteristics in multiple sclerosis: A retrospective study. *Lancet Neurol* November 2012;**11**(11):963–72.
50. Brar M, Yuson R, Kozak I, Mojana F, Cheng L, Bartsch DU, et al. Correlation between morphologic features on spectral-domain optical coherence tomography and angiographic leakage patterns in macular edema. *Retina* March 2010;**30**(3):383–9.
51. Sotirchos ES, Saidha S, Byraiah G, Mealy MA, Ibrahim MA, Sepah YJ, et al. In vivo identification of morphologic retinal abnormalities in neuromyelitis optica. *Neurology* April 9, 2013;**80**(15):1406–14.

52. Kaufhold F, Zimmermann H, Schneider E, Ruprecht K, Paul F, Oberwahrenbrock T, et al. Optic neuritis is associated with inner nuclear layer thickening and microcystic macular edema independently of multiple sclerosis. *PLoS One* August 6, 2013;**8**(8):e71145.
53. Barboni P, Carelli V, Savini G, Carbonelli M, La Morgia C, Sadun AA. Microcystic macular degeneration from optic neuropathy: Not inflammatory, not trans-synaptic degeneration. *Brain* July 2013; **136**(Pt 7):e239.
54. Wolff B, Basdekidou C, Vasseur V, Mauget-Faysse M, Sahel JA, Vignal C. Retinal inner nuclear layer microcystic changes in optic nerve atrophy: A novel spectral-domain OCT finding. *Retina* November–December 2013;**33**(10):2133–8.
55. Gills JP,Jr, Wadsworth JA. Degeneration of the inner nuclear layer of the retina following lesions of the optic nerve. *Trans Am Ophthalmol Soc* 1966;**64**:66–88.
56. Engell T, Hvidberg A, Uhrenholdt A. Multiple sclerosis: Periphlebitis retinalis et cerebro-spinalis. A correlation between periphlebitis retinalis and abnormal technetium brain scintigraphy. *Acta Neurol Scand* May 1984;**69**(5):293–7.
57. Sepulcre J, Murie-Fernandez M, Salinas-Alaman A, Garcia-Layana A, Bejarano B, Villoslada P. Diagnostic accuracy of retinal abnormalities in predicting disease activity in MS. *Neurology* May 2007;**68**(18):1488–94.
58. Ortiz-Perez S, Martinez-Lapiscina EH, Gabilondo I, Fraga-Pumar E, Martinez-Heras E, Saiz A, et al. Retinal periphlebitis is associated with multiple sclerosis severity. *Neurology*. September 3, 2013;**81**(10):877–81.
59. Donaldson MJ, Pulido JS, Herman DC, Diehl N, Hodge D. Pars planitis: A 20-year study of incidence, clinical features, and outcomes. *Am J Ophthalmol* December 2007;**144**(6):812–7.
60. Gordon-Lipkin E, Chodkowski B, Reich DS, Smith SA, Pulicken M, Balcer LJ, et al. Retinal nerve fiber layer is associated with brain atrophy in multiple sclerosis. *Neurology* October 16, 2007;**69**(16):1603–9.
61. Grazioli E, Zivadinov R, Weinstock-Guttman B, Lincoff N, Baier M, Wong JR, et al. Retinal nerve fiber layer thickness is associated with brain MRI outcomes in multiple sclerosis. *J Neurol Sci* May 15, 2008;**268** (1–2):12–7.
62. Siger M, Dziegielewski K, Jasek L, Bieniek M, Nicpan A, Nawrocki J, et al. Optical coherence tomography in multiple sclerosis: Thickness of the retinal nerve fiber layer as a potential measure of axonal loss and brain atrophy. *J Neurol* October 2008;**255**(10):1555–60.
63. Dorr J, Wernecke KD, Bock M, Gaede G, Wuerfel JT, Pfueller CF, et al. Association of retinal and macular damage with brain atrophy in multiple sclerosis. *PLoS One* April 8, 2011;**6**(4):e18132.
64. Reich DS, Smith SA, Gordon-Lipkin EM, Ozturk A, Caffo BS, Balcer LJ, et al. Damage to the optic radiation in multiple sclerosis is associated with retinal injury and visual disability. *Arch Neurol* August 2009;**66** (8):998–1006.
65. Pfueller CF, Brandt AU, Schubert F, Bock M, Walaszek B, Waiczies H, et al. Metabolic changes in the visual cortex are linked to retinal nerve fiber layer thinning in multiple sclerosis. *PLoS One* April 6, 2011;**6**(4):e18019.
66. Syc SB, Warner CV, Hiremath GS, Farrell SK, Ratchford JN, Conger A, et al. Reproducibility of high-resolution optical coherence tomography in multiple sclerosis. *Multiple Sclerosis*. July 2010;**16**(7):829–39.
67. Warner CV, Syc SB, Stankiewicz AM, Hiremath G, Farrell SK, Crainiceanu CM, et al. The impact of utilizing different optical coherence tomography devices for clinical purposes and in multiple sclerosis trials. *PLoS One* 2011;**6**(8):e22947.
68. Young KL, Brandt AU, Petzold A, Reitz LY, Lintze F, Paul F, et al. Loss of retinal nerve fibre layer axons indicates white but not grey matter damage in early multiple sclerosis. *Eur J Neurol*. May 2013;**20**(5): 803–11.
69. Zimmermann H, Freing A, Kaufhold F, Gaede G, Bohn E, Bock M, et al. Optic neuritis interferes with optical coherence tomography and magnetic resonance imaging correlations. *Multiple Sclerosis* April 2013;**19** (4):443–50.
70. Saidha S, Sotirchos ES, Oh J, Syc SB, Seigo MA, Shiee N, et al. Relationships between retinal axonal and neuronal measures and global central nervous system pathology in multiple sclerosis. *JAMA Neurol* January 2013;**70**(1):34–43.
71. Gabilondo I, Martinez-Lapiscina EH, Martinez-Heras E, Fraga-Pumar E, Llufriu S, Ortiz S, et al. Trans-synaptic axonal degeneration in the visual pathway in multiple sclerosis. *Ann Neurol* October 2, 2013;
72. Shiee N, Bazin PL, Zackowski KM, Farrell SK, Harrison DM, Newsome SD, et al. Revisiting brain atrophy and its relationship to disability in multiple sclerosis. *PLoS One* 2012;7(5):e37049

Chapter

11 Optical coherence tomography in neurodegenerative and other neurologic diseases

Friedemann Paul and Alexander Ulrich Brandt

Introduction

In recent years, OCT has been used in studies across a wide range of neurodegenerative diseases, from highly prevalent conditions such as Alzheimer's disease to rare diseases like spinocerebellar ataxias. OCT assessment was initially introduced in response to clinical observation of symptoms and paraclinical findings (e.g., visual evoked potentials, brain MRI) suggesting that the visual system was involved in many of these conditions, and was also first studied to examine validity for clinical visual outcome measures such as low-contrast letter acuity for clinical trials and research in multiple sclerosis (MS; see Chapter 6). Since then, its easy applicability and noninvasiveness have also contributed to its increasing popularity. However, our understanding of retinal pathology measured by OCT in most neurodegenerative diseases is still lacking compared to the plethora of literature published on MS and optic neuritis (ON) over the past 15 years. Many studies are limited by small cohort sizes, lack of reproducibility by independent research groups, and the unassessed influence of comorbidities such as glaucoma, diabetic retinopathy, and macular disease, which all may be present in elderly patients with neurodegenerative diseases.

Neuromyelitis optica

Neuromyelitis optica (NMO) is a rare autoimmune inflammatory CNS disease that predominantly presents with clinical attacks of optic neuritis and myelitis [1, 2]. Following the detection of a highly specific biomarker, a serum antibody to the most abundant CNS water channel aquaporin-4 (AQP4), in 60–80% of patients with NMO, the latter was classified as an autoimmune condition distinct from MS but with substantial overlaps in clinical presentation and paraclinical findings. In NMO, the disease course is usually more aggressive and irreversible neurological disability accrues more rapidly than in MS [3]. Considering that it is less common than MS, yet may have worse visual consequences, the number of OCT studies on NMO is impressive, and several groups have published similar and consistent data on the disease's retinal pathology [4]. Previous research has focused on quantifying retinal damage in comparison to MS – the most relevant clinical differential diagnosis – and healthy subjects, on the one hand, and the suitability of OCT as a differential diagnosis tool for distinguishing between NMO and MS, on the other.

Based on long-standing clinical experience, NMO-induced ON is understood to cause more severe visual impairment than a "classical" MSON attack and tends to show poorer recovery, even after treatment with high-dose corticosteroids or plasma exchange. In an NMO cohort characterized at the Mayo Clinic, 60% of relapsing patients were functionally blind (acuity 20/200 or worse) in at least one eye after a mean disease duration of 7.7 years [5].

In line with this, some studies have reported more pronounced thinning of the retinal nerve fiber layer (RNFL) in NMO-ON eyes compared to MSON eyes [6]. Naismith and colleagues found RNFL thicknesses in ON eyes from NMO patients to be on average 10 μm or more thinner (depending on the statistical model) than those from MS patients, and 39% of NMO eyes versus 10% of MS eyes had RNFL values < = 39 μm, indicating that NMO leads to more pronounced axonal damage in the optic nerve. Similarly, Ratchford and colleagues reported substantial RNFL thinning in NMO-ON eyes versus MSON eyes and healthy controls (63.6 μm, 88.3 μm, and 102.4 μm, respectively) [7]. In this study, a first episode of ON

Optical Coherence Tomography in Neurological Disease, ed. Peter A. Calabresi, Laura J. Balcer, and Elliot M. Frohman. Published by Cambridge University Press.

was assumed to lead to 24 μm more RNFL loss than in MS, and visual impairment was more severe. Similar results were found for macular volume. A French study reported a strong inverse correlation between visual field defects and RNFL thickness and between the Expanded Disability Status Scale (EDSS) as a global measure of neurological disability and RNFL thickness [8]. More recent studies have applied modern spectral-domain (SD) technology that offers higher resolution at reduced scan times [9] and allows segmentation of the different intra-retinal layers [10] (see Chapter 13). Both Syc et al. [11] and Sotirchos et al. [12] reported thinning of the ganglion cell layer (GCL) and inner plexiform layer (IPL) in NMO-ON eyes versus MS-ON eyes or healthy controls, which confirmed earlier data suggesting a more severe retinal involvement in NMO. Similar results are reported by Monteiro et al. and Fernandes et al. [13,14]. Schneider et al. detected a more pronounced thinning of the RNFL and the GCL in NMO-ON eyes as opposed to MS and, interestingly, a more pronounced association of structural morphological damage and impaired visual function: GCL thickness was a stronger predictor of visual acuity, including low-contrast acuity, in NMO than in MS [15]. This may indicate that, below a certain threshold of neuroaxonal loss, retinal neurons and axons are no longer able to sufficiently maintain visual function. The latter study also suggested that the pattern of retinal damage may differ between NMO and MS. While MS-ON eyes tended to show the typical preponderance of damage localized to the temporal quadrant, which is in line with clinical observations of optic disc pallor and optic atrophy predominantly in this sector, NMO-ON eyes exhibited a broader distribution of RNFL thinning across all quadrants, albeit with the highly salient observation that the nasal quadrant RNFL thickness was more strongly affected than the temporal quadrant (Figure 11.1). Notwithstanding the differentiated patterns of retinal tissue damage when considering MS vs NMO, the construct validity of these observations has yet to be confirmed, thereby precluding the application of these pattern differences as an objective criterion for differential diagnosis.

In 2012, microcystic macular edema (MME) was reported in both MS and NMO in association with reduced visual acuity and retinal nerve fiber layer thinning [12, 15–17]. MME presents as a microcystic pattern with lower reflectance (Figure 11.2) and is mainly located in the inner nuclear layer (INL) in small, discrete patches [16]. Both the pathogenesis and association with various nosologic entities have yet to be clarified. One possibility is that MME is a symptom of chronic inflammation in the INL, because this layer was shown to be a prominent site of inflammation and microglia activation in a recent autopsy study [18]. A further argument for an inflammatory pathogenesis is provided by Saidha et al., who showed that the INL thickening, which usually accompanies MME, may be indicative of a more severe disease progression in MS, as indicated by a higher number of inflammatory lesions on brain MRI, accelerated EDSS progression, and a higher frequency of relapses [19]. A study by our group further revealed that MME is not specific to MS or NMO, but is strongly linked to a history of ON: 95% of eyes with MME (in total 22 eyes) from a cohort of 255 patients with MS or clinically isolated syndrome (CIS), 20 NMO spectrum disorder patients, and 9 patients with chronic inflammatory optic neuropathy had previously experienced ON. In all three groups, patients with unilateral ON and without visible MME showed an increased INL thickness of the ON-affected eyes compared to the contralateral eyes, suggesting that INL thickening and MME may both be symptoms of underlying retinal inflammation [20]. Additionally, Gelfand et al. only detected MME in eyes with a prior history of ON in a cohort of 25 NMO patients [17]. Both studies showed that MME may be more frequent in NMO (approx. 20%) as compared to MS (approx. 5%); however, this finding has to be interpreted with caution given the low number of the subjects characterized in the two NMO cohorts. In contradistinction to the premise that MME represents a cardinal feature of retinal edema and inflammation restricted to a few diagnostic entities, recent case reports on a patient with optic nerve glioma and a patient with Leber's hereditary optic neuropathy (LHON), both of whom exhibited MME, strongly contested the idea that MME has an inflammatory pathogenesis, and instead suggested that MME may be a consequence of any optic nerve pathology, irrespective of their pathobiological basis. [21–23]

The literature to date is inconclusive regarding the detection of retinal damage by OCT in NMO non-ON eyes. In some studies, NMO non-ON eyes exhibited

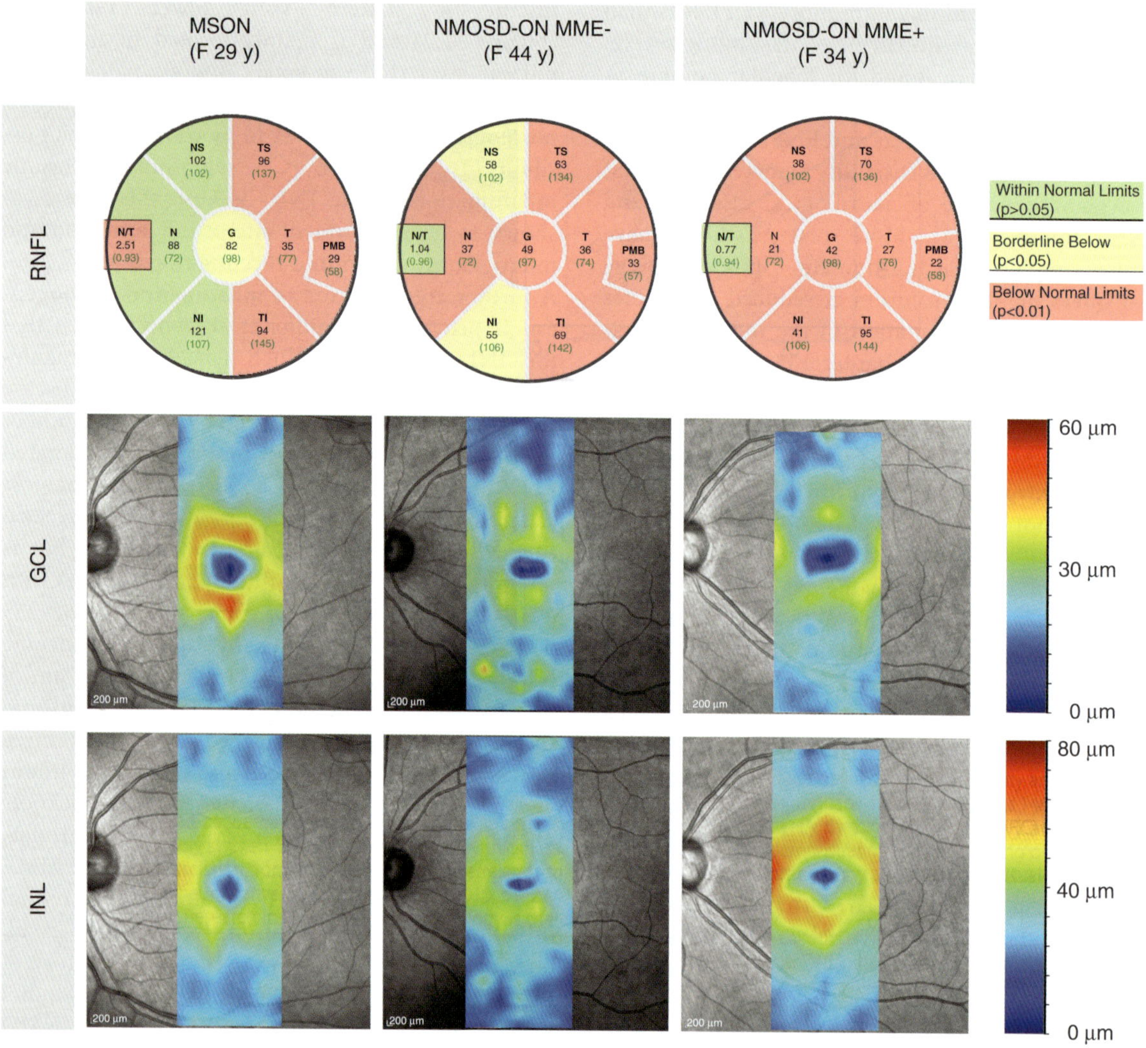

Figure 11.1 RNFL thinning in NMO vs. MS.

Three examples of OCT findings from an MS patient's eye with previous ON (left), a neuromyelitis optica spectrum disorder (NMOSD) patient's eye with previous ON without microcystic macular edema (MME) (center), and an NMOSD patient's eye with previous ON and MME (right). The first row shows peripapillary RNFL thickness data for average RNFL (G) and sectors. The second and third rows show thickness maps of the retinal ganglion cell layer (GCL) and inner nuclear layer (INL) (adapted from [15]).

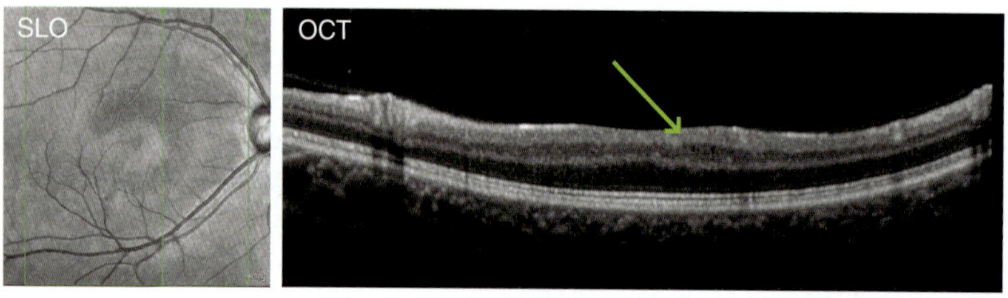

Figure 11.2 Microcystic macular edema (MME) in NMO

Examples of images from one NMO patient's eye showing MME. In the scanning laser ophthalmoscopy (SLO) image on the left, MME is visible as the darker crescent around the fovea. In the OCT B-scan on the right, MME can be identified by the small hypointense lesions exclusively in the INL (green arrow).

no apparent retinal damage, as all OCT measurements closely approximated those derived from healthy control subjects [7, 8, 15]. This supports the notion that retinal damage in NMO is linked to clinically manifest ON attacks, and does not occur progressively or as a consequence of subclinical optic neuropathy, as may be the case in many MS patients [15]. Accordingly, NMO has rarely been found to exhibit features that would confirm the presence of a secondary progressive course [24]. However, Sotirchos et al. and Syc et al. have reported both GCL and IPL thinning in NMO non-ON eyes, a highly conspicuous and controversial finding that must be confirmed or refuted in future studies [11,12].

In summary, OCT data on morphological retinal damage in NMO-ON eyes and analysis of the correlation between this damage and poor visual function are abundant and largely consistent. In contrast, the pathophysiology of retinal damage in a disease characterized by serum antibodies against the CNS water channel AQP4 has not been fully elucidated. Mechanistic studies have shown that AQP4-antibodies not only serve as a biomarker for an NMO diagnosis, but also are pathogenically relevant in terms of binding to astrocytic membranes, the putative scaffolding upon which targeted damage to the aquaporin water channel can materialize [25, 26]. Could an inflammatory attack targeting the AQP4-expressing myelinated retrolaminar optic nerve conceivably cause retinal atrophy via a dying-back mechanism. A further and perhaps more intriguing scientific question arises from evidence that the retina also contains a plethora of astrocytes that express AQP4 at high levels (e.g., Müller cells are but one of a number of astrocytic subtypes capable of cell-surface expression of this key target antigen within the retina). Taken together, the evidence would suggest that the retinal Müller cell represents a bona fide second ocular target of pathogenic AQP4 antibodies [27]. Confirmation of this potentially seminal observation represents a formidable challenge, particularly given that adequate animal models for human NMO have yet to be developed.

In the clinical setting, the use of OCT in the diagnosis and treatment of NMO is proliferating throughout the neurological and ophthalmological communities, with the powerful advent of performing a simple, rapid, convenient, reproducible, and noninvasive assessment of an elegantly eloquent CNS compartment, with compelling ramifications for longitudinal ascertainment of retinal damage, and its corresponding relationship to clinical disability, along with emerging utility as a tool for differentiating those pathophysiologic mechanisms that help distinguish NMO from MS and other conditions. Not surprisingly, the features that characterize high precision, high-speed, high-definition spectral-domain OCT have ushered in a new and exciting era, one where this powerful technique may have utility in helping to advance treating neuroinflammatory and neurodegenerative disorders by being endowed with the capability to detect and monitor preventative, protective, and even restorative properties of novel neurotherapeutic agents.

Parkinson's disease

Parkinson's disease (PD) is a neurodegenerative condition that typically presents with motor symptoms such as akinesia, tremor, and rigidity, and olfactory dysfunction. However, PD has also been widely reported to include visual symptoms like decreased contrast sensitivity and color discrimination, visuospatial deficits, visual hallucinations [28–30], and some electrophysiological studies of visual evoked potentials (VEPs) and pattern electroretinograms suggest pathological signatures within the retina and/or the anterior visual pathways [30–32]. While PD has long been associated with a neuropathological hallmark, the accelerated loss of dopaminergic (DA) neurons within the substantia nigra, dopaminergic neurons (amacrine cells) have also been detected in the INL and IPL of the human retina, thereby suggesting that the pathobiological basis for PD involves, at least in part, the specific targeting of DA neurons by disease-specific injury cascades [33].

Retinal DA deficiency may contribute to visual impairment in PD, as DA is involved in visual processing by modulating the organization of receptive fields of the retinal ganglion cell neurons, whose axons ultimately coalesce into the optic nerve [34, 35]. A post-mortem study showed decreased DA in retinas from PD patients who had *not been treated* with levodopa [36], whereas an in vivo study involving PD patients reported improvement of spatial contrast sensitivity after treatment with levodopa [37].

Several OCT studies have investigated retinal atrophy in patients with PD with diverging results, probably as a result of differences between the cohorts and the OCT devices used. The validity of most OCT studies in PD is hampered by small cohort size and the insufficient or ambiguous consideration of confounding factors prevalent among PD patients, including glaucoma and diabetic retinopathy, to name a few. Altintas et al. found a significant reduction in average RNFL thickness and TMV in 17 PD patients vs. healthy controls, and an inverse correlation between foveal retinal thickness and the Unified Parkinson Disease Rating Scale (UPDRS), a clinical scale to assess neurological impairment in PD [38]. In another investigation, Inzelberg et al. reported a reduction of RNFL thickness in inferior and temporal quadrants in 10 PD patients [39], while a another study found a decreased foveal thickness in 9 PD patients [40]. Hajee et al. demonstrated significant thinning of the inner retinal layers in 24 PD patients [41], and Aaker et al. found differences in macular thickness (thinning and thickening), but no differences in RNFL thickness in 9 PD patients vs. 16 controls [42]. Shrier et al. found increased intraocular differences in macular volume between 23 PD patients and 18 controls [43]. In contrast, Archibald et al. did not find any alteration in RNFL thickness or TMV in 37 PD patients [44]. Likewise, application of modern SD OCT technology in another study showed no differences in RNFL and TMV between 40 PD patients and 25 healthy controls [45]. Interestingly, manual intra-retinal segmentation revealed a thicker INL in PD vs. controls in this study. No correlation between OCT measures and visual acuity, disease duration, or disease severity according to the UPDRS was observed. In a recent study using SD OCT, Garcia-Martin et al. investigated 75 PD patients in comparison with 75 matched healthy controls and found subtle RNFL reduction using three different RNFL scan protocols [46].

Our group recently completed a spectral-domain OCT study on 97 patients with idiopathic PD and 32 healthy controls [47]. Intra-retinal segmentation revealed significant thinning of the combined outer nuclear (ONL) and photoreceptor layer (PRL) in PD vs. controls (118.6 vs. 123.5 μm, $p = 0.001$). Neither RNFL thickness nor TMV or any of the other layers differed from those of controls. We investigated whether retinal damage is associated with impaired color vision, as assessed by the Farnsworth-Munsell color discrimination test (FMT), as color perception has been reported to be altered in PD, a salient feature that may be associated with disease progression [48]. We identified no correlation between performance in the FMT, and any of the OCT measures. Furthermore, no association was found between OCT measures and clinical parameters such as UPDRS or disease duration. Despite the heterogeneity of previous OCT results, our study, in which we had applied modern SD OCT technology with intra-retinal segmentation, as previously used in numerous studies [49], clearly showed that retinal DA deficiency may cause structural retinal damage beyond the RNFL that is detectable by OCT. The cause for this observation remains largely unexplained, and we have already formulated strategic plans to fully characterize this pathological substrate. For example, the PRL contains rods and cones that receive input from dopaminergic interplexiform and amacrine cells via the inner and outer plexiform layers [50, 51]. Thus, we may assume a process of transsynaptic degeneration of ONL neurons as a consequence of altered synaptic input from dopaminergic neurons. The fact that atrophy of the ONL/PRL was not associated with deficits in color discrimination may be – at least in part – explained by the observation that FMT is prone to various confounding elements such as motor and cognitive impairment as well as dopaminergic treatment.

In summary, OCT data in PD are highly heterogeneous, and the value of OCT in the clinical assessment of patients with PD remains to be established. A complicating factor is that many PD patients have difficulties complying with the experimental requirements of OCT examination (thereby leading to a clear acquisition bias) due to head or neck tremor, axial rigidity, or cognitive impairment. Recognizing these important and test-limiting factors may represent at least part of the bases for the discrepant outcomes across previous studies. Ultimately, OCT image quality from PD patients has been demonstrated to be of lower than the image characteristics derived from healthy controls. Image quality cannot be ignored, especially given that OCT generated data can easily be skewed in the setting of poor-quality images [52].

Alzheimer's disease

Alzheimer's disease (AD), which predominantly affects episodic memory, is the most common neurodegenerative cause of dementia in the elderly. The pathophysiological cause is unclear, but the deposition of Aβ plaques in the brain has been suggested as having a major role and is linked – along with other biomarkers – to clinical disease severity [53]. Recently, the presence of Aβ plaques in the retina was reported in a murine Alzheimer's disease model, and confirmed in postmortem tissue from Alzheimer's patients. Importantly, retinal Aβ plaques correlated with brain pathology and clinical severity, and were detectable in suspected AD patients [54]. These recent observations might lead to AD-specific retinal imaging, once labeling of the pathognomonic Aβ plaque becomes feasible in human subjects. The authors of this study (ref 54) have provided the first in vivo data in mice using systemically administered curcumin for the specific labeling of Aβ plaques.

Currently, researchers and clinicians seeking to focus on the retina of AD patients face two challenges. First, although visual symptoms in AD patients are widely reported, they could easily be the result of impairment to higher cognitive functions necessary for visual processing [55, 56]. Second, the high coincidence of other pathologies commonly associated with the aging retina problematizes analysis. Age-related macular dystrophy (AMD), vascular changes, wide-angle glaucoma, cataract, and diabetic retinopathy are common comorbidities that partially account for the reported visual dysfunction in AD (see also below). Consequently, distinguishing between retinal changes that are potentially AD-related and those caused by comorbidities is difficult.

Studies investigating retinal changes in AD have yielded conflicting results: A reduction of retinal ganglion cells (RGC) in comparison to healthy controls was reported in an early postmortem study investigating 10 AD patients [57], as well as in a further study comprised of 9 AD patients with matched healthy subjects [58]. RGC reduction was confirmed by investigating postmortem optic nerve tissue from AD patients, what showed prominent loss of M-cells, the largest class of RGCs contributing large calibre fibers to the optic nerve [59]. Other histopathological studies reported no differences in the layout in the AD patient's retina [60–62]. The latter is supported by several studies using scanning laser polarimetry, retina tomography, and pattern electroretinography [62–66].

Several studies have applied OCT to investigate retinal changes in AD patients. Iseri and colleagues investigated 14 AD patients vs. 15 matched healthy subjects. They reported a reduction of RNFL (AD, average RNFL 87±24 μm (mean ± standard deviation) vs. controls, average RNFL 113 ±7 μm) and total macula volume (AD, TMV 6.8 ±0.4 mm^3 vs. controls, TMV 7.1 ±0.2 mm^3). Reduction in TMV correlated with clinical severity expressed by minimental state examination [67]. Paquet et al., who in addition to AD patients also investigated cohorts with mild cognitive impairment (a precursor symptom of AD), reported a similar finding in 49 cognitively impaired patients. Here, RNFL reduction was more prominent in the more severely affected patients [68]. Lu et al. reported RNFL thinning in the superior and inferior quadrants in 22 patients compared to age-matched healthy controls [69]. Berisha and colleagues studied nine early stage AD patients vs. matched healthy subjects and found that the AD patients showed significant RNFL reduction in the superior quadrant (AD, superior RNFL 92 ±22 μm compared to the controls' superior 114 ±1 μm) [70]. In one of the largest AD cohorts investigated to date, which included 40 patients and 40 well-matched healthy subjects, Kirbas and colleagues reported significant RNFL reductions (AD, average RNFL 65 ±6 μm vs. average RNFL 75±4 μm). Again, RNFL thinning was predominantly located in the superior quadrant [71].

In summary, these OCT studies suggest significant RNFL reduction is a common feature of AD. As in PD, owing to comorbid physical and cognitive symptoms, performing OCT examinations reliably on AD patients can represent a formidable challenge, one that markedly limits obtaining data of acceptable quality, whether used in clinical practice or as outcome measures in clinical research. The recognized high standard deviations of the data collected from small cohorts of patients afflicted by neurodegenerative disease may reflect the broad pathological heterogeneity across patients carrying the same diagnosis. Further, the age matching in most of the referenced studies lacked stringency, adding age as a potentially important confounder.

Of note in this regard is another important finding in AD: the high co-occurrence with open-angle glaucoma (OAG). In comparison to healthy subjects, AD patients show a higher occurrence of OAG [72], and subjects with OAG show a higher risk to develop AD in later life [73]. The link between OAG and AD is currently unclear and needs to be investigated further in the future. Conspicuously, the preponderance of RNFL loss in the superior quadrant in most of the studies interrogated may also represent a potential confounding effect, namely, undiagnosed glaucoma, which also tends to affect the superior quadrant [74].

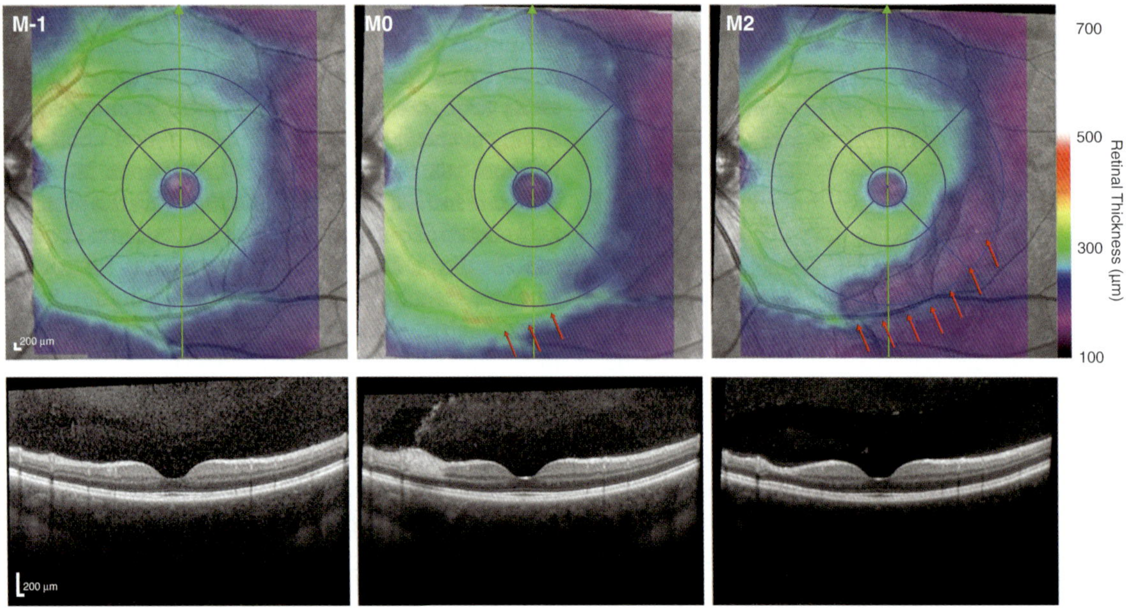

Figure 11.3 Formation of a Susac syndrome retinal lesion.

Examples of findings from a Susac syndrome patient's eye. One month prior to the acute lesion (M-1 on the left), the retina appears mostly normal in the nasal-inferior area around the macula. During the acute event (M0), massive swelling can be observed around the retinal branch vessel directly inferior to the macula, indicated by the red arrows. After two months (M2 on the right), the swelling has decreased and the inner retinal layers at the site of prior inflammation and in all of the area supplied by this vessel are almost completely degenerated, indicated by the red arrows.

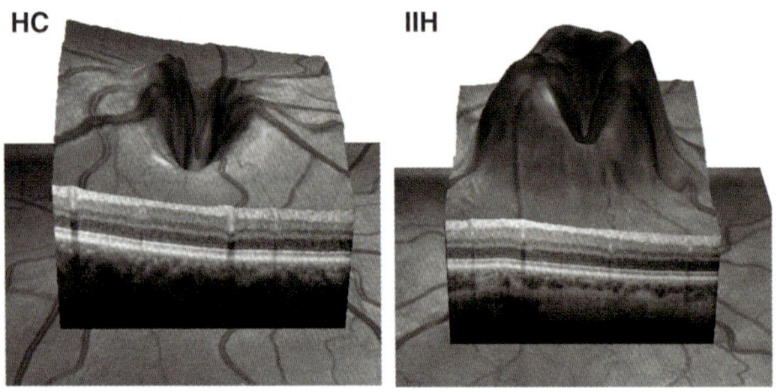

Figure 11.4 Papilledema in idiopathic intracranial hypertension.

Comparison of a 3-D optic nerve head scan from a healthy subject (HC on the left) and a patient with idiopathic intracranial hypertension (IIH) with increased ICP (adapted from [79]).

Other neurologic diseases

Susac syndrome

Susac syndrome presents as a combination of encephalopathy, hearing loss, and visual deficits due to acute branch retinal artery occlusions [75]. The etiology of this rare disease and its exact prevalence are unknown [76]. Differentiating it from MS can be challenging since the corresponding clinical presentation and diagnostic findings may significantly overlap. However, in OCT, eyes from patients with Susac syndrome show sectorial damage that can be distinguished from MS patients [77]. During an acute event of Susac syndrome, the affected areas show profound swelling, which later leads to almost complete loss of all inner retinal layers supplied by the occluded branch artery (Figure 11.3). This presentation during the acute phase of visual symptoms clearly differentiates Susac syndrome from optic neuritis resulting from MS or NMO, where acute and chronic damage is much more broadly distributed and certainly not a consequence of a single vessel distribution of localized tissue damage.

Table 11.1

	Susac	FRDA		SCA-1		SCA-2
Study	Brandt et al. [77]	Fortuna et al. [84]	Noval et al. [86]	Stricker et al. [89]	Pula et al. [90]	Pula et al. [90]
Year	2011	2009	2012	2010	2011	2011
Device	Stratus TD-OCT	Stratus TD-OCT	Stratus TD-OCT	Spectralis SD-OCT	Spectralis SD-OCT	Spectralis SD-OCT
Cohort (age, F/M)	9 (33±11 y, 6/3)	26 (32±8 y, 8/18)	23 (25±7 y)	9 (52±9 y, 4/5)	7 (n=29, 58 y, 18/11)*	7 (n=29, 58 y, 18/11)*
Matched cohorts (age F)/M	matched HC and MS	48 HC (33±8 y, 20/28)	none	9 HC (51±9 y, 4/5)	27 HC (56 y, 18/9)*	27 HC (56 y, 18/9)*
Main results	Significant RNFL reduction (81±18 μm) vs. HC (107 ±9 μm). in comparison to MS sectorial damage both in RNFL and TMV.	Significant RNFL reduction (76 ±12 μm) vs. HC (100±9 μm). Description of 3 distinct loss types correlating visual dysfunction.	RNFL reduction in comparison to normative data and with good correlation to visual function tests.	Significant reduction of average RNFL (84±13 μm) and temporal RNFL (62±8 μm) vs. HC average RNFL (97±8 μm) and temporal RNFL (74±9 μm).	Non-significant RNFL reduction (93±8 μm) vs. HC (98±9 μm).	Significant RNFL reduction (84±12 μm) vs. HC (98±9 μm).
Summary	Sectorial damage separates Susac retinal damage from ON related retinal damage.	RNFL reduction in 3 distinct types correlating with visual function.	RNFL reduction.	RNFL reduction with temporal quadrant focus.	No changes in RNFL.	Significant RNFL reduction.

In differential diagnosis – for example, when acute visual symptoms present in combination with cognitive changes or hearing loss – OCT should always be performed to exclude possible Susac syndrome. A suspected diagnosis of Susac syndrome can then be substantiated using fluorescence angiography (FAG).

Intracranial hypertension

Elevated intracranial pressure can present as papilledema. This edema of the optic nerve head (ONH), long familiar to neurology and ophthalmology clinicians, can also be measured using OCT (Figure 11.4) [78]. In idiopathic intracranial hypertension (IIH), our group could show that ONH volume measurements can reliably quantify the papilledema and discriminate between healthy subjects, IIH patients undergoing clinically effective therapy but who nevertheless exhibited increased ONH volume, and untreated patients, who showed the largest ONH volume [79]. This parameter (i.e., ONH volume) correlated highly with intracranial pressure (ICP), suggesting that OCT is also of benefit in the diagnosis and monitoring of patients affected by other

SCA-3	SCA-6	SCA-7	MSA-C	ARSACS	ALS	Wilson's Disease
Pula et al. [90]	Pula et al. [90]	Manrique et al. [91]	Pula et al. [90]	Vingolo et al. [95]	Roth et al. [101]	Albrecht et al.
2011	2011	2009	2011	2011	2013	2012
Spectralis SD-OCT	Spectralis SD-OCT	Stratus TD-OCT	Spectralis SD-OCT	not reported	Cirrus HD-OCT	Spectralis SD-OCT
5 (n=29, 58 y, 18/11)*	6 (n=29, 58 y, 18/11)*	7 (5 from one family)	5 (n=29, 58 y, 18/11)*	5 (34±8 y, 5/3)	76 (56±11 y, 26/50)	42 (40±14 y, 24/18)
27 HC (56 y, 18/9)*	27 HC (56 y, 18/9)*	none	27 HC (56 y, 18/9)*	5 HC (62±8 y, 4/1)	54 HC (56 ±11 y, 26/28)	76 HC (43 ±13 y, 35/29)
Significant RNFL reduction (85±9 µm) vs. HC (98 ±9 µm).	Non-significant RNFL reduction (95±5 µm) vs. HC (98±9 µm). Significant reduction of macular thickness (310±5 µm vs. HC (339 ±17 µm).	Case-wise discussion. RNFL reduction with focus on the superior and in more severe cases also on nasal and inferior quadrants.	Non-significant RNFL changes (100±11 µm) vs. HC (98±9 µm). Significant reduction of macular thickness (314±12 µm) vs. HC (339 ±17 µm).	Case-wise discussion. RNFL thickening with myelinated appearance.	No changes in RNFL (94 ±9 µm) vs. HC (93±10). No differences in GCL, INL/OPL and ONL/PRL. Only 15 definite ALS according to El Escorial criteria.	Significant RNFL reduction (95±9 µm) vs. HC (97 ±10). Reduction in GCL and INL.
Significant RNFL reduction.	Significant macular thickness reduction but no changes in RNFL.	Mild to severe RNFL loss focussed on superior, nasal and inferior quadrants.	No changes.	RNFL thickening with myelinated appearance.	No changes.	RNFL, RGC and INL thinning.

* Pula et al [90]. only reported cohort statistics for the full cohort, not for disease subtypes

diseases with elevated ICP. Another study using the Frisén scale, which quantifies edema using fundus photography, also showed good correlation between an alternative ONH quantification approach and Frisén scale derived papilledema grades [80]. Currently, further studies are needed on the temporal dynamics in conjunction with inter- and intra-individual changes in ONH volume, and visual function loss and ICP. Such studies will determine whether OCT has satisfactory utility as a surrogate biomarker in the assessment of ICP.

Hereditary and other rare neurodegenerative diseases

OCT has been applied in several other hereditary or rare neurodegenerative diseases. With a few exceptions, most published OCT studies show varying levels of RNFL reduction in the peripapillary ring scan that is often accentuated in the temporal quadrant. Fibers of the temporal quadrant RNFL comprise primarily parvo-cellular axons from the papillo-macular bundle. These axons consist of small and thinly myelinated axons with rapid firing rates that connect macular ganglion cells via the lateral geniculate nucleaus with the visual cortex. As such, they are highly relevant to high-resolution visual acuity and high spatial frequency of contrast sensitivity and color vision. Degeneration of these macular fibers has a much greater effect on visual quality of life than defects in the peripheral visual areas. Unfortunately, precisely these fibers are affected by neurodegeneration in many mitochondriopathies and other optic neuropathies, such as Leber's hereditary optic neuropathy (LHON) and OPA1-related dominant optic nerve atrophy (DOA) [81]. One reason for this may be their small volume and fast firing, which might make them more susceptible to energy depletion by defective cellular metabolism and, thus, neurodegeneration [82]. Consequently, OCT assessment of RNFL focuses on the peripapillary ring rather than the macula. An overview of current OCT studies is given in Table 11.1, and a summary of key findings is provided in the following paragraphs.

Friedreich's ataxia

One of the first hereditary ataxias investigated in detail using OCT was Friedreich's ataxia (FRDA) [83]. Visual symptoms and optic neuropathy are regularly found in FRDA [84] and mitrochondriopathy is likely to directly contribute to the disease pathophysiology [85]. In OCT, FRDA patients present with widespread RNFL reduction. Notably, visually asymptomatic patients also show optic neuropathy, the level of which correlates to general clinical severity and progression [84, 86, 87]. Fortuna et al. proposed three different types of RNFL degeneration in FRDA: Type 1 with diffuse and severe reduction of RNFL thickness in all quadrants, Type 2 with diffuse RNFL reduction that is more marked in the superior quadrant, and Type 3 with diffuse but mild reduction of RNFL thickness in all quadrants [84]. However, the clinical and pathophysiological significance of the individual categories remains to be elucidated.

Spinocerebellar ataxias

Spinocerebellar ataxias (SCAs) comprise a group of over 30 genetically distinct hereditary ataxias with similar clinical features. They are mostly numbered according to the date of their first description. Differential diagnosis of these disorders can be challenging because patients often present with only a subset of the symptoms known for SCA diseases as a whole [88]. OCT can aid in differential diagnosis by identifying patients with optic nerve atrophy especially without apparent visual symptoms. However, in many diseases OCT changes might be statistically significant but hardly relevant on an individual level.

Retinal changes identified by OCT have been reported in SCA patients with and without visual symptoms. SCA-1 presents with a mild and temporally focused RNFL reduction, and exhibits features similar to other mitochondria-related optic neuropathies [89]. SCA-2, SCA-3 and SCA-6 patients also show RNFL or macular thickness reductions [90]. The focal distribution of changes in many SCAs is currently unclear, as is a potential correlation with clinical scores, because most studies have involved only a few patients, especially in the rare SCAs, which limits their usefulness for detailed review.

Of the forms of SCA, SCA-7 is unique in having a high prevalence of retinal photoreceptor abnormalities that appear to be directly related to disease pathology. Consequently, SCA-7 patients regularly present with visual symptoms. However, current OCT technology can only detect these photoreceptor anomalies with difficulty and primarily in advanced disease stages when RGCs and retinal axons in the RNFL undergo secondary neurodegeneration [91]. In contrast to the temporal quadrant RNFL effect usually found in mitochondria-related disorders and other SCAs [92, 93], in SCA-7 patients' eyes, the superior, inferior, and nasal quadrants are preferentially affected, whereas the temporal quadrant is mainly affected during late stages of disease [91].

Preliminary data on OCT findings further exist in SCA-14. In the largest cohort of SCA-14 patients investigated to date (n = 15) – a SCA that does not commonly present with visual symptoms – there were no SCA-14 specific retinal changes detectable on testing (unpublished data).

Autosomal recessive spastic ataxia of Charlevoix-Saguenay

Autosomal recessive spastic ataxia of Charlevoix-Saguenay (ARSACS) is a rare disorder that was first identified in the Quebec region but can today be found throughout Northern America and Europe

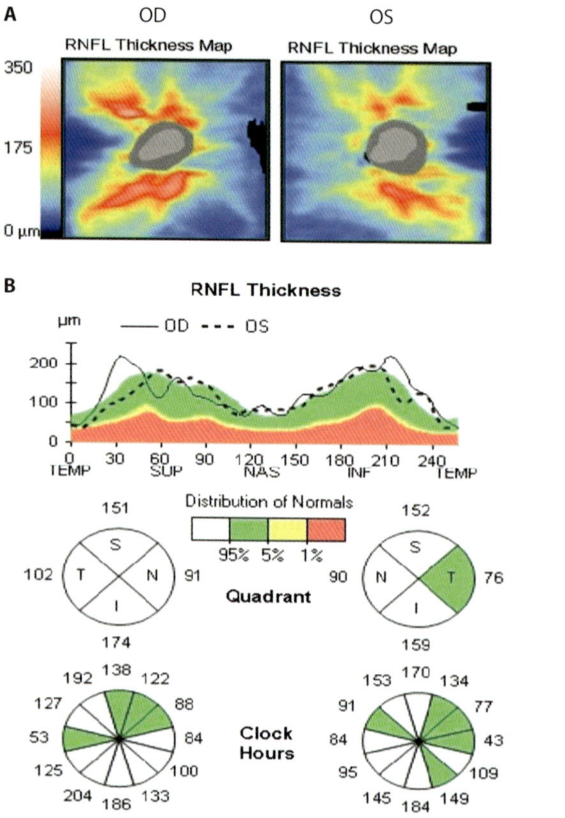

Figure 11.5 OCT findings in ARSACS.
Examples of an OCT report from an ARSACS patient. (A) RNFL thickness maps around the optic nerve head show RNFL thickening; (B) RNFL thickening can also be detected using the peripapillary RNFL ring scan. Comparison to RNFL distribution of normal controls shows elevated RNFL thickness in the inferior and superior quadrants (kindly provided by Dr. Elena Garcia-Martin, Zaragoza, Spain).

[94]. In OCT, patients with ARSACS present with increased RNFL thickness [95], which has been proposed as due to pathological myelination of retinal axons [96] or axonal hypertrophy (Figure 11.5) [97].

Hereditary spastic paraplegia

Hereditary spastic paraplegias (HSPs) are progressive neurodegenerative disorders with several distinct genetic phenotypes [98]. Common features are a dysfunction of axonal transport, predominantly leading to axonal length-dependent neurodegeneration of corticospinal tracts. Visual symptoms are rarely reported and mostly are limited to complex forms of the disease [99]. OCT shows RNFL reduction in temporal quadrants in clinically complex forms of the disease but not in clinically pure forms [100].

Amyotrophic lateral sclerosis

Amyotrophic lateral sclerosis (ALS) is a neurodegenerative disorder affecting upper and lower motor neuron tracts. Although visual symptoms are uncommon, VEP abnormalities have been reported. However, there is currently no evidence that OCT can detect retinal involvement in amyotrophic lateral sclerosis (ALS) [101]. This requires confirmation in further studies, because genetically distinct subtypes of this heterogeneous disease, which has several different clinical phenotypes, might lend themselves to assessment by OCT.

Wilson's disease

Wilson's disease (WD) is a hereditary disorder of copper accumulation that leads to hepatic damage and neurodegeneration [102]. Although only few patients report visual symptoms, many patients show pathological findings in electroretinography and VEP [103]. In OCT, patients with WD show reduction in RNFL and RGC thickness [104].

Limitations

While OCT is likely helpful to further elucidate the natural or treated history of neurodegenerative disease, or to complete models of structure–function correlation for treatment, OCT measurements are not specific for any particular disorder.

First, RNFL changes with age. In healthy subjects, annual RNFL decrease is reported as between −0.16 µm/year [105] and −0.44 µm/year [106]. However, this decrease is not evenly distributed over age but is initially slow and accelerates after the age of 50 [105, 106]. A similar process takes place in the macula and affects mainly the RNFL, RGC, IPL, and INL but not, it appears, the outer plexiform and nuclear layers, including the photoreceptors [107]. Age-related accelerated loss of RNFL and macular thickness in older patients makes OCT assessment of optic nerve or retinal neurodegeneration in neurodegenerative diseases more suitable in younger patients. In clinical research, exact age matching of cohorts is, therefore, essential to ensure the validity of results. Minor differences in age can produce differences in results unrelated to the neuropathology being studied.

Additionally, the coincidence of other eye diseases, particularly glaucoma (GD) but also diabetic retinopathy (DR) and AMD, increases with age. Above all, the risk of GD and here open-angle glaucoma rises considerably after the age of 50 [108]. While open-angle glaucoma prevalence among 50-year-olds is only 0–3%, in 80-year-olds it rises to 5–15%. Its incidence is also strongly ethnicity-dependent, with the disorder being more common among African, Asian, and Latin American groups than Caucasians [109]. Moreover, GD often also remains undiagnosed [110] because retinal changes due to GD are sometimes difficult to differentiate from reported findings in several neurodegenerative diseases. This makes GD an important confounder that should be considered in both research and clinical routine. Although some OCT studies discussed here went to considerable lengths to minimize potential confounder effects especially all of the studies investigating older cohorts should be interpreted with these limitations in mind.

Second, the majority of existing studies, especially in rarer neurodegenerative diseases, are cross-sectional studies, which often included only a small number of subjects. Only in very few diseases, such as NMO and SCA-1, have findings been reported and confirmed by several independent groups. In all cases, the cross-sectional nature of the studies makes validating the disease specificity of many findings difficult. Longitudinal studies are urgently required to better implement disease-specific and neurodegeneration-generic OCT findings into clinical routine.

Finally, OCT examinations are more demanding in severely clinically affected patients, who have difficulty complying with the needs of the experimental setting due to cognitive or motor impairment. In clinical routine, and especially in research, strictly adhering to the quality guidelines given in literature is vital to preventing artifacts and diagnostic errors [111]. Any significant variation in image quality should be investigated and reported [52].

Summary

OCT has potential benefit in the assessment of several neurodegenerative diseases. In routine clinical practice, OCT is highly recommended for both differential diagnosis and follow-up of patients with (suspected) MS and related neuroimmunologic diseases like NMO or Susac syndrome. Above all, OCT should always be performed as part of the differential diagnosis of patients presenting with symptoms indicating acute optic neuritis [112].

Furthermore, using OCT to detect optic nerve atrophy, which is characteristic of some, but not all, neurodegenerative diseases is of benefit in the differential diagnosis of other complex, often-related diseases. It provides an objective means of detecting visual system involvement, which is challenging to assess and often overlooked, particularly in patients with cognitive impairment. In our experience, OCT is a means of tracing visual symptoms in these patients to retinal or optic nerve abnormalities. Therefore, we suggest routinely performing OCT if at least one important differential diagnosis involving the retina is under discussion for a patient. Moreover, several rare diseases show distinct retinal pathologies that can easily be identified by means of OCT.

The current value of OCT in AD and PD is far more difficult to assess. Both diseases show clear retinal pathologies – in the case of AD the formation of possible retinal Aβ plaques and in the case of PD neurodegeneration of dopaminergic ganglion cells and potentially also photoreceptors. However, state-of-the-art OCT is currently unable to trace these changes, which are probably simply too subtle. Higher imaging resolution or functional OCT macular scan applications that specifically target the affected structures in these diseases might well solve this limitation in the future.

Currently, both diseases show a high co-occurrence with other diseases or changes of the aging retina, such as GD DR, AMD, and vascular changes. This makes applying OCT challenging, particularly when attempting to track disease-specific changes. More importantly, such confounders increase the quality requirements for OCT studies on AD and PD tremendously and hamper assessing the validity of published studies. Current data do suggest OCT is a valuable tool for studying AD and PD in research settings. However, clinician researchers should interpret possible findings cautiously, keeping the preceding issues in mind.

We expect OCT will prove a valuable follow-up marker in many of the diseases discussed previously.

However, more research is required into its role as a disease monitoring tool before we can support its integration into everyday routine clinical practice.

Acknowledgments

We thank Ella Maria Kadas and Timm Oberwahrenbrock for assistance with preparing the figures. This work was supported by the German Research Council (DFG Exc 257 to FP) and the German Ministry for Education and Research (KKNMS Competence Network Multiple Sclerosis to FP).

References

1. Jarius S, Ruprecht K, Wildemann B, Kuempfel T, Ringelstein M, Geis C, et al. Contrasting disease patterns in seropositive and seronegative neuromyelitis optica: A multicentre study of 175 patients. *J Neuroinflammation* 2012;**9**:14.
2. Wingerchuk DM, Lennon VA, Pittock SJ, Lucchinetti CF, Weinshenker BG. Revised diagnostic criteria for neuromyelitis optica. *Neurology* May 23, 2006;**66**(10):1485–9.
3. Jarius S, Paul F, Franciotta D, Waters P, Zipp F, Hohlfeld R, et al. Mechanisms of disease: aquaporin-4 antibodies in neuromyelitis optica. *Nat Clin Pract Neurol* April 2008;**4**(4):202–14.
4. Bennett JL, Seze J de, Lana-Peixoto M, Palace J, Waldman A, Schippling S, et al. Neuromyelitis optica and multiple sclerosis: Seeing differences through optical coherence tomography. *Mult Scler* February 6, 2015. pii: 1352458514567216.
5. Wingerchuk DM, Hogancamp WF, O'Brien PC, Weinshenker BG. The clinical course of neuromyelitis optica (Devic's syndrome). *Neurology* September 22, 1999;**53**(5):1107–14.
6. Naismith RT, Tutlam NT, Xu J, Klawiter EC, Shepherd J, Trinkaus K, et al. Optical coherence tomography differs in neuromyelitis optica compared with multiple sclerosis. *Neurology*. March 24, 2009;**72**(12):1077–82.
7. Ratchford JN, Quigg ME, Conger A, Frohman T, Frohman EM, Balcer LJ, et al. Optical coherence tomography helps differentiate neuromyelitis optica and MS optic neuropathies. *Neurology* July 28, 2009;**73**(4):302–8.
8. De Seze J, Blanc F, Jeanjean L, Zéphir H, Labauge P, Bouyon M, et al. Optical coherence tomography in neuromyelitis optica. *Arch Neurol* July 2008;**65**(7):920–3.
9. Bock M, Brandt AU, Dörr J, Pfueller CF, Ohlraun S, Zipp F, et al. Time domain and spectral domain optical coherence tomography in multiple sclerosis: a comparative cross-sectional study. *Mult Scler Houndmills Basingstoke Engl.* July 2010;**16**(7):893–6.
10. Oberwahrenbrock T, Ringelstein M, Jentschke S, Deuschle K, Klumbies K, Bellmann-Strobl J, et al. Retinal ganglion cell and inner plexiform layer thinning in clinically isolated syndrome. *Mult Scler* December 2013;**19**(14): 1885–95. doi: 10.1177/1352458513489757. Epub May 23, 2013.
11. Syc SB, Saidha S, Newsome SD, Ratchford JN, Levy M, Ford E, et al. Optical coherence tomography segmentation reveals ganglion cell layer pathology after optic neuritis. Brain J Neurol [Internet]. October 17, 2011 [cited December 6, 2011]; Available from: http://www.ncbi.nlm.nih.gov/pubmed/22006982
12. Sotirchos ES, Saidha S, Byraiah G, Mealy MA, Ibrahim MA, Sepah YJ, et al. In vivo identification of morphologic retinal abnormalities in neuromyelitis optica. *Neurology* April 9, 2013;**80**(15):1406–14.
13. Monteiro MLR, Fernandes DB, Apóstolos-Pereira SL, Callegaro D. Quantification of retinal neural loss in patients with neuromyelitis optica and multiple sclerosis with or without optic neuritis using Fourier-domain optical coherence tomography. *Invest Ophthalmol Vis Sci* 2012;**53**(7):3959–66.
14. Fernandes DB, Raza AS, Nogueira RGF, Wang D, Callegaro D, Hood DC, et al. Evaluation of inner retinal layers in patients with multiple sclerosis or neuromyelitis optica using optical coherence tomography. *Ophthalmology*. October 17, 2012;
15. Schneider E, Zimmermann H, Oberwahrenbrock T, Kaufhold F, Kadas EM, Petzold A, et al. Optical coherence tomography reveals distinct patterns of retinal damage in neuromyelitis optica and multiple sclerosis. *PLoS ONE*. June 21, 2013;**8**(6):e66151.
16. Gelfand JM, Nolan R, Schwartz DM, Graves J, Green AJ. Microcystic macular edema in multiple sclerosis is associated with disease severity. *Brain* [Internet]. April 25, 2012 [cited May 30, 2012]; Available from: http://brain.oxfordjournals.org/content/early/2012/04/25/brain.aws098
17. Gelfand JM, Cree BA, Nolan R, Arnow S, Green AJ. Microcystic inner nuclear layer abnormalities and neuromyelitis optica. *JAMA Neurol*. March 25, 2013;**1**–5.
18. Green AJ, McQuaid S, Hauser SL, Allen IV, Lyness R. Ocular pathology in multiple sclerosis: retinal

atrophy and inflammation irrespective of disease duration. *Brain J Neurol* June 2010;**133** (Pt 6):1591–601.

19. Saidha S, Sotirchos ES, Ibrahim MA, Crainiceanu CM, Gelfand JM, Sepah YJ, et al. Microcystic macular edema, thickness of the inner nuclear layer of the retina, and disease characteristics in multiple sclerosis: a retrospective study. *Lancet Neurol* October 4, 2012;
20. Kaufhold F, Zimmermann H, Schneider E, Ruprecht K, Paul F, Oberwahrenbrock T, et al. Optic Neuritis Is Associated with Inner Nuclear Layer Thickening and Microcystic Macular Edema Independently of Multiple Sclerosis. *PLoS ONE* Aug 6, 2013;**8**(8): e71145.
21. Barboni P, Carelli V, Savini G, Carbonelli M, La Morgia C, Sadun AA. Microcystic macular degeneration from optic neuropathy: not inflammatory, not trans-synaptic degeneration. *Brain J Neurol* February 8, 2013;
22. Abegg M, Zinkernagel M, Wolf S. Microcystic macular degeneration from optic neuropathy. *Brain J Neurol* September 7, 2012;
23. Brandt AU, Oberwahrenbrock T, Kadas EM, Lagrèze WA, Paul F. Dynamic formation of macular microcysts independent of vitreous traction changes. *Neurology* July 1, 2014;**83**(1):73–7. doi: 10.1212/WNL.0000000000000545. Epub May 23, 2014.
24. Wingerchuk DM, Pittock SJ, Lucchinetti CF, Lennon VA, Weinshenker BG. A secondary progressive clinical course is uncommon in neuromyelitis optica. *Neurology* February 20, 2007;**68**(8):603–5.
25. Jarius S, Wildemann B, Paul F. Neuromyelitis optica: clinical features, immunopathogenesis and treatment. *Clin Exp Immunol* May 2014;**176**(2):149–64. doi: 10.1111/cei.12271. Review.
26. Hinson SR, Pittock SJ, Lucchinetti CF, Roemer SF, Fryer JP, Kryzer TJ, et al. Pathogenic potential of IgG binding to water channel extracellular domain in neuromyelitis optica. *Neurology* December 11, 2007;**69**(24):2221–31.
27. Levin MH, Bennett JL, Verkman AS. Optic neuritis in neuromyelitis optica. *Prog Retin Eye Res* March 30, 2013;
28. Biousse V, Skibell BC, Watts RL, Loupe DN, Drews-Botsch C, Newman NJ. Ophthalmologic features of Parkinson's disease. *Neurology* January 27, 2004;**62**(2):177–80.
29. Archibald NK, Clarke MP, Mosimann UP, Burn DJ. The retina in Parkinson's disease. *Brain J Neurol.* May 2009;**132**(Pt 5):1128–45.
30. Bodis-Wollner I, Marx MS, Mitra S, Bobak P, Mylin L, Yahr M. Visual dysfunction in Parkinson's disease. *Loss in spatiotemporal contrast sensitivity.* Brain J Neurol December 1987;**110** (Pt 6):1675–98.
31. Nightingale S, Mitchell KW, Howe JW. Visual evoked cortical potentials and pattern electroretinograms in Parkinson's disease and control subjects. *J Neurol Neurosurg Psychiatry* November 1986;**49**(11):1280–7.
32. Tagliati M, Bodis-Wollner I, Yahr MD. The pattern electroretinogram in Parkinson's disease reveals lack of retinal spatial tuning. *Electroencephalogr Clin Neurophysiol* January 1996;**100**(1):1–11.
33. Frederick JM, Rayborn ME, Laties AM, Lam DM, Hollyfield JG. Dopaminergic neurons in the human retina. *J Comp Neurol* September 1, 1982;**210**(1):65–79.
34. Djamgoz MB, Hankins MW, Hirano J, Archer SN. Neurobiology of retinal dopamine in relation to degenerative states of the tissue. *Vision Res* December 1997;**37**(24):3509–29.
35. Jackson GR, Owsley C. Visual dysfunction, neurodegenerative diseases, and aging. *Neurol Clin* August 2003;**21**(3):709–28.
36. Harnois C, Di Paolo T. Decreased dopamine in the retinas of patients with Parkinson's disease. *Invest Ophthalmol Vis Sci* November 1990;**31**(11):2473–5.
37. Hutton JT, Morris JL, Elias JW. Levodopa improves spatial contrast sensitivity in Parkinson's disease. *Arch Neurol* July 1993;**50**(7):721–4.
38. Altintaş O, Işeri P, Ozkan B, Cağlar Y. Correlation between retinal morphological and functional findings and clinical severity in Parkinson's disease. *Doc Ophthalmol Adv Ophthalmol* March 2008;**116**(2):137–46.
39. Inzelberg R, Ramirez JA, Nisipeanu P, Ophir A. Retinal nerve fiber layer thinning in Parkinson disease. *Vision Res* November 2004;**44**(24):2793–7.
40. Cubo E, Tedejo RP, Rodriguez Mendez V, López Peña MJ, Trejo Gabriel Y Galán JM. Retina thickness in Parkinson's disease and essential tremor. *Mov Disord Off J Mov Disord Soc.* October 30, 2010;**25**(14):2461–2.
41. Hajee ME, March WF, Lazzaro DR, Wolintz AH, Shrier EM, Glazman S, et al. Inner retinal layer thinning in Parkinson disease. *Arch Ophthalmol.* June 2009;**127**(6):737–41.
42. Aaker GD, Myung JS, Ehrlich JR, Mohammed M, Henchcliffe C, Kiss S. Detection of retinal changes in Parkinson's disease with spectral-domain optical

coherence tomography. *Clin Ophthalmol Auckl NZ* 2010;**4**:1427–32.

43. Shrier EM, Adam CR, Spund B, Glazman S, Bodis-Wollner I. Interocular asymmetry of foveal thickness in Parkinson disease. *J Ophthalmol* 2012;**2012**:728457.
44. Archibald NK, Clarke MP, Mosimann UP, Burn DJ. Retinal thickness in Parkinson's disease. *Parkinsonism Relat Disord* July 2011;**17**(6):431–6.
45. Albrecht P, Müller A-K, Südmeyer M, Ferrea S, Ringelstein M, Cohn E, et al. Optical coherence tomography in parkinsonian syndromes. *PloS One* 2012;**7**(4):e34891.
46. Garcia-Martin E, Satue M, Fuertes I, Otin S, Alarcia R, Herrero R, et al. Ability and reproducibility of Fourier-domain optical coherence tomography to detect retinal nerve fiber layer atrophy in Parkinson's disease. *Ophthalmology* October 2012;**119**(10):2161–7.
47. Roth NM, Saidha S, Zimmermann H, Brandt AU, Isensee J, Benkhellouf-Rutkowska A, et al. Photoreceptor layer thinning in idiopathic Parkinson's disease. *Mov Disord* April 1, 2014;n/a–n/a.
48. Müller T, Woitalla D, Peters S, Kohla K, Przuntek H. Progress of visual dysfunction in Parkinson's disease. *Acta Neurol Scand* April 2002;**105**(4):256–60.
49. Saidha S, Syc SB, Durbin MK, Eckstein C, Oakley JD, Meyer SA, et al. Visual dysfunction in multiple sclerosis correlates better with optical coherence tomography derived estimates of macular ganglion cell layer thickness than peripapillary retinal nerve fiber layer thickness. *Mult Scler J* [Internet] August 24, 2011 [cited September 12, 2011]; Available from: http://www.ncbi.nlm.nih.gov/pubmed/21865411
50. Nguyen-Legros J. Functional neuroarchitecture of the retina: hypothesis on the dysfunction of retinal dopaminergic circuitry in Parkinson's disease. *Surg Radiol Anat SRA* 1988;**10**(2):137–44.
51. Wulle I, Wagner HJ. GABA and tyrosine hydroxylase immunocytochemistry reveal different patterns of colocalization in retinal neurons of various vertebrates. *J Comp Neurol* June 1, 1990;**296**(1):173–8.
52. Wu Z, Huang J, Dustin L, Sadda SR. Signal strength is an important determinant of accuracy of nerve fiber layer thickness measurement by optical coherence tomography. *J Glaucoma* March 2009;**18**(3):213–6.
53. Jack CR Jr, Knopman DS, Jagust WJ, Petersen RC, Weiner MW, Aisen PS, et al. Tracking pathophysiological processes in Alzheimer's disease: an updated hypothetical model of dynamic biomarkers. *Lancet Neurol* February 2013;**12**(2):207–16.
54. Koronyo-Hamaoui M, Koronyo Y, Ljubimov AV, Miller CA, Ko MK, Black KL, et al. Identification of amyloid plaques in retinas from Alzheimer's patients and noninvasive in vivo optical imaging of retinal plaques in a mouse model. *NeuroImage* January 2011;**54** Suppl 1:S204–217.
55. Cronin-Golomb A, Rizzo JF, Corkin S, Growdon JH. Visual function in Alzheimer's disease and normal aging. *Ann N Y Acad Sci* 1991;**640**:28–35.
56. Rizzo JF 3rd, Cronin-Golomb A, Growdon JH, Corkin S, Rosen TJ, Sandberg MA, et al. Retinocalcarine function in Alzheimer's disease. A clinical and electrophysiological study. *Arch Neurol* January 1992;**49**(1):93–101.
57. Hinton DR, Sadun AA, Blanks JC, Miller CA. Optic-nerve degeneration in Alzheimer's disease. *N Engl J Med* August 21, 1986;**315**(8):485–7.
58. Blanks JC, Torigoe Y, Hinton DR, Blanks RH. Retinal pathology in Alzheimer's disease. I. Ganglion cell loss in foveal/parafoveal retina. *Neurobiol Aging* June 1996;**17**(3):377–84.
59. Sadun AA, Bassi CJ. Optic nerve damage in Alzheimer's disease. *Ophthalmology* January 1990;**97**(1):9–17.
60. Curcio CA, Drucker DN. Retinal ganglion cells in Alzheimer's disease and aging. *Ann Neurol* March 1993;**33**(3):248–57.
61. Davies DC, McCoubrie P, McDonald B, Jobst KA. Myelinated axon number in the optic nerve is unaffected by Alzheimer's disease. *Br J Ophthalmol* June 1995;**79**(6):596–600.
62. Justino L, Kergoat M, Bergman H, Chertkow H, Robillard A, Kergoat H. Neuroretinal function is normal in early dementia of the Alzheimer type. *Neurobiol Aging* August 2001;**22**(4):691–5.
63. Danesh-Meyer HV, Birch H, Ku JY-F, Carroll S, Gamble G. Reduction of optic nerve fibers in patients with Alzheimer disease identified by laser imaging. *Neurology* November 28, 2006;**67**(10):1852–4.
64. Kergoat H, Kergoat MJ, Justino L, Robillard A, Bergman H, Chertkow H. Normal optic nerve head topography in the early stages of dementia of the Alzheimer type. *Dement Geriatr Cogn Disord* December 2001;**12**(6):359–63.
65. Kergoat H, Kergoat MJ, Justino L, Chertkow H, Robillard A, Bergman H. An evaluation of the

retinal nerve fiber layer thickness by scanning laser polarimetry in individuals with dementia of the Alzheimer type. *Acta Ophthalmol Scand* April 2001;**79**(2):187–91.

66. Kergoat H, Kergoat M-J, Justino L, Chertkow H, Robillard A, Bergman H. Visual retinocortical function in dementia of the Alzheimer type. *Gerontology* August 2002;**48**(4):197–203.

67. Iseri PK, Altinaş O, Tokay T, Yüksel N. Relationship between cognitive impairment and retinal morphological and visual functional abnormalities in Alzheimer disease. *J Neuro-Ophthalmol Off J North Am Neuro-Ophthalmol Soc* March 2006;**26**(1):18–24.

68. Paquet C, Boissonnot M, Roger F, Dighiero P, Gil R, Hugon J. Abnormal retinal thickness in patients with mild cognitive impairment and Alzheimer's disease. *Neurosci Lett* June 2007;**420**(2):97–9.

69. Lu Y, Li Z, Zhang X, Ming B, Jia J, Wang R, et al. Retinal nerve fiber layer structure abnormalities in early Alzheimer's disease: evidence in optical coherence tomography. *Neurosci Lett* August 9, 2010;**480**(1):69–72.

70. Berisha F, Feke GT, Trempe CL, McMeel JW, Schepens CL. Retinal abnormalities in early Alzheimer's disease. *Invest Ophthalmol Vis Sci* May 2007;**48**(5):2285–9.

71. Kirbas S, Turkyilmaz K, Anlar O, Tufekci A, Durmus M. Retinal nerve fiber layer thickness in patients with Alzheimer disease. *J Neuro-Ophthalmol Off J North Am Neuro-Ophthalmol Soc* March 2013;**33**(1):58–61.

72. Bayer AU, Ferrari F, Erb C. High occurrence rate of glaucoma among patients with Alzheimer's disease. *Eur Neurol* 2002;**47**(3):165–8.

73. Helmer C, Malet F, Rougier M-B, Schweitzer C, Colin J, Delyfer M-N, et al. Is there a link between open-angle glaucoma and dementia? The 3C-alienor cohort. *Ann Neurol* May 18, 2013;

74. Bock M, Brandt AU, Dörr J, Kraft H, Weinges-Evers N, Gaede G, et al. Patterns of retinal nerve fiber layer loss in multiple sclerosis patients with or without optic neuritis and glaucoma patients. *Clin Neurol Neurosurg* October 2010;**112**(8):647–52.

75. Dörr J1, Radbruch H, Bock M, Wuerfel J, Brüggemann A, Wandinger KP, Zeise D, Pfueller CF, Zipp F, Paul F. Encephalopathy, visual disturbance and hearing loss-recognizing the symptoms of Susac syndrome. *Nat Rev Neurol* December 2009;**5**(12):683–8. doi: 10.1038/nrneurol.2009.176.

76. Dörr J, Krautwald S, Wildemann B, Jarius S, Ringelstein M, Duning T, et al. Characteristics of Susac syndrome: a review of all reported cases. *Nat Rev Neurol* June 2013;**9**(6):307–16.

77. Brandt AU, Zimmermann H, Kaufhold F, Promesberger J, Schippling S, Finis D, et al. Patterns of retinal damage facilitate differential diagnosis between Susac syndrome and MS. *PloS One* 2012;7(6):e38741.

78. Scott CJ, Kardon RH, Lee AG, Frisén L, Wall M. Diagnosis and grading of papilledema in patients with raised intracranial pressure using optical coherence tomography vs clinical expert assessment using a clinical staging scale. *Arch Ophthalmol* June 2010;**128**(6):705–11.

79. Kaufhold F, Kadas EM, Schmidt C, Kunte H, Hoffmann J, Zimmermann H, et al. Optic nerve head quantification in idiopathic intracranial hypertension by spectral domain OCT. *PloS One* 2012;7(5):e36965.

80. Wang J-K, Kardon RH, Kupersmith MJ, Garvin MK. Automated quantification of volumetric optic disc swelling in papilledema using spectral-domain optical coherence tomography. *Invest Ophthalmol Vis Sci* June 2012;**53**(7):4069–75.

81. Carelli V, Ross-Cisneros FN, Sadun AA. Optic nerve degeneration and mitochondrial dysfunction: genetic and acquired optic neuropathies. *Neurochem Int* May 2002;**40**(6):573–84.

82. Carelli V, Ross-Cisneros FN, Sadun AA. Mitochondrial dysfunction as a cause of optic neuropathies. *Prog Retin Eye Res* January 2004;**23**(1):53–89.

83. Harding AE. Friedreich's ataxia: a clinical and genetic study of 90 families with an analysis of early diagnostic criteria and intrafamilial clustering of clinical features. *Brain J Neurol* September 1981;**104**(3):589–620.

84. Fortuna F, Barboni P, Liguori R, Valentino ML, Savini G, Gellera C, et al. Visual system involvement in patients with Friedreich's ataxia. *Brain J Neurol* January 2009;**132**(Pt 1):116–23.

85. Alldredge CD, Schlieve CR, Miller NR, Levin LA. Pathophysiology of the optic neuropathy associated with Friedreich ataxia. *Arch Ophthalmol* November 2003;**121**(11):1582–5.

86. Noval S, Contreras I, Sanz-Gallego I, Manrique RK, Arpa J. Ophthalmic features of Friedreich ataxia. *Eye Lond Engl* February 2012;**26**(2):315–20.

87. Seyer LA, Galetta K, Wilson J, Sakai R, Perlman S, Mathews K, et al. Analysis of the visual system in Friedreich ataxia. *J Neurol* June 18, 2013;

88. Klockgether T. The clinical diagnosis of autosomal dominant spinocerebellar ataxias. *Cerebellum Lond Engl* 2008;7(2):101–5.

89. Stricker S, Oberwahrenbrock T, Zimmermann H, Schroeter J, Endres M, Brandt AU, et al. Temporal retinal nerve fiber loss in patients with spinocerebellar ataxia Type 1. *PLoS ONE* July 29, 2011;**6**(7):e23024.

90. Pula JH, Towle VL, Staszak VM, Cao D, Bernard JT, Gomez CM. Retinal nerve fibre layer and macular thinning in spinocerebellar ataxia and cerebellar multisystem atrophy. *Neuro-Ophthalmol Aeolus Press* Jun 2011;**35**(3):108–14.

91. Manrique RK, Noval S, Aguilar-Amat MJ, Arpa J, Rosa I, Contreras I. Ophthalmic features of spinocerebellar ataxia type 7. *J Neuro-Ophthalmol Off J North Am Neuro-Ophthalmol Soc* September 2009;**29**(3):174–9.

92. Hugosson T, Gränse L, Ponjavic V, Andréasson S. Macular dysfunction and morphology in spinocerebellar ataxia type 7 (SCA 7). *Ophthalmic Genet.* March 2009;**30**(1):1–6.

93. Miller RC, Tewari A, Miller JA, Garbern J, Van Stavern GP. Neuro-ophthalmologic features of spinocerebellar ataxia type 7. *J Neuro-Ophthalmol Off J North Am Neuro-Ophthalmol Soc* September 2009;**29**(3):180–6.

94. Bouchard JP, Barbeau A, Bouchard R, Bouchard RW. Autosomal recessive spastic ataxia of Charlevoix-Saguenay. *Can J Neurol Sci J Can Sci Neurol* February 1978;**5**(1):61–9.

95. Vingolo EM, Di Fabio R, Salvatore S, Grieco G, Bertini E, Leuzzi V, et al. Myelinated retinal fibers in autosomal recessive spastic ataxia of Charlevoix-Saguenay. *Eur J Neurol Off J Eur Fed Neurol Soc* September 2011;**18**(9):1187–90.

96. Desserre J, Devos D, Sautière BG, Debruyne P, Santorelli FM, Vuillaume I, et al. Thickening of peripapillar retinal fibers for the diagnosis of autosomal recessive spastic ataxia of Charlevoix-Saguenay. *Cerebellum Lond Engl* December 2011;**10**(4):758–62.

97. Garcia-Martin E, Pablo LE, Gazulla J, Polo V, Ferreras A, Larrosa JM. Retinal nerve fibre layer thickness in ARSACS: myelination or hypertrophy? *Br J Ophthalmol* February 2013;**97**(2):238–41.

98. Blackstone C, O'Kane CJ, Reid E. Hereditary spastic paraplegias: membrane traffic and the motor pathway. *Nat Rev Neurosci* January 2011;**12**(1):31–42.

99. Carelli V, La Morgia C, Valentino ML, Barboni P, Ross-Cisneros FN, Sadun AA. Retinal ganglion cell neurodegeneration in mitochondrial inherited disorders. *Biochim Biophys Acta* May 2009;**1787**(5):518–28.

100. Wiethoff S, Zhour A, Schöls L, Fischer MD. Retinal nerve fibre layer loss in hereditary spastic paraplegias is restricted to complex phenotypes. *BMC Neurol* 2012;**12**:143.

101. Roth NM, Saidha S, Zimmermann H, Brandt AU, Oberwahrenbrock T, Maragakis NJ, et al. Optical coherence tomography does not support optic nerve involvement in amyotrophic lateral sclerosis. *Eur J Neurol Off J Eur Fed Neurol Soc* April 14, 2013;

102. Ala A, Walker AP, Ashkan K, Dooley JS, Schilsky ML. Wilson's disease. *Lancet* February 3, 2007;**369** (9559):397–408.

103. Satishchandra P, Ravishankar Naik K. Visual pathway abnormalities Wilson's disease: an electrophysiological study using electroretinography and visual evoked potentials. *J Neurol Sci* May 1, 2000;**176**(1):13–20.

104. Albrecht P, Müller A-K, Ringelstein M, Finis D, Geerling G, Cohn E, et al. Retinal neurodegeneration in Wilson's disease revealed by spectral domain optical coherence tomography. *PloS One* 2012;7(11): e49825.

105. Parikh RS, Parikh SR, Sekhar GC, Prabakaran S, Babu JG, Thomas R. Normal Age-Related Decay of Retinal Nerve Fiber Layer Thickness. *Ophthalmology* May 2007;**114**(5):921–6.

106. Alamouti B, Funk J. Retinal thickness decreases with age: an OCT study. *Br J Ophthalmol* July 2003;**87**(7):899–901.

107. Ooto S, Hangai M, Tomidokoro A, Saito H, Araie M, Otani T, et al. Effects of age, sex, and axial length on the three-dimensional profile of normal macular layer structures. *Invest Ophthalmol Vis Sci* 2011;**52**(12):8769–79.

108. Rudnicka AR, Mt-Isa S, Owen CG, Cook DG, Ashby D. Variations in primary open-angle glaucoma prevalence by age, gender, and race: a Bayesian meta-analysis. *Invest Ophthalmol Vis Sci* October 2006;**47**(10):4254–61.

109. Quigley HA, Broman AT. The number of people with glaucoma worldwide in 2010 and 2020. *Br J Ophthalmol* March 2006;**90**(3):262–7.

110. Varma R, Ying-Lai M, Francis BA, Nguyen BB-T, Deneen J, Wilson MR, et al. Prevalence of open-angle glaucoma and ocular hypertension in Latinos: the Los Angeles Latino Eye Study. *Ophthalmology* August 2004;**111**(8):1439–48.

111. Tewarie P, Balk L, Costello F, Green A, Martin R, Schippling S, et al. The OSCAR-IB Consensus Criteria for Retinal OCT Quality Assessment. *PLoS ONE* April 19, 2012;7(4):e34823.

112. Petzold A, Wattjes MP, Costello F, Flores-Rivera J, Fraser CL, Fujihara K, et al. The investigation of acute optic neuritis: a review and proposed protocol. *Nat Rev Neurol* August 2014;**10**(8):447–58. doi: 10.1038/nrneurol.2014.108. Epub Jul 8, 2014.

Chapter 12

Optical coherence tomography pathologies to know about in clinical practice

Scott D. Newsome and John N. Ratchford

Introduction

In neurology, OCT has primarily been used as a research tool to quantitatively assess the peripapillary retinal nerve fiber layer (RNFL) and macular volume in patients with inflammatory optic neuropathies and demyelinating disorders. However, more recently OCT is being used in neurology clinical practices to help aid with specific neurological diagnoses (i.e., optic neuritis vs. macular disease) and determine to what extent an individual's anterior visual pathway is structurally compromised (as in multiple sclerosis or neuromyelitis optica). Neurologists utilizing OCT for research and clinical purposes should be aware of the more common retinal abnormalities that may be detected, many of which will be reviewed in this chapter. These incidental findings are important to recognize since detailed ophthalmologic evaluation may be warranted to further characterize these abnormalities; this differential of optic nerve vs. retinal disease is one of the most important potential uses of OCT in neurological practice.

Epiretinal membrane

Epiretinal membranes (ERM), also known as macular pucker, typically occur as a response to changes within the vitreous humor and proliferation of glial tissue within the RNFL [1]. The underlying retinal structures are affected by traction forces from ERM and appear thicker than the normal fellow eyes [2]. Macular degeneration usually does not occur with ERM because photoreceptor, rod, and cone cells are not damaged. However, in rare instances the ERM can become very thick and hard, resulting in damage to these cells.

On OCT, an ERM can be identified as a thin hyperreflective band that lies between the vitreous and retina (Figure 12.1). This is one of the more common findings on OCT, especially in older populations. Cystic-like gaps between the RNFL and inner limiting membrane (ILM) often occur with ERM (Figure 12.2) [1]. In addition, ERM often accompanies a posterior vitreous detachment.

Common predisposing factors for ERM include aging and diabetes. Even though ERM does not

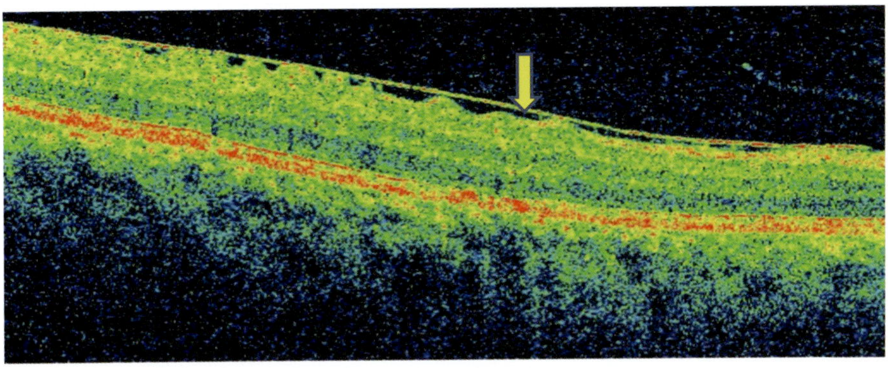

Figure 12.1 OCT image of a patient with a simple epiretinal membrane (arrow).

Optical Coherence Tomography in Neurological Disease, ed. Peter A. Calabresi, Laura J. Balcer, and Elliot M. Frohman. Published by Cambridge University Press.

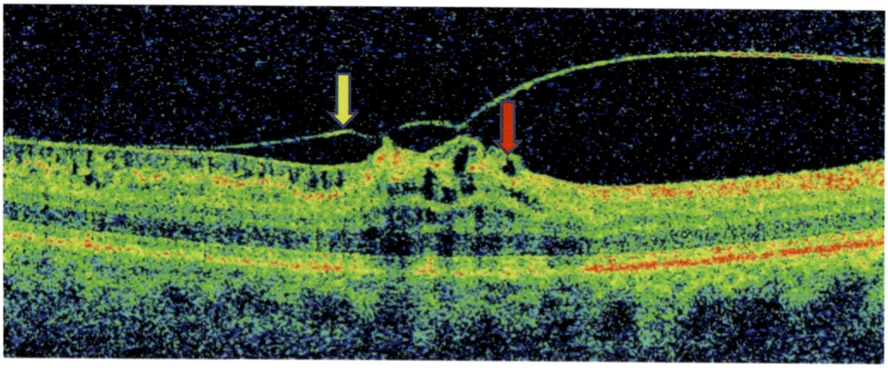

Figure 12.2 OCT image of a patient with an epiretinal membrane (yellow arrow) with cystic gaps (red arrow) and vitreomacular traction.

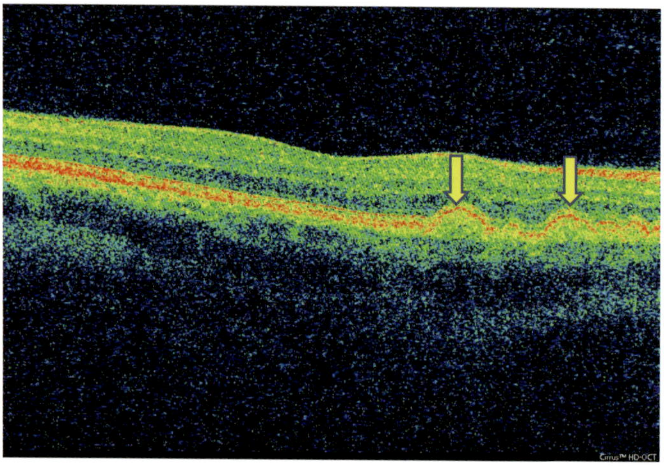

Figure 12.3 OCT images of a patient with retinal drusen (arrow).

threaten vision loss, in severe cases it can cause a decrease in visual acuity and metamorphopsia (i.e., distorted vision). Surgical intervention is usually not warranted in ERM unless visual symptoms are impeding individuals' daily activities.

Drusen

Drusen typically occur in eyes due to accumulations of extracellular substances between Bruch's membrane and the retinal pigment epithelium (RPE) [3]. It is suspected that drusen decrease oxygen and nutrients to the RPE and photoreceptor cells, which in turn leads to the pathologies discussed in the paragraph below.

Drusen most commonly occur with aging and, when severe, are associated with macular degeneration. Rarely, drusen are related to dominant familial drusen, which is a comparatively benign condition. In contrast, the presence of large, soft, and numerous drusen appear to increase an individual's risk for progressing more rapidly to advanced age-related macular degeneration (AMD) and is an early clinical manifestation of AMD [3–5]. Age-related drusen are distinct from optic disc drusen, which result in calcific degeneration in some of the axons of the optic nerve. Both of these entities can be seen via ophthalmoscopy and visualized with OCT.

On OCT, retinal drusen are visualized as hyperreflective protuberances underneath the RPE layer (Figure 12.3). The retinal tissue can be displaced if the drusen are large enough. Optic disc drusen can displace the RNFL, which can be associated with a thickening of the disc tissue (Figure 12.4).

Most patients with drusen are asymptomatic; however, it can mimic symptoms of papilledema and is associated with AMD [6, 7]. Optic disc drusen can ultimately lead to loss of visual field due to displacement of the nerve fiber layers. OCT is a useful tool to monitor the progression of drusen over time.

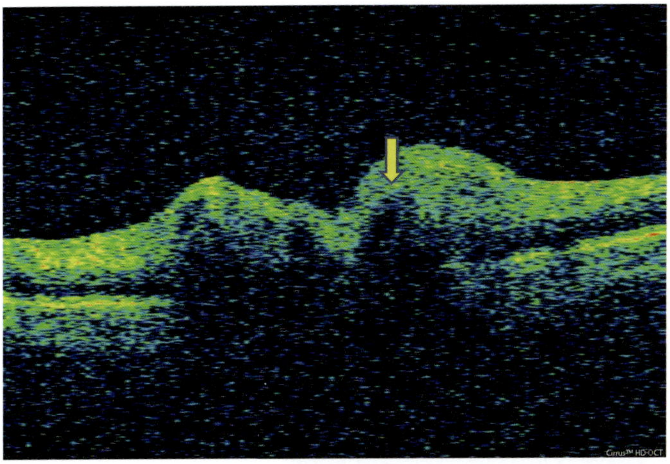

Figure 12.4 OCT images of a patient with optic disc drusen (arrow).

Central serous chorioretinopathy

Central serous chorioretinopathy (CSR) develops when a leakage of fluid occurs in the subretinal space or in conjunction with a pigment epithelium detachment (PED). This fluid leakage is thought to develop due to dysfunction of the RPE and/or choroid. Fluid accumulation can involve the central macula which can ultimately lead to vision loss that mimics acute optic neuritis.

CSR is most commonly seen in young and middle-aged patients, with a higher proportion of men being affected. The majority of CSR cases are idiopathic in nature; however, there are several potential triggering factors. Specifically, previous studies have noted that stress, Cushing's syndrome, corticosteroid therapy, and anti-anxiety medications are independent risk factors for developing CSR [8–10].

CSR is best detected by OCT and fluorescein angiography. On OCT, CSR is identified as subretinal clear fluid accumulation in the macular region, which leads to elevation of the retinal layers above (Figure 12.5). If the RPE is intact then there is a hyperreflective band at the base of the fluid cavity (Figure 12.5). However, if the RPE is detached then a hyperreflective band is seen over the fluid cavity (Figure 12.6).

The majority of patients with CSR will experience some form of visual disturbance. It can be acute in onset with a visual acuity as severe as 20/200 with accompanying central and paracentral relative scotomas. An urgent evaluation is needed to rule out retinal detachment, which requires a detailed ophthalmological evaluation, including OCT. However, upon resolution of the subretinal fluid collection, visual acuity can improve almost back to patients' pre-CSR baseline, although some individuals will have permanent impaired night vision, color desaturation, metamorphosis, and poor contrast sensitivity [11] CSR can reoccur, resulting in progressive vision loss, and can be associated with subretinal neovascularization and pigment epitheliopathy.

CSR treatment should be considered if it has not spontaneously resolved in a few months and especially if an individual is still symptomatic. The therapy chosen depends on whether there is fluid leakage into the central macula. Laser photocoagulation is done if the CSR is distant from the central macula because of risk for causing permanent central vision loss with this treatment. In CSR cases involving or within close proximity of the central macula, transpupillary thermotherapy is preferred [12]. There are other treatments that demonstrate promise with minimal complications that are becoming more popular [13].

Pigment epithelium detachment

Pigment epithelium detachment (PED) occurs when there is disruption of the normal junction between the basement membrane of the RPE and Bruch's membrane. Subretinal fluid accumulates from the choriocapillaries, resulting in PED. This fluid collection and the resultant separation of membranes can also occur in conjunction with a CSR and retinal detachment.

PEDs are most commonly seen in males between the ages of 20 and 60 years. There are several conditions

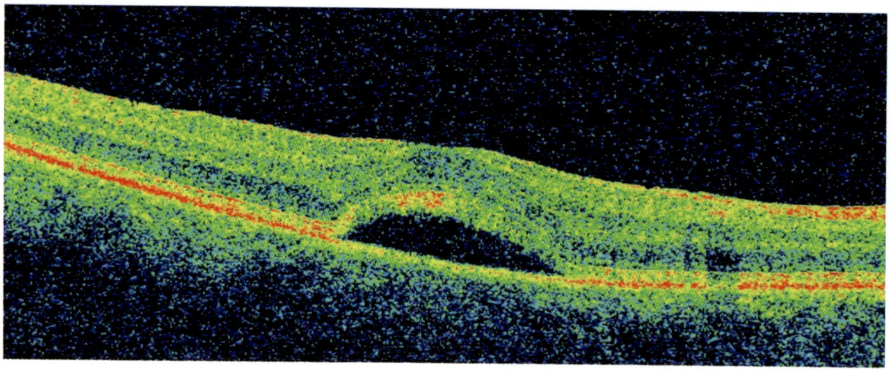

Figure 12.5 OCT image of a patient with central serous chorioretinopathy.

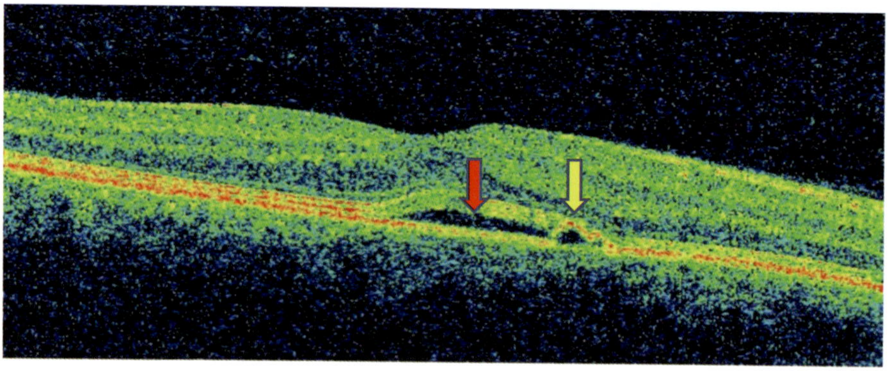

Figure 12.6 OCT image of a patient with central serous chorioretinopathy (red arrow) with retinal pigment epithelium detachment (yellow arrow).

that predispose individuals to developing PEDs, including AMD, choroidal tumors, high myopia, choroidal neovascular membranes (CNM), ocular histoplasmosis, and hereditary choroidal degeneration [14]. In some cases, PEDs are idiopathic in nature. However, in clinical practice PEDs are mostly seen in association with eyes that are treated for neovascular AMD [15].

PEDs can be seen ophthalmoscopically in the posterior fundus, although they are best visualized with fluorescein angiography and OCT. On OCT, PEDs appear as a dome-shaped elevation with a hyperreflective red band overlying the dome (Figure 12.7). The PED causes shadowing of the choroid below, which is not seen in CSR without accompanying PED.

The majority of patients are < 55 years old with PED present with small detachments that are not associated with other chorio-retinal disease processes. In these cases, the prognosis is excellent and the patient requires no specific intervention, especially if the fovea is not involved. If the fovea is involved patients may report blurred vision, visual distortion, micropsia, or metamorphopsia [14]. In older patients with PED that does not have accompanying CNM, close monitoring is required because these membranes can develop, resulting in significant visual impairment, including loss of central vision and less than 20/200 visual acuity [16]. Older patients with PEDs that are associated with CNM have a poor visual prognosis; therefore, focal laser photocoagulation therapy is warranted in these patients. Serious retinal detachments will often occur concurrently with PEDs which requires treating the underlying precipitating disease process.

Macular edema

Macular edema occurs when deposits of protein and fluid accumulate within or under the macula. The macula is located near the center of the retina, where the cones are located, which become affected with macular edema.

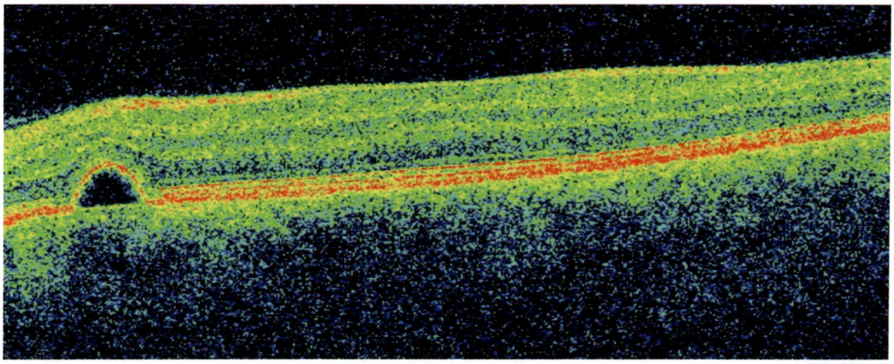

Figure 12.7 OCT image of a patient with pigment epithelium detachment.

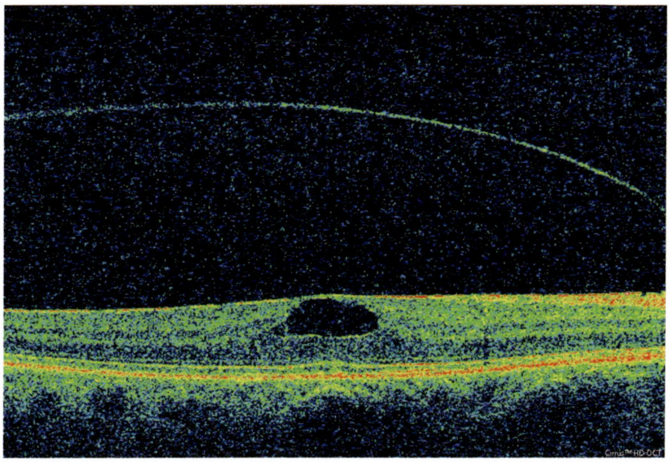

Figure 12.8 OCT image of a patient with macular edema.

There are two main categories of macular edema: cystoid macular edema and diabetic macular edema. Both types appear to occur due to abnormal retinal/macular capillary permeability. There are several causes of cystoid macular edema, including diabetes, pars planitis, specific medications (i.e., fingolimod), post-cataract or retinal detachment surgery, retinitis pigmentosa, and venous occlusion, among other causes. Diabetic macular edema leads to the most common cause of vision loss in diabetic retinopathy.

Macular edema is well visualized on OCT. On OCT, macular edema results in thickening of the retina and loss of the normal foveal contour, which is best seen on the macular tomograms (Figure 12.8). Continued intraretinal fluid accumulation eventually leads to the visible cystic spaces in cystic macular edema.

The presence of macular edema from any cause can result in central vision distortion. The initial symptoms of macular edema can manifest as just blurred vision or result in severe central vision loss. Colors can also appear altered or washed out. Peripheral vision is spared with macular edema, which in combination with central vision loss and changes in color can be mistaken as acute optic neuritis.

The treatment for macular edema varies depending on the cause and severity of the condition. The primary goal of treating macular edema in diabetic patients is to stabilize their vision with focal laser treatment. This treatment seals off the leaky blood vessels that are causing disruption in macular function. More recently, novel medications, including anti-VEGF, are being used to help slow the leakage and growth of abnormal blood vessels [17]. Cystoid macular edema may need nonsteroidal anti-inflammatory or steroid eye drops and, in more refractory cases, intraocular steroid injections, vitrectomy, or lens replacement.

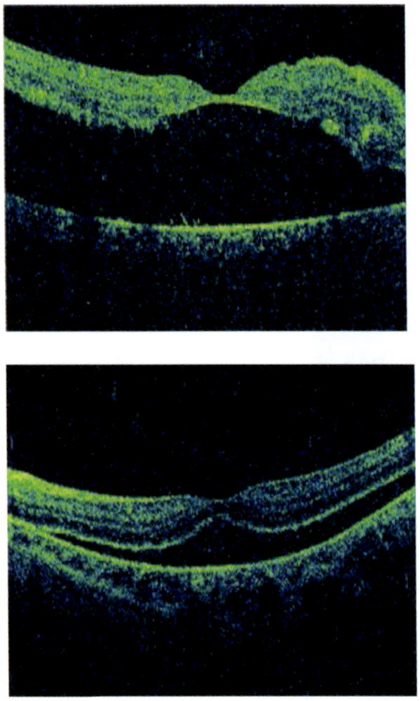

Figure 12.9 OCT images of the macula in two patients with rhegmatogenous retinal detachments. Vitreous fluid is present in the subretinal space [30].

Retinal detachment

Retinal detachment occurs when the neurosensory retina separates from the retinal pigment epithelium (RPE). This separation creates a potential space where subretinal fluid accumulates. There are several types of retinal detachment: rhegmatogenous, serous, and traction.

A rhegmatogenous retinal detachment occurs when a full thickness retinal break allows vitreous fluid to access the subretinal space. It will typically present with photopsias, floaters, a curtain across the visual field, or decreased visual acuity, or it could rarely be asymptomatic. OCT will show a hyporeflective dark space under the neurosensory retina (Figure 12.9). A rhegmatogenous retinal detachment is treated with urgent surgery (within 24 hours if central vision is threatened), so if there is a suspicion of this, urgent referral to a retina specialist is recommended.

A serous retinal detachment is caused by subretinal transudation of fluid without a retinal break. Fluid can be from an inflammatory condition, vascular lesion, tumor, or degenerative process. Predisposing conditions include Vogt–Koyanagi–Harada syndrome, Harada's disease, idiopathic uveal effusion syndrome, choroidal tumors, central serous retinopathy, posterior scleritis, hypertensive retinopathy, Coats' disease, optic nerve pit, retinal coloboma, and toxemia of pregnancy [18]. A serous retinal detachment can be asymptomatic until it involves the macula. Symptoms include photopsias, floaters, a curtain across the visual field, or decreased vision. OCT will show a fluid collection between the neurosensory retina and the RPE without a break in the retina (Figure 12.10). This may manifest as an area of elevated macular thickness when the macula is involved. Treatment is focused on the underlying cause, and surgery is usually not needed.

A traction retinal detachment occurs when a fibrotic proliferation causes the retina to pull off of the RPE without evidence of a retinal break. Predisposing etiologies include diabetic retinopathy, sickle cell retinopathy, retinopathy of prematurity, venous occlusions, proliferative vitreoretinopathy, toxocariasis, and familial exudative vitreoretinopathy.[18] When a traction retinal detachment involves the macula, symptoms are similar to other types of retinal detachment. Though often managed conservatively, surgery is considered if it threatens the macula.

Posterior vitreous detachment and vitreomacular traction syndrome

A posterior vitreous detachment occurs when the vitreous separates from the retina throughout the peripheral fundus but remains adherent to it posteriorly. This can produce traction on the region containing the macula and optic nerve. This syndrome is called vitreomacular traction syndrome. Vitreomacular traction is believed to contribute to multiple macular diseases, including cystoid macular edema and macular holes [19]. Vitreomacular traction syndrome is almost invariably accompanied by an epiretinal membrane, suggesting that the membrane contributes to the pathogenesis (Figure 12.11) [20].

The individual OCT findings of the various manifestations of vitreomacular traction syndrome are described individually below. OCT is used by ophthalmologists to evaluate the macula in detail in order to determine the type of maculopathy in vitreomacular traction syndrome.

Macular hole

A macular hole is a full-thickness hole in the retina that involves the fovea. It can be distinguished clinically from a macular pseudohole or lamellar hole by

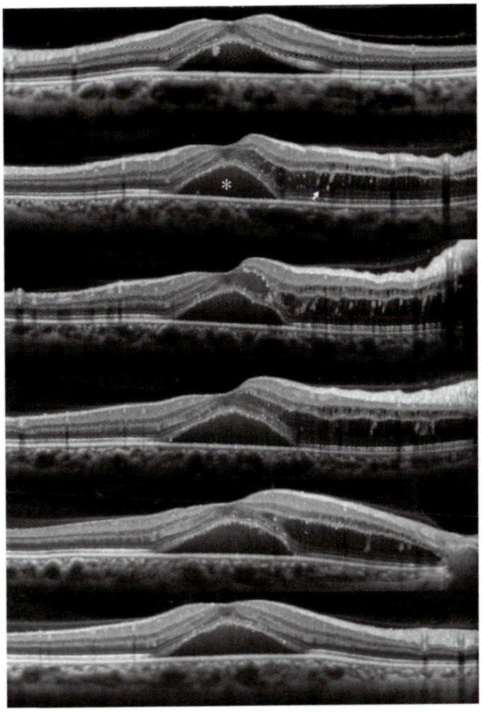

Figure 12.10 OCT image of a patient with serous retinal detachment

the presence of significant central vision loss and by other testing methods such the Watzke-Allen and laser aiming beam tests.

Macular holes are often idiopathic, but risk factors include cystoid macular edema, vitreomacular traction, inflammation, trauma, ocular surgery, and laser treatment [18]. Presenting symptoms typically include a sudden-onset metamorphopsia (i.e., abnormal Amsler grid test), decreased vision, and, less commonly, central scotoma.

An isolated foveal cyst can be seen as an early stage of the development of a macular hole (Figure 12.12). With a macular hole, OCT will typically show a full-thickness retinal defect involving the fovea on a macular scan (Figure 12.13). Treatment depends on the severity of the hole and visual defect. An impending hole is followed conservatively, but more significant macular holes are typically treated by a retina specialist with vitrectomy, detachment of the posterior vitreous cortex, peeling of any epiretinal membrane around the hole, gas–fluid exchange, and postoperative prone positioning [21, 22].

Macular pseudoholes

A macular pseudohole can resemble a full-thickness macular hole clinically, but it does not have loss of foveal tissue (Figure 12.14). The pathogenesis is different, because these lesions have been attributed to the centripetal contraction of a surrounding epiretinal membrane. Since they appear similar to lamellar macular holes on biomicroscopy, OCT can help distinguish the two entities. Vision typically remains relatively good with macular pseudoholes.

On OCT, pseudoholes are found to have a steepened foveal pit with thickened edges contracted by an epiretinal membrane, reduced foveal pit diameter, and normal or slightly increased central foveal thickness [23]. Most pseudoholes are followed conservatively [24].

Lamellar macular hole

The term *lamellar macular hole* was first used to describe a macular lesion resulting from the opening of the central cyst of a cystoid macular edema [25]. This term is also used to describe a macular lesion that results from the same process that leads to a full-thickness macular hole when the process does not go to completion. By definition, a lamellar macular hole is a partial thickness macular hole where the inner layers of the fovea are detached from the underlying cellular layers of the fovea (Figure 12.15). Patients with lamellar holes have relatively well-preserved vision, and the macula contains a round, well-circumscribed reddish lesion [26].

Proposed OCT criteria for diagnosis of a lamellar hole include an irregular foveal contour, a break in the inner fovea separation of the inner from the outer foveal retinal layers leading to an intraretinal split, and absence of a full-thickness foveal defect with intact photoreceptors posterior to the area of foveal dehiscence [26]. OCT will show a high central foveal thickness. Epiretinal membranes are present in 50–89% of lamellar macular holes [26, 27], suggesting that they may be involved in the pathogenesis of some lamellar macular holes. Many patients are followed conservatively, but surgery with vitrectomy and epiretinal membrane peeling has also been used with success [28, 29].

Conclusion

OCT is becoming more widely used by neurologists in clinical practice for the evaluation of suspected or established neurological disease. This technology is

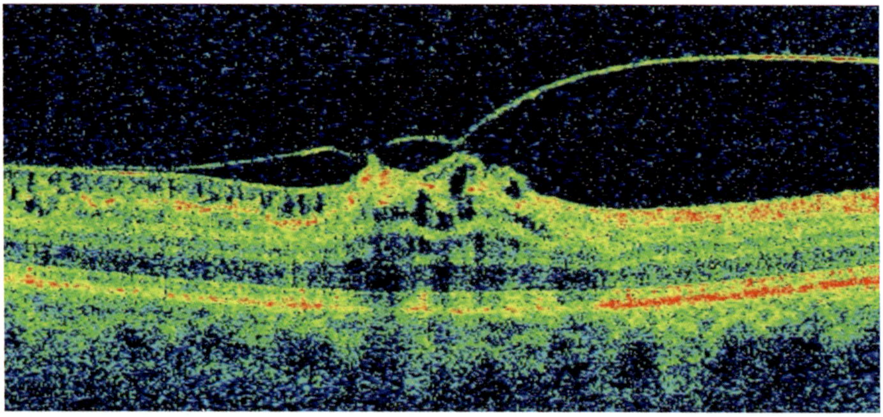

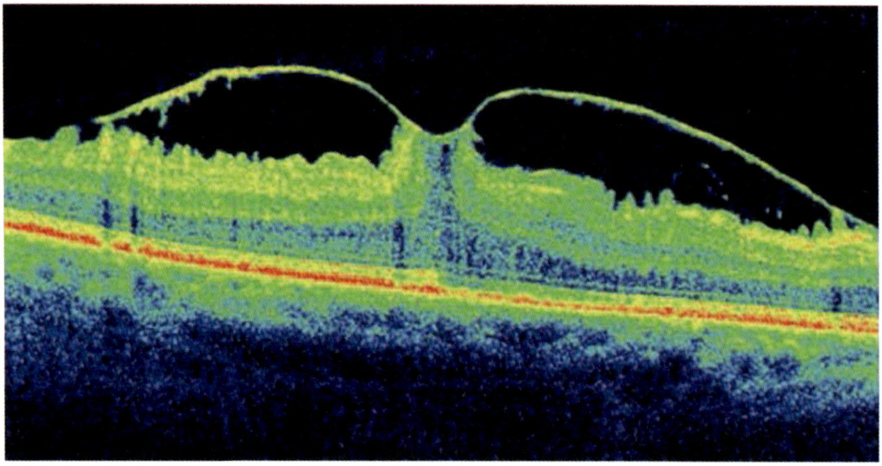

Figure 12.11 Two examples of vitreomacular traction with associated epiretinal membranes. [31, 32]

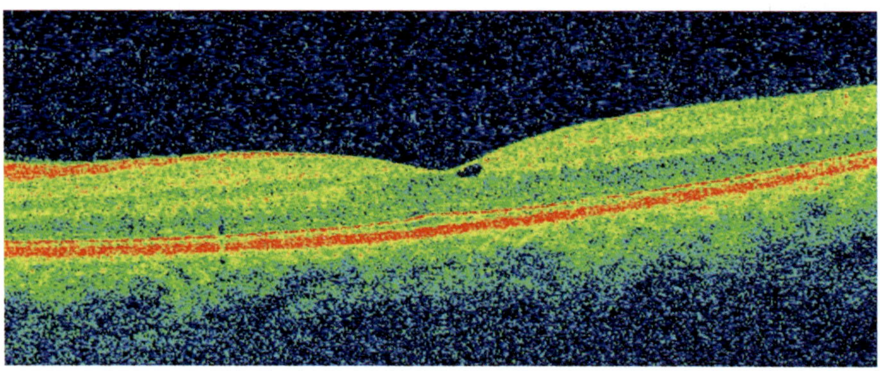

Figure 12.12 OCT image of a patient with a foveal cyst. [31]

generating great interest in clinical practice because it is noninvasive, relatively inexpensive, and quickly acquires quantitative information that has structure-function correlations.

It is crucial for neurologists using OCT to be aware of the common qualitative retinal abnormalities that can be detected with these devices. More importantly, neurologists need to know which incidental findings

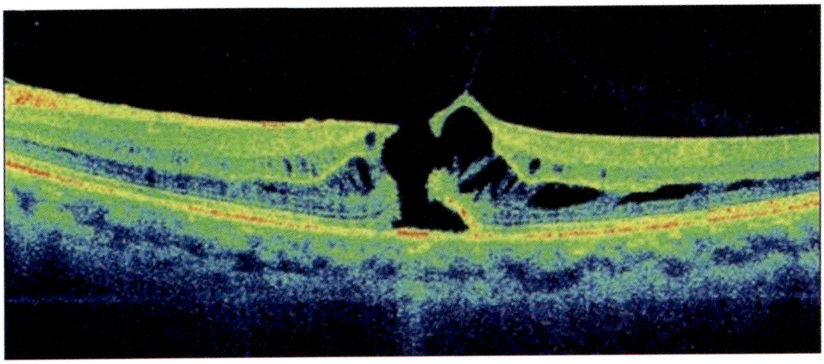

Figure 12.13 OCT image of a patient with a macular hole. [32]

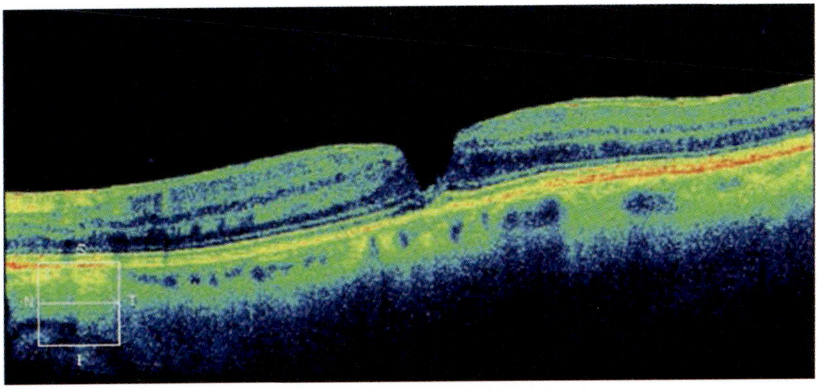

Figure 12.14 OCT image of a patient with a macular pseudohole with a steepened foveal contour. [32]

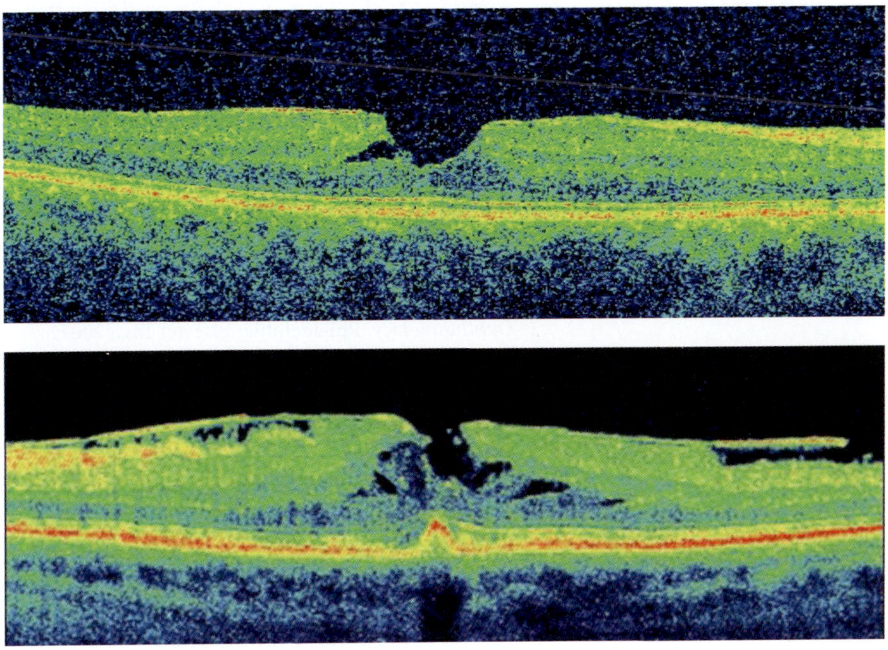

Figure 12.15 OCT image of two examples of lamellar macular holes. [31, 32]

Table 12.1 Common retinal abnormalities needing ophthalmological/retinal referral

Complicated epiretinal membrane
Central serous chorioretinopathy
Pigment epithelium detachment
Macular edema
Retinal detachment
Macular hole
Macular pseudohole
Lamellar macular hole
Any incidentally identified condition that may be associated with visual dysfunction

need appropriate referral to an ophthalmologist and/or retinal specialist (Table 12.1). Independent of these referrals, it is typically also recommended for patients with diseases that can affect the anterior visual pathway to undergo yearly ophthalmological evaluation as part of their general care. Moreover, thorough review of research OCT scans is vitally important since unexpected retinal pathologies can impact accurate data acquisition.

References

1. Reed B, Glabe D, and Yudcovitch L. Ocular Coherence Tomography Guide. *Faculty Scholarship* 2011; Paper 12.
2. Koo H, Rhim W, and Lee E. Morphologic and functional association of retinal layers beneath the epiretinal membrane with spectral-domain optical coherence tomography in eyes without photoreceptor abnormality. *Graefes Arch Clin Exp Ophthalmol* 2012; **250**: 491–8.
3. Garcia-Garcia J, Ruiz-Moreno J, Holm K, et al. Macular dysfunction in drusen maculopathy assessed with multifocal electroretinogram and optical coherence tomography. *Clinical Ophthalmology* 2013: **7**; 1303–9.
4. Klein R, Klein B, Tomany S, et al. Ten-Year incidence and progression of age-related maculopathy; The Beaver Dam Eye study. *Ophthalmology* 2002; **109**: 1767–79.
5. Klein R, Peto T, Bird A, et al. The Epidemiology of Age-Related Macular Degeneration. *Am J Ophthalmol* 2004; **137**: 486–95.
6. Sahin A, Cingü AK, Ari S, et al. Bilateral optic disc drusen mimicking papilledema. *J Clin Neurol* 2012; **8**(2): 151–4.
7. Kinori M, Moroz I, Zolf R, et al. Pseudopapilledema–optic disc drusen. *Harefuah* 2013; **152**(3): 154–7.
8. Carvalho-Recchia C, Yannuzzi L, Negra˜o S, et al. Corticosteroids and central serous chorioretinopathy. *Ophthalmology* 2002; **109**: 1834–7.
9. Tsai D-C, Chen S-J, Huang C-C, et al. Epidemiology of idiopathic central serous chorioretinopathy in Taiwan, 2001–2006: A population-based study. *PLoS ONE* 2013; **8**(6): e66858.
10. Haimovici R, Koh S, Gagnon D, et al. Risk factors for central serous chorioretinopathy: a case–control study. *Ophthalmology* 2004; **111**: 244–9.
11. Baran N, Gürlü V, and Esgin H. Long-term macular function in eyes with central serous chorioretinopathy. *Clinical and Experimental Ophthalmology* 2005; **33**: 369–72.
12. Wei SY and Yang CM. Transpupillary thermotherapy in the treatment of central serous chorioretinopathy. *Ophthalmic surgery, lasers & imaging* 2005; **36**(5): 412–5.
13. Karakus SH, Basarir B, Pinarci EY, et al. Long-term results of half-dose photodynamic therapy for chronic central serous chorioretinopathy with contrast sensitivity changes. *Eye* 2013; **27**: 612–20.
14. Zayit-Soudry S, Moroz I, and Loewenstein A. Retinal pigment epithelial detachment. *Surv Ophthalmol* 2007; **52**: 227–43.
15. Nagiel A, Bailey Freund K, et al. Mechanism of retinal pigment epithelium tear formation following intravitreal anti–vascular endothelial growth factor therapy revealed by spectral-domain optical coherence tomography. *Am J Ophthalmol* 2013 [Epub ahead of print].
16. Chang L and Sarraf D. Tears of the retinal pigment epithelium. *RETINA* 2007; **27**: 523–4.
17. Kiire CA, Porta M, and Chong V. Medical management for the prevention and treatment of diabetic macular edema. *Surv Ophthalmol* 2013; **58**(5): 459–65.
18. Friedman NJ and Kaiser PK. *Essentials of Ophthalmology*. Philadelphia: Elsevier Inc., 2007.
19. Shechtman DL and Dunbar MT. The expanding spectrum of vitreomacular traction. *Optometry* 2009; **80**: 681–7.
20. Smiddy W. Vitreomacular traction syndrome. In: Yanoff M., Duker J.S., eds. *Ophthalmology*. Third Ed. Philadelphia: Elsevier, Inc., 2009.
21. Kelly NE and Wendel RT. Vitreous surgery for idiopathic macular holes. Results of a pilot study. *Arch Ophthalmol* 1991; **109**: 654–9.
22. Wendel RT, Patel AC, Kelly NE, et al. Vitreous surgery for macular holes. *Ophthalmology* 1993; **100**: 1671–6.

23. Haouchine B, Massin P, Tadayoni R, et al. Diagnosis of macular pseudoholes and lamellar macular holes by optical coherence tomography. *Am J Ophthalmol* 2004; **138**: 732–9.

24. Garcia-Fernandez M, Navarro JC, Sanz AF, et al. Long-term evolution of idiopathic lamellar macular holes and macular pseudoholes. *Can J Ophthalmol* 2012; **47**: 442–7.

25. Gass JD. Lamellar macular hole: a complication of cystoid macular edema after cataract extraction: a clinicopathologic case report. *Trans Am Ophthalmol Soc* 1975; **73**: 231–50.

26. Witkin AJ, Ko TH, Fujimoto JG, et al. Redefining lamellar holes and the vitreomacular interface: an ultrahigh-resolution optical coherence tomography study. *Ophthalmology* 2006; **113**: 388–97.

27. Chen JC and Lee LR. Clinical spectrum of lamellar macular defects including pseudoholes and pseudocysts defined by optical coherence tomography. *Br J Ophthalmol* 2008; **92**: 1342–6.

28. Sanisoglu H, Elbay A, Sevim S, et al. Surgical therapy versus observation for lamellar macular hole: a retrospective comparison study. *Clin Ophthalmol* 2013; **7**: 1843–8.

29. Sun JP, Chen SN, Chuang CC, et al. Surgical treatment of lamellar macular hole secondary to epiretinal membrane. *Graefes Arch Clin Exp Ophthalmol* 2013 May 17 (Epub).

30. Huang C, Fu T, Zhang T, et al. Scleral buckling versus vitrectomy for macula-off rhegmatogenous retinal detachment as accessed with spectral-domain optical coherence tomography: a retrospective observational case series. *BMC Ophthalmol* 2013; **13**: 12.

31. Sotirchos ES, Vidal-Jordana A, Saidha S, et al. Unexpected retinal abnormalities detected upon evaluation for neurological disease. Abstract, presented at the 2013 American Committee for Treatment and Research in Multiple Sclerosis meeting, p. 47.

32. Yong SO and Lam WC. Differential diagnosis of macular holes and pseudoholes. *Retinal Physician* 2011; **8**: 30–4.

Chapter 13

Optical coherence tomography and retinal segmentation in neurological diseases

Elias S. Sotirchos and Shiv Saidha

Introduction

The advent of optical coherence tomography (OCT) has provided the ability to rapidly and noninvasively acquire micrometer-resolution cross-sectional or 3-D images of the retina. OCT has revolutionized the study, diagnosis, and monitoring of retinal disease by providing both qualitative (morphology) and quantitative (thickness and volume) information. The ability to easily and cost-effectively acquire images of a component of the central nervous system is especially attractive for neurologists and has spurred significant interest in the potential research and clinical applications of retinal imaging with OCT in neurological diseases. The main focus of interest in OCT in neurology has been on quantitative retinal measures, since neurological conditions are predominantly thought to be associated with atrophy of retinal structures rather than morphologic abnormalities, although emerging evidence suggests that qualitative aberrations may also occur in neurological disease.

OCT images are generated by scanning the retina with a beam of near-infrared light and analyzing the backscattered light, in a fashion analogous to ultrasonography [1]. Contrast between retinal layers is generated by differences in their optical properties, which result from their varying histological composition. High-reflectivity layers correspond to areas where retinal elements are arranged horizontally, such as the retinal nerve fiber layer (RNFL) and plexiform layers, whereas the nuclear layers exhibit relatively lower reflectivity [2]. In order to derive quantitative measures from OCT scans, post-acquisition processing is required and involves the identification of boundaries between areas of interest, thus allowing the partitioning of the acquired images into specific regions that may subsequently be measured; this process is known as *segmentation*. Furthermore, in the case of multiple adjacent cross-sectional images (i.e., B-scans), such as in the case of a macular cube scan, three-dimensional reconstructions can be created from the segmentation-derived boundaries by interpolating them to the unsampled areas between B-scans. The quantitative OCT measures that predominantly have been utilized include borders that can be easily and reliably detected due to significant differences in the reflectivity of tissues at their interface; these measures have mainly included the peripapillary retinal nerve fiber layer (RNFL) thickness and the average macular thickness or total macular volume.

Advances in segmentation algorithms and the development of modern, spectral-domain OCT that allows for the three-dimensional acquisition of ultra-high-resolution images have vastly expanded the potential of OCT by enabling the isolation of more specific regions of interest, including individual retinal layers. In contrast to gross quantitative measures, such as the average macular thickness, this refined approach generates quantitative information about specific neuronal and axonal subpopulations of the retina and provides the possibility of pinpointing specific retinal areas and structures that are differentially affected by disease processes. The study of these measures is currently an area of intensive research and holds promise for the development of novel biomarkers of neurological disease and for promoting our understanding of the pathological mechanisms underlying various neurological diseases.

Retinal layers and cell populations

The retina is structured in a multilayered fashion and is traditionally described as being composed of the

Optical Coherence Tomography in Neurological Disease, ed. Peter A. Calabresi, Laura J. Balcer, and Elliot M. Frohman. Published by Cambridge University Press.

following ten layers (beginning from the inner portion of the retina, i.e., closest to the vitreous):

1. **Inner limiting membrane (ILM):** This layer constitutes the boundary between the retina and the vitreous and is formed primarily by end-feet of the Müller cells, which are located in the inner nuclear layer.
2. **Retinal nerve fiber layer (RNFL):** This layer consists of unmyelinated axons of the ganglion cells that coalesce at the optic disc to form the optic nerve, which becomes myelinated posterior to the lamina cribrosa. In addition to the nerve fibers, fibrous astrocytes are present in the RNFL.
3. **Ganglion cell layer (GCL):** This layer contains primarily the cell bodies of the ganglion cells.
4. **Inner plexiform layer (IPL):** This layer contains the synaptic connections between ganglion cell dendrites, bipolar cell axons, and axons and/or dendrites of amacrine cells.
5. **Inner nuclear layer (INL):** This layer comprises the cell bodies of the bipolar cells, horizontal cells, amacrine cells, and Müller cells (primary glial cell of the retina).
6. **Outer plexiform layer (OPL):** This layer is the location of synaptic connections between the photoreceptors and the dendrites of the bipolar cells.
7. **Outer nuclear layer (ONL):** This layer consists of the cell bodies of the photoreceptors (rods and cones).
8. **External limiting membrane (ELM):** This is a line of intercellular junctions between photoreceptor cells and Müller cells that separates the photoreceptor segments from the cell bodies.
9. **Photoreceptor layer:** This layer contains the inner and outer (photosensitive) segments of the rods and cones.
10. **Retinal pigment epithelium (RPE):** This is a single layer of pigmented hexagonal cells that plays a multifunctional supportive role, including absorption of excess light, synthesis of growth factors, and phagocytosis of photoreceptor waste products, among other roles. Beneath the RPE lies Bruch's membrane, which separates the RPE from the choroid.

The layers of the retina can be easily discerned in images acquired with SD-OCT (Figures 13.1 and 13.2).

Functionally, the retina may be considered as being composed of three nuclear layers (where the cell bodies of the retinal neurons are located) that are separated by the two plexiform layers, where the synaptic connections between the retinal neurons are located. The flow of information occurs in the following direction: Photoreceptors -> Bipolar Cells -> Ganglion Cells. Furthermore, retinal interneurons include the horizontal and amacrine cells, which modify the signals between the photoreceptors and bipolar cells, and bipolar and ganglion cells, respectively.

Retinal segmentation

The discussion of the technical details of segmentation is beyond the scope of this chapter, but in general this process may be performed either manually by an individual visually identifying the boundaries between retinal layers and using specialized software in order to trace them, or by applying computerized algorithms that automatically detect retinal boundaries. Manual techniques have been employed in small-scale studies and for the validation of automated segmentation algorithms, and have provided important information in studies of retinal involvement in neurological disease. As can be expected, however, manual segmentation is an extremely tedious and time-consuming process and, thus, cannot be used for large-scale clinical studies or in everyday clinical practice. Automated segmentation algorithms have been commercially available for many years and have primarily focused on the segmentation of the RNFL in a ring scan around the optic disc; thus, the peripapillary RNFL thickness has been the most extensively utilized OCT measure in both research studies and clinical practice. Other measures that may be quantified with commercially available software include the average macular thickness and total macular volume. These measures have been shown to demonstrate excellent reproducibility, especially with modern spectral-domain OCT, and their reliability can be maximized by ensuring optimal scan acquisition. [3, 4].

All quantitative OCT measures are obviously derived from segmentation of OCT images; however, we make the distinction between "conventional" OCT measures, which include the

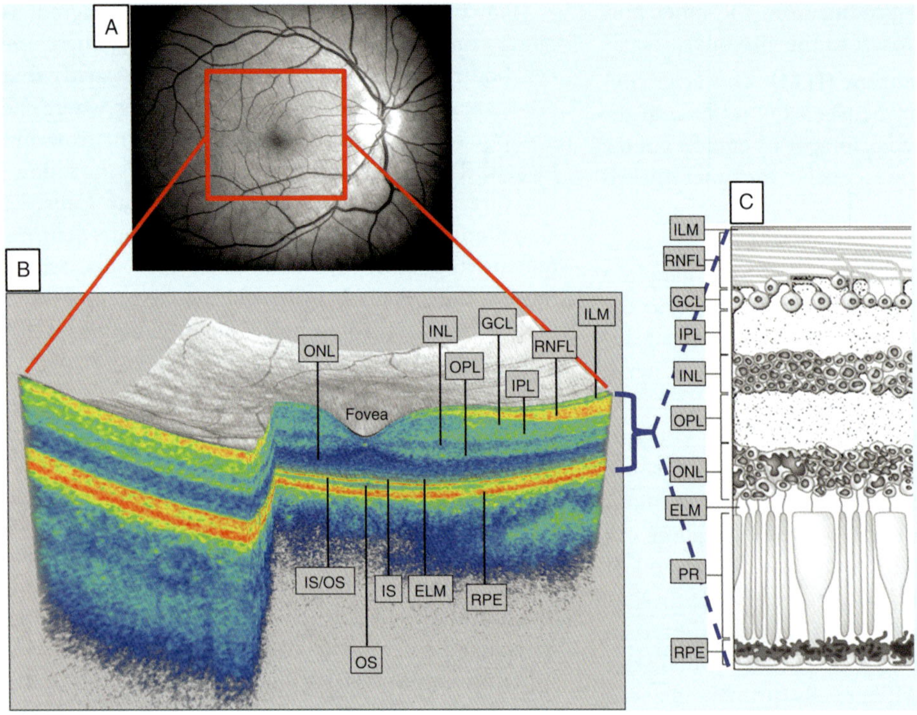

Figure 13.1 Eye of a healthy control subject.
(A) Fundus photograph from a healthy control subject. (B) A three-dimensional macular volume cube generated by spectral-domain OCT (Cirrus HD-OCT) from the macular region denoted by the red box in panel A from the same healthy control subject. Note the individual layers of the retina are readily discernible, except for the ganglion cell layer (GCL) and inner plexiform layer (IPL), which are difficult to distinguish. During the segmentation process (performed in 3-dimension), the segmentation software identifies the outer boundaries of the macular retinal nerve fiber layer (RNFL), IPL, and outer plexiform layer (OPL), as well as the inner boundary of the retinal pigment epithelium (RPE), which is identified by the conventional Cirrus HD-OCT algorithm. The identification of these boundaries facilitates OCT segmentation, enabling determination of the thicknesses of the macular RNFL, GCL+IPL, the inner nuclear layer (INL) + OPL, and the outer nuclear layer (ONL), including the inner and outer photoreceptor segments. (C) Illustration of the cellular composition of the retinal layers depicted in panel B. ELM indicates the external limiting membrane; ILM, the inner limiting membrane; IS, the inner photoreceptor segments; and OS, the outer photoreceptor segments.

Reproduced with permission from Saidha, Shiv, Sotirchos, Elias S., et al. Relationships Between Retinal Axonal and Neuronal Measures and Global Central Nervous System Pathology in Multiple Sclerosis Retinal Measures and Global CNS Pathology in MS. American Medical Association, Archives of Neurology, 2012.

peripapillary RNFL thickness, the average macular thickness and the total macular volume, and "intra-retinal segmentation derived" measures, which include the thicknesses of individual or composite layers in the macular area. Intra-retinal segmentation has been made possible by advances in scan acquisition with the advent of high-resolution spectral-domain OCT and also by the development of sophisticated automated algorithms. As previously mentioned, contrast is generated between retinal layers on OCT by differences in their optical properties, which result from their varying histological composition, and high reflectivity layers correspond to areas where retinal elements are arranged horizontally, such as the RNFL and plexiform layers, whereas the nuclear layers exhibit relatively lower reflectivity. Of note, however, is the fact that the contrast difference between the GCL and IPL is small, and consequently the boundary between these layers is difficult to assess (Figure 13.2) [5, 6]. The same, but to a lesser extent, is also true of the INL and OPL. Thus, distinguishing these layers has been challenging and the vast majority of studies utilizing intra-retinal segmentation in the study of neurological disease have utilized composite measures, including the combined GCL and IPL (GCL+IPL) and combined INL and OPL (INL+OPL). In addition to these composite measures, the macular RNFL and the ONL, including the photoreceptor segments, have also been utilized, and all these layers may now be isolated with great accuracy and reliability with fully automated segmentation algorithms.

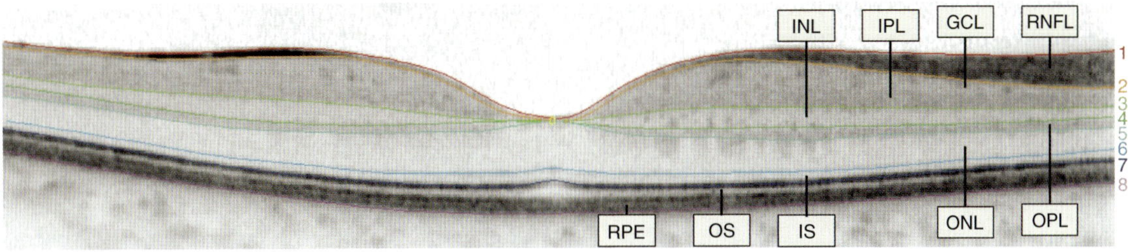

Figure 13.2 Example of a manually segmented spectral-domain OCT (Spectralis) macular B-scan traversing the fovea.
(1) inner limiting membrane, (2) outer boundary of retinal nerve fiber layer, (3) outer boundary of inner plexiform layer, (4) outer boundary of inner nuclear layer, (5) outer boundary of outer plexiform layer, (6) external limiting membrane, (7) inner/outer photoreceptor segment junction, (8) Bruch's membrane. Layers: (1–2) = RNFL; (2–3) = GCL+IPL (note the minimal difference in contrast between the two layers, the border has not been segmented); (3–4) = INL; (4–5) = OPL; (5–6) = ONL; (6–7) = IS; and (7–8) = OS + RPE (OS/RPE border has not been segmented)

Reproduced with permission from Siego, Micahaela A., In vivo assessment of retinal neuronal layers in multiple sclerosis with manual and automated optical coherence tomography segmentation techniques. *Journal of Neurology*; Volume 259, Issue 10, pp 2119–2130.

Retinal segmentation in demyelinating diseases of the central nervous system

Multiple sclerosis

Multiple sclerosis (MS) is an inflammatory disorder of the central nervous system that has a predilection to affect the optic nerves clinically and subclinically. Acute optic neuritis (ON) is the initial demyelinating event in 15–20% of patients with MS and occurs at some time during the course of the disease in 50% of patients [7]. Moreover, postmortem studies have revealed that 94–99% of MS patients have demyelinating plaques in their optic nerves, irrespective of ON history [8, 9]. Retinal pathology is thought to occur primarily secondary to optic nerve involvement in MS; optic nerve inflammation and demyelination results in axonal transection and retrograde degeneration of its constituent fibers, leading to atrophy of the RNFL, the innermost retinal layer, where these axons originate. Degeneration of the retinal nerve fibers in turn leads to death of retinal ganglion cells (the neurons from which these axons are derived) via apoptotic mechanisms [10]. Pathologic studies examining the retinas of patients with MS have demonstrated atrophy of the inner retinal layers (RNFL and GCL) in 71–79% of eyes of patients with MS [11, 12].

In addition to the inner retinal layer pathology observed in MS, evidence exists that deeper retinal layers may also be affected in MS, with extensive qualitative atrophy of the INL identified in over 40% of MS eyes [12]. Also, studies employing electroretinography have identified abnormalities suggestive of INL and ONL dysfunction in MS [13–15]. Furthermore, retinal perivascular inflammation (periphlebitis), suggesting disruption of the blood–retina barrier, occurs in up to 20% of patients with MS. Active retinal periphlebitis tends to occur simultaneously with disruption of the blood–brain barrier in these patients, and may be a risk factor for relapses and gadolinium-enhancing lesions [16, 17]. Intermediate uveitis, especially pars planitis, also occurs in up to 15% of patients with MS [12]. Consistent with these clinical observations, postmortem analyses show retinal inflammation with activated microglia in the eyes of people with MS [12].

Collectively, these findings show that the retina is a common site of inflammation, disruption of the blood-retina barrier, and neuronal-axonal loss in MS. Thus, in the study of MS the retina represents a unique, unmyelinated, and easily accessible part of the CNS within which to study the neurodegeneration and inflammation associated with the disease. This has fueled extensive interest in utilization of OCT with macular intra-retinal segmentation in order to study in vivo the effects of MS-related disease processes in the retina.

The primary OCT measure that has been utilized in the study of MS eyes is the peripapillary RNFL thickness. The use of macular intra-retinal segmentation has also allowed the measurement of the macular RNFL and GCL+IPL thicknesses, measures that in general are considered to convey similar information. These measures have been shown across OCT platforms and segmentation algorithms to exhibit excellent reproducibility, and both measures have been shown to be decreased in MS eyes relative to healthy controls irrespective of ON history, but the decreases are significantly greater in eyes with a clinical history of ON [5, 6, 18–20].

Following ON, the thickness of the peripapillary RNFL and GCL + IPL have been shown to exhibit a decrease over time, with most thinning occurring during the first three months and continuing for six months to one year after onset [21, 22]. During the initial phase of ON, however, the two measures exhibit different characteristics: the GCL + IPL thickness appears to be unaffected initially, whereas the peripapillary RNFL thickness may exhibit increased thickness, most likely due to axonal edema. Thus, when utilizing peripapillary RNFL measurements in acute ON to follow patients longitudinally, it is inherently difficult to differentiate between resolution of edema versus true atrophy of the peripapillary RNFL. Approaches to this problem have included utilizing the fellow "unaffected" eye to establish baseline measures; however, this approach has significant shortcomings due to the fact that often patients with multiple sclerosis have experienced ON in their fellow eye and also since it is known that, even in the absence of a clinical episode of ON, peripapillary RNFL thinning occurs in MS. This is an important factor and makes the GCL + IPL appear to be a more useful measure in acute ON since establishing with confidence a baseline measurement, since establishing with confidence a baseline measurement that can be followed longitudinally is extremely important in order to reliably employ a measure in clinical practice as well as in research studies.

Multiple studies have demonstrated the functional relevance of RNFL and GCL + IPL atrophy by showing that thinning of these layers correlates with visual dysfunction in MS, as measured by assessment of high- and low-contrast visual acuity [6, 19, 23]. Additionally, these layers have been shown to correlate with the Expanded Disability Status Scale (EDSS; a global measure of disability in MS) and with MRI measures of brain atrophy, correlations that are predominantly observed in the absence of a history of ON, suggesting that the atrophy of inner retinal layers observed in non-ON eyes may reflect global neurodegenerative processes in MS [18, 24, 25]. Longitudinal studies in MS have shown that the peripapillary RNFL exhibits accelerated thinning in MS compared to healthy controls, even in the absence of ON, and this has been shown to correlate with clinically significant visual loss and with relapses during follow-up [26, 27]. However, data are conflicting and other studies have been unable to recapitulate these findings [28–30]. One longitudinal study utilizing macular intra-retinal segmentation showed that accelerated thinning of the GCL + IPL also occurs in MS in the absence of clinical episodes of ON and that the rate of thinning is significantly increased in those patients with more active disease, as defined by clinical relapses, presence of gadolinium-enhancing lesions and/or new T2-hyperintense lesions [30].

As previously mentioned, abnormalities of deeper retinal layers have also been reported in MS on the basis of pathologic and electrophysiologic studies [12–15]. Quantitative abnormalities of deeper retinal layers in OCT studies utilizing macular intra-retinal segmentation have also been reported in MS; however, results vary. In one study, thinning of the deeper retinal layers (INL + OPL and ONL + PR) was demonstrated to occur in a subset of MS patients in eyes without a history of ON that had normal peripapillary RNFL thickness [5]. Patients with eyes exhibiting these characteristics were determined to exhibit a macular thinning predominant (MTP) retinal phenotype and were shown to have accelerated accumulation of global disability, as demonstrated by higher Multiple Sclerosis Severity Scores (MSSS), a measure of disability adjusted for disease duration. It was suggested that these retinal abnormalities may be due to a primary retinal process that occurs independent of optic nerve pathology, but this thinning of deeper retinal layers has not been consistently shown to occur in other studies. Furthermore, an entity that has been termed microcystic macular edema (MME; Figure 13.3), which predominantly affects the INL, has been recently described in association with optic neuropathies of various etiologies, including MS, NMO, CRION, optic nerve glioma associated with neurofibromatis type I, and Leber's and Tanzanian hereditary optic neuropathy [31–38]. MME was first described in association with MS, and in studies that have systematically examined for the presence of MME in MS (of which one employed macular intra-retinal segmentation), this pathology was reported to occur in 4.7–6% of MS patients [15, 31, 32]. MME eyes had more frequently experienced a prior episode of symptomatic ON, had worse letter acuity at both high- and low-contrast and correspondingly more severe thinning of the RNFL and GCL + IPL, and patients exhibiting MME had experienced more rapid progression of their disease (i.e., higher MSSS scores). MME was found to be related to increased INL + OPL thickness, which was detectable

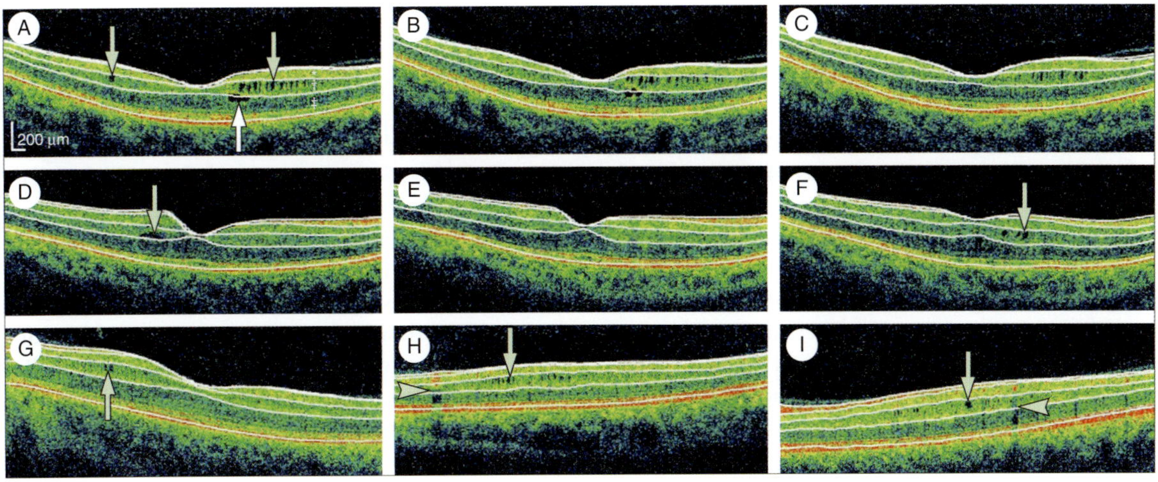

Figure 13.3 Microcystic macular edema of the inner nuclear layer as identified by spectral-domain optical coherence tomography, with automated segmentation lines displayed.

Optical coherence tomography (OCT) segmentation done in three dimensions shows the inner limiting membrane, the outer boundaries of the retinal nerve fiber layer (RNFL), inner plexiform layer, outer plexiform layer, and the inner boundary of the retinal pigment epithelium. The identification of these retinal boundaries enables the determination of the thicknesses of the macular RNFL, the ganglion cell layer and inner plexiform layer (GCL + IPL; labeled * in panel A), the INL (including the outer plexiform layer; labeled † in panel A), and the ONL (including the inner and outer photoreceptor segments; labeled ‡ in panel A). For panels A to C, all images were acquired from the same patient during a three-year period and are presented in chronological order. Microcystic macular edema (MME; green arrows) of the INL was present at baseline, as well as a foveal cyst of the outer nuclear layer (ONL; white arrow A). The ONL cyst progressively resolved during follow-up (B–C). For panels D to F, all images were acquired from the same patient during a two-year period and are presented in chronological order. A single INL cyst (green arrow) was present at baseline (D). The cyst spontaneously resolved after one year (E). After fingolimod treatment (initiated after scan E), the patient developed new cystic changes of the INL (green arrow; F). Panels G to I show three different patients with MME of the INL (green arrows). Vessel artifacts (arrow heads) are shown for comparison.

Reproduced with permission from *Lancet Neurology*

in eyes prior to the development of visible MME, highlighting the potential for earlier and broader identification of this process with utilization of OCT segmentation [32]. Additionally, increased INL thickness has been shown to occur in MS eyes after ON in the absence of MME, and this increase has been shown to correlate with the atrophy observed in the GCL + IPL, suggesting that MME may represent the extreme end of a spectrum of INL pathology [32, 39]. Interestingly, one cross-sectional study showed that in RRMS the INL + OPL thickness exhibits a positive correlation with T2 lesion volume and an inverse correlation with normal appearing white matter [24]. Moreover, in the one longitudinal study of MME that employed macular intra-retinal segmentation, increased INL thickness at baseline was associated with increased clinico-radiological disease activity during follow-up (relapses, EDSS progression, new T2 and contrast-enhancing lesions) [32]. This finding must be validated by further studies but highlights the potential of OCT segmentation for identifying novel biomarkers for neurological disease.

Neuromyelitis optica

Neuromyelitis optica (NMO) is an inflammatory disorder of the central nervous system, the cardinal manifestations of which are ON and longitudinally extensive transverse myelitis (LETM). Autoantibodies (NMO-immunoglobulin G [IgG]) targeting aquaporin-4 are found in the sera of the majority of patients with NMO. In approximately 50% of NMO patients isolated ON is the initial manifestation of the disease. ON associated with NMO carries a worse prognosis than in MS with 60% of NMO patients experiencing unilateral or bilateral blindness at a median of 7.7 years after disease onset, compared with 4% of MS patients with ON at 15-year follow-up [40]. Histopathologically, NMO lesions are not uncommonly associated with necrosis and cavitation, features that are not typically encountered in MS [41]. Unfortunately, retinal pathologic studies have not been performed in NMO and the data regarding retinal involvement in NMO is almost exclusively derived from studies utilizing OCT.

OCT studies utilizing conventional OCT measures have shown that the decrease that occurs in the peripapillary RNFL and macular volume following NMO-associated ON is substantially greater than in MS, and this has been proposed as an important differentiating factor between the two conditions [42–44]. Also, the pattern of peripapillary RNFL atrophy appears to differ, with NMO-ON resulting in severe thinning of all quadrants, whereas MSON is predominantly associated with temporal thinning [42, 44]. Intra-retinal segmentation has allowed for more specific observations to be made and studies have shown that not only the peripapillary RNFL, but also the macular-RNFL and GCL + IPL are more severely affected in NMO [22, 45].

Furthermore, MME of the INL has been shown to occur in 18–26% of patients with NMO-spectrum disorders, a prevalence substantially greater than that observed in MS (~5%).[33, 34, 45] Moreover, MME in NMO appears to be more closely linked with ON, with MME being exclusively identified in eyes with a history of symptomatic ON. As in MS, MME in NMO has been shown to be associated with increased thickness of the INL and poor visual function and is present in eyes that have severe retinal axonal and neuronal loss, as demonstrated by greater decreases in the thickness of the RNFL (peripapillary and macular) and GCL + IPL when compared to NMO-ON eyes that have not developed MME.

The etiology of the higher prevalence of MME in NMO relative to MS has been proposed to be due to the increased severity of NMO-ON, with MME representing a marker of axonal and neuronal injury. Alternatively, it has been thought that a primary retinal process occurring in conjunction with ON may be responsible. Aquaporin-4 (the target of the immune response in NMO) is highly expressed in the retina by Müller glial cells (the cell bodies of which are located in the INL), especially in end-feet membranes facing blood vessels [40]. Thus, a plausible and intriguing hypothesis is that following acute ON and breakdown of the blood–retinal barrier, an immune response directed against aquaporin-4 in the retina may contribute to the development of MME and account in part for the poor visual outcomes in NMO-ON. In any case, further studies and characterization of MME is necessary in order to clarify the pathogenesis of this retinal phenotype.

Additionally, subclinical involvement of the visual pathway has been suggested to occur in NMO spectrum disorders, with some studies identifying decreased RNFL and GCL + IPL thicknesses in NMO non-ON eyes, but data are conflicting [22, 33, 42, 43, 46–48].

Retinal segmentation in other neurological diseases

Alzheimer's disease

Visual dysfunction may occur early in Alzheimer's disease (AD) and includes deficits in visual acuity, contrast sensitivity, color vision, motion perception, visuospatial construction and visual memory [49]. Furthermore, histopathologic studies have found axonal degeneration in the optic nerves, and reductions in the number of retinal ganglion cells and in RNFL thickness in eyes of patients with AD. Studies utilizing OCT have confirmed in vivo that thinning of the peripapillary RNFL and reduction of macular volume occurs in AD eyes; however, OCT studies employing intra-retinal segmentation have not been conducted and this is an important future direction for retinal research in AD [49, 50].

Parkinson's disease

Visual symptomatology is common in Parkinson's disease (PD), as demonstrated by reports of abnormal visual acuity, contrast sensitivity, color vision motion perception, and the presence of visual hallucinations [51]. Furthermore, of interest is the fact that some of these abnormalities have been shown to improve with L-dopa administration. Electrophysiologic studies, including electroretinograms and visual evoked potentials, have also identified abnormalities in PD. The preceding evidence has provided the impetus for OCT studies to be performed in PD. Decreases of the peripapillary RNFL and macular thickness have been identified in some studies in PD; however, other studies have been unable to reproduce these findings. Larger-scale studies employing high-definition OCT with intra-retinal segmentation are indicated in order to further study retinal involvement in PD [51, 52].

Amyotrophic lateral sclerosis

Although visual disturbances are not recognized to occur in amyotrophic lateral sclerosis (ALS), growing evidence supports that non-motor systems may be involved in amyotrophic lateral sclerosis. One study has utilized OCT with automated intra-retinal segmentation to examine the eyes of ALS patients, but no differences were found relative to healthy controls in the macular GCL + IPL, INL + OPL, ONL + PR and peripapillary RNFL thicknesses [53].

References

1. Frohman EM, Fujimoto JG, Frohman TC, Calabresi PA, Cutter G, Balcer LJ. Optical coherence tomography: a window into the mechanisms of multiple sclerosis. *Nat Clin Pract Neurol* 2008; **4**:664–75.
2. Debuc DC. A review of algorithms for segmentation of retinal image data using optical coherence tomography. In: Ho P-G, editor. *Image Segmentation: InTech*; 2011.
3. Cettomai D, Pulicken M, Gordon-Lipkin E, Salter A, Frohman TC, Conger A, et al. Reproducibility of optical coherence tomography in multiple sclerosis. *Arch Neurol* 2008; **65**:1218–22.
4. Syc SB, Warner CV, Hiremath GS, Farrell SK, Ratchford JN, Conger A, et al. Reproducibility of high-resolution optical coherence tomography in multiple sclerosis. *Mult Scler* 2010; **16**:829–39.
5. Saidha S, Syc SB, Ibrahim MA, Eckstein C, Warner CV, Farrell SK, et al. Primary retinal pathology in multiple sclerosis as detected by optical coherence tomography. *Brain* 2011; **134**:518–33.
6. Seigo MA, Sotirchos ES, Newsome S, Babiarz A, Eckstein C, Ford E, et al. In vivo assessment of retinal neuronal layers in multiple sclerosis with manual and automated optical coherence tomography segmentation techniques. *J Neurol* 2012; **259**:2119–30.
7. Balcer LJ. Clinical practice. Optic neuritis. *N Engl J Med* 2006; **354**:1273–80.
8. Toussaint D, Perier O, Verstappen A, Bervoets S. Clinicopathological study of the visual pathways, eyes, and cerebral hemispheres in 32 cases of disseminated sclerosis. *J Clin Neuroophthalmol* 1983; **3**:211–20.
9. Ikuta F, Zimmerman HM. Distribution of plaques in seventy autopsy cases of multiple sclerosis in the United States. *Neurology* 1976; **26**:26–8.
10. Shindler KS, Ventura E, Dutt M, Rostami A. Inflammatory demyelination induces axonal injury and retinal ganglion cell apoptosis in experimental optic neuritis. *Exp Eye Res* 2008; **87**:208–13.
11. Kerrison JB, Flynn T, Green WR. Retinal pathologic changes in multiple sclerosis. *Retina* 1994; **14**:445–51.
12. Green AJ, McQuaid S, Hauser SL, Allen IV, Lyness R. Ocular pathology in multiple sclerosis: retinal atrophy and inflammation irrespective of disease duration. *Brain* 2010; **133**:1591–601.
13. Papakostopoulos D, Fotiou F, Hart JC, Banerji NK. The electroretinogram in multiple sclerosis and demyelinating optic neuritis. *Electroencephalogr Clin Neurophysiol* 1989; **74**:1–10.
14. Forooghian F, Sproule M, Westall C, Gordon L, Jirawuthiworavong G, Shimazaki K, et al. Electroretinographic abnormalities in multiple sclerosis: possible role for retinal autoantibodies. *Doc Ophthalmol* 2006; **113**:123–32.
15. Gundogan FC, Demirkaya S, Sobaci G. Is optical coherence tomography really a new biomarker candidate in multiple sclerosis?–A structural and functional evaluation. *Invest Ophthalmol Vis Sci* 2007; **48**:5773–81.
16. Engell T, Hvidberg A, Uhrenholdt A. Multiple sclerosis: periphlebitis retinalis et cerebro-spinalis. A correlation between periphlebitis retinalis and abnormal technetium brain scintigraphy. *Acta Neurol Scand* 1984; **69**:293–7.
17. Sepulcre J, Murie-Fernandez M, Salinas-Alaman A, Garcia-Layana A, Bejarano B, Villoslada P. Diagnostic accuracy of retinal abnormalities in predicting disease activity in MS. *Neurology* 2007; **68**:1488–94.
18. Petzold A, de Boer JF, Schippling S, Vermersch P, Kardon R, Green A, et al. Optical coherence tomography in multiple sclerosis: a systematic review and meta-analysis. *Lancet Neurol* 2010; **9**:921–32.
19. Walter SD, Ishikawa H, Galetta KM, Sakai RE, Feller DJ, Henderson SB, et al. Ganglion cell loss in relation to visual disability in multiple sclerosis. *Ophthalmology* 2012; **119**:1250–7.
20. Warner CV, Syc SB, Stankiewicz AM, Hiremath G, Farrell SK, Crainiceanu CM, et al. The impact of utilizing different optical coherence tomography devices for clinical purposes and in multiple sclerosis trials. *PLoS ONE* 2011; **6**:e22947.
21. Henderson AP, Altmann DR, Trip AS, Kallis C, Jones SJ, Schlottmann PG, et al. A serial study of retinal changes following optic neuritis with sample size estimates for acute neuroprotection trials. *Brain* 2010; **133**:2592–602.
22. Syc SB, Saidha S, Newsome SD, Ratchford JN, Levy M, Ford E, et al. Optical coherence tomography segmentation reveals ganglion cell layer pathology after optic neuritis. *Brain* 2012; **135**:521–33.
23. Saidha S, Syc SB, Durbin MK, Eckstein C, Oakley JD, Meyer SA, et al. Visual dysfunction in multiple sclerosis correlates better with optical coherence tomography derived estimates of macular ganglion cell layer thickness than peripapillary retinal nerve fiber layer thickness. *Mult Scler* 2011; **17**:1449–63.
24. Saidha S, Sotirchos ES, Oh J, Syc SB, Seigo MA, Shiee N, et al. Relationships between retinal axonal and neuronal measures and global central nervous system pathology in multiple sclerosis. *JAMA Neurol* 2013; **70**:34–43.
25. Zimmermann H, Freing A, Kaufhold F, Gaede G, Bohn E, Bock M, et al. Optic neuritis interferes with optical coherence tomography and magnetic resonance imaging correlations. *Mult Scler* 2013; **19**:443–50.
26. Talman LS, Bisker ER, Sackel DJ, Long DA, Jr., Galetta KM, Ratchford JN, et al. Longitudinal study of vision and retinal nerve fiber layer thickness in multiple sclerosis. *Ann Neurol* 2010; **67**:749–60.

27. Garcia-Martin E, Pueyo V, Almarcegui C, Martin J, Ara JR, Sancho E, et al. Risk factors for progressive axonal degeneration of the retinal nerve fibre layer in multiple sclerosis patients. *Br J Ophthalmol* 2011; **95**:1577–82.
28. Henderson AP, Trip SA, Schlottmann PG, Altmann DR, Garway-Heath DF, Plant GT, et al. A preliminary longitudinal study of the retinal nerve fiber layer in progressive multiple sclerosis. *J Neurol* 2010; **257**:1083–91.
29. Serbecic N, Aboul-Enein F, Beutelspacher SC, Vass C, Kristoferitsch W, Lassmann H, et al. High resolution spectral domain optical coherence tomography (SD-OCT) in multiple sclerosis: the first follow up study over two years. *PLoS ONE* 2011; **6**:e19843.
30. Ratchford JN, Saidha S, Sotirchos ES, Oh JA, Seigo MA, Eckstein C, et al. Active MS is associated with accelerated retinal ganglion cell/inner plexiform layer thinning. *Neurology* 2013; **80**:47–54.
31. Gelfand JM, Nolan R, Schwartz DM, Graves J, Green AJ. Microcystic macular edema in multiple sclerosis is associated with disease severity. *Brain* 2012; **135**:1786–93.
32. Saidha S, Sotirchos ES, Ibrahim MA, Crainiceanu CM, Gelfand JM, Sepah YJ, et al. Microcystic macular edema, thickness of the inner nuclear layer of the retina, and disease characteristics in multiple sclerosis: a retrospective study. *Lancet Neurol* 2012; **11**:963–72.
33. Sotirchos ES, Saidha S, Byraiah G, Mealy MA, Ibrahim MA, Sepah YJ, et al. In vivo identification of morphologic retinal abnormalities in neuromyelitis optica. *Neurology* 2013; **80**:1406–14.
34. Gelfand JM, Cree BA, Nolan R, Arnow S, Green AJ. Microcystic inner nuclear layer abnormalities and neuromyelitis optica. *JAMA Neurol* 2013; **70**:629–33.
35. Balk LJ, Killestein J, Polman CH, Uitdehaag BM, Petzold A. Microcystic macular edema confirmed, but not specific for multiple sclerosis. *Brain* 2012; **135**:e226.
36. Abegg M, Zinkernagel M, Wolf S. Microcystic macular degeneration from optic neuropathy. *Brain* 2012; **135**:e225.
37. Barboni P, Carelli V, Savini G, Carbonelli M, La Morgia C, Sadun AA. Microcystic macular degeneration from optic neuropathy: not inflammatory, not trans-synaptic degeneration. *Brain* 2013; **136**:e239.
38. Kisimbi J, Shalchi Z, Mahroo OA, Mhina C, Sanyiwa AJ, Mabey D, et al. Macular spectral domain optical coherence tomography findings in Tanzanian endemic optic neuropathy. *Brain* 2013.
39. Kaushik M, Wang CY, Barnett MH, Garrick R, Parratt J, Graham SL, et al. Inner Nuclear Layer Thickening Is Inversley Proportional to Retinal Ganglion Cell Loss in Optic Neuritis. *PLoS ONE* 2013; **8**:e78341.
40. Levin MH, Bennett JL, Verkman AS. Optic neuritis in neuromyelitis optica. *Prog Retin Eye Res* 2013.
41. Lucchinetti CF, Mandler RN, McGavern D, Bruck W, Gleich G, Ransohoff RM, et al. A role for humoral mechanisms in the pathogenesis of Devic's neuromyelitis optica. *Brain* 2002; **125**:1450–61.
42. Naismith RT, Tutlam NT, Xu J, Klawiter EC, Shepherd J, Trinkaus K, et al. Optical coherence tomography differs in neuromyelitis optica compared with multiple sclerosis. *Neurology* 2009; **72**:1077–82.
43. Ratchford JN, Quigg ME, Conger A, Frohman T, Frohman E, Balcer LJ, et al. Optical coherence tomography helps differentiate neuromyelitis optica and MS optic neuropathies. *Neurology* 2009; **73**:302–8.
44. Green AJ, Cree BA. Distinctive retinal nerve fibre layer and vascular changes in neuromyelitis optica following optic neuritis. *J Neurol Neurosurg Psychiatry* 2009; **80**:1002–5.
45. Schneider E, Zimmermann H, Oberwahrenbrock T, Kaufhold F, Kadas EM, Petzold A, et al. Optical coherence tomography reveals distinct patterns of retinal damage in neuromyelitis optica and multiple sclerosis. *PLoS ONE* 2013; **8**:e66151.
46. de Seze J, Blanc F, Jeanjean L, Zephir H, Labauge P, Bouyon M, et al. Optical coherence tomography in neuromyelitis optica. *Arch Neurol* 2008; **65**:920–3.
47. Merle H, Olindo S, Donnio A, Richer R, Smadja D, Cabre P. Retinal peripapillary nerve fiber layer thickness in neuromyelitis optica. *Invest Ophthalmol Vis Sci* 2008; **49**:4412–7.
48. Monteiro ML, Fernandes DB, Apostolos-Pereira SL, Callegaro D. Quantification of retinal neural loss in patients with neuromyelitis optica and multiple sclerosis with or without optic neuritis using optical coherence tomography. *Invest Ophthalmol Vis Sci* 2012.
49. Ikram MK, Cheung CY, Wong TY, Chen CP. Retinal pathology as biomarker for cognitive impairment and Alzheimer's disease. *J Neurol Neurosurg Psychiatry* 2012; **83**:917–22.
50. He XF, Liu YT, Peng C, Zhang F, Zhuang S, Zhang JS. Optical coherence tomography assessed retinal nerve fiber layer thickness in patients with Alzheimer's disease: a meta-analysis. *Int J Ophthalmol* 2012; **5**:401–5.
51. Archibald NK, Clarke MP, Mosimann UP, Burn DJ. The retina in Parkinson's disease. *Brain* 2009; **132**:1128–45.
52. Archibald NK, Clarke MP, Mosimann UP, Burn DJ. Retinal thickness in Parkinson's disease. *Parkinsonism Relat Disord* 2011; **17**:431–6.
53. Roth NM, Saidha S, Zimmermann H, Brandt AU, Oberwahrenbrock T, Maragakis NJ, et al. Optical coherence tomography does not support optic nerve involvement in amyotrophic lateral sclerosis. *Eur J Neurol* 2013; **20**:1170–6.

Chapter

14 Optical coherence tomography and retinal pathology in neurologic diseases

Ari J. Green

Pathology is the foundation of clinical medicine. Since the nineteenth century, diseases have come to be understood not simply in the context of the symptoms they produce but in consideration of the cellular disruption that accompanies them. We, therefore, define diseases in reference to their particular pattern of cellular injury and molecular dysfunction. Knowledge concerning cellular pathology guides our understanding of the biological mechanisms that underpin disease development and progression. In the age of immunohistochemistry, histopathology has been extended to help unfold the specific molecular pathways that are dysregulated in each disease process.

The principal limitation of standard pathology is that it only provides a window on the specific aberrant cellular and molecular processes at a single point in time (when the tissue is obtained). In diseases outside of the central nervous system, the capacity to clinically analyze biopsy specimens allows for the study of cellular dysregulation on a semi-dynamic scale. However, in tissues where maintenance of intact cellular architecture is crucial to retained organ function (such as in the central nervous system [CNS]) biopsy has a limited role for diagnosing disease and essentially no role for monitoring and tracking pathological progression. This is an obvious limitation in the brain – where critical periods of highly dynamic development hardwire the system's functionality – and dysfunction caused by disruption from tissue acquisition would be difficult to recover. This circumstance is accentuated in the retina because the complex cellular architecture of the retina is engraved on a tissue that is paper thin and not amenable to easy tissue sampling. Therefore biopsies of the brain to diagnose neurological disease are the exception rather than the rule, and tissue samples from the living retina are exceptionally uncommon indeed.

As a consequence, our understanding of the pathological underpinnings of neurodegenerative conditions comes principally from pathological specimens obtained at the end of life – and not from tissue samples obtained when the disease is developing or is most active. Even these end-of-life samples are in short supply because of a combination of cultural and social considerations and the difficulty with procuring neuronal tissues in a timely manner before tissue degradation associated with death has significantly compromised tissue quality. This poses a challenge for our understanding of these disease processes because the end stage of tissue injury may not reflect the mechanisms that led to this ultimate state. In some instances, by the time tissue can be obtained, the distortion caused by the disease leaves us without insights regarding the mechanisms and processes that resulted in that injury. As a field, this has left us with [1] a limited supply of tissue with [2] a restricted view of disease processes reflecting the end result of years or even decades of disease progression.

Biomedical imaging provides the capacity to study pathological processes more dynamically, especially in the tissue types that cannot be sampled without disrupting critical cellular function. However, findings from biomedical imaging must be grounded in a pathology-based understanding of the disease under study. Therefore, imaging is principally useful in reference to known pathological processes, which allow us to contextualize our observations in regard to the standard methods for categorizing and understanding disease. This is particularly true for imaging methods that are optimized in terms of scale and resolution for

Optical Coherence Tomography in Neurological Disease, ed. Peter A. Calabresi, Laura J. Balcer, and Elliot M. Frohman. Published by Cambridge University Press.

monitoring tissue morphology. Although their relative resolutions differ substantially, this limitation applies across a broad selection of biomedical imaging techniques including standard radiography, computerized tomography, magnetic resonance imaging, and even optical coherence tomography.

This condition constitutes the principal challenge in using retinal imaging to understand and track diseases of the central nervous system. Namely, we must demonstrate that we have identified the specific significance of any imaging abnormality identified. For example, we must determine if volume loss detected on imaging reflects cell loss, tissue atrophy, or loss of tissue water. Furthermore, in a pathological state we don't know that volume loss per se reflects tissue injury to a particular class of cells unless we know the cell types that inhabit that tissue in both health and disease. The second major assumption of retinal imaging in CNS diseases is that retinal manifestations of the disease meaningfully represent some broader aspect of the disease process. It has been suggested that retinal imaging must recapitulate all the features of the broader CNS disease to be useful. While desirable to some degree, this contention is not true. For example, in multiple sclerosis, a single lesion in the subcortical white matter may not reflect all the elements of the broader disease, but studying it in detail is still profoundly valuable – especially if we possess the capacity to study lesion dynamics at a cellular level. The same is true of retinal manifestations of neurological disease. Understanding the disease in the retina has the potential to provide us important insights about the disease in general if it represents some fundamental aspect of pathogenesis or progression– it does not necessarily need to manifest the full spectrum of the disease process.

Unfortunately, given the challenges posed with obtaining tissue, much of what we know about retinal manifestations of brain diseases is based on a limited sample. Very few cases of neurological disease have undergone ophthalmic pathological analysis. Furthermore, in many of the cases that have come to autopsy there is limited data to determine if these cases constitute typical examples of disease. Even fewer have received systematic ophthalmic pathological review – meaning that certain pathological processes may have been missed or overlooked, especially if they are not evident in all patients with the disease. Therefore, new discoveries on retinal imaging may need to be contextualized by returning to human pathological tissue or at least by reference to animal models of disease with fidelity for the disease feature under study.

MRI and to a lesser extent CT scans have come to prominence in clinical neuroscience in large part because the images can be represented in such a way that they show good fidelity for known gross pathology of brain substructures and disease pathology (i.e., lesions in MS and localized atrophy in neurodegeneration). There is, therefore, tremendous value to correlative studies between pathology and biomedical imaging. At the spatial resolution of OCT, that association would best be represented by histopathology.

In total, imaging is most meaningful in reference to known underlying histopathology, but advancing the field is likely an iterative process requiring human subject imaging, acquisition, and analysis of carefully ascertained human tissue samples when available, and additional cautious reference to animal tissue samples with matched imaging acquired for further refinement.

Multiple sclerosis

Multiple sclerosis is a common neurodegenerative disease of the central nervous system, characterized by robust inflammation with an adaptive immune response that appears to target myelin. It effects nearly 2.5 million people worldwide and frequently leads to the development of relentless disability within a few decades of disease onset. The disease is pathologically manifested by a number of principal features. These include lymphocyte and monocyte infiltration into the central nervous system, especially in the area around blood vessels, microglial activation, substantial myelin loss – with less pronounced loss of neurons and their axons – and an astrocytic response with gliosis and scarring. As it is the most common acquired disease involving CNS myelin and given that the principal adaptive immune response appears to target myelin, it is considered the canonical demyelinating disease of the central nervous system.

Under normal circumstances the human retina does not contain any myelin. Therefore, it may be surprising that the retina could serve as a model for understanding or studying MS. However, the retinal ganglion cell – which processes visual information transmitted from the outer retinal layers and transmits it the brain (including targets in the thalamus, midbrain tectum and hypothalamus) – is myelinated along most of its distal portion (through the optic nerve, chiasm, and tract). The pathology detailed below highlights that all the canonical features of MS other than demyelination can be detected in the retina [1–7, 10–13]. This includes axonal and neuronal loss, microglial and astroglial activation, lymphocyte infiltration with perivascular cuffing, and gliosis. In fact, the presence of the injury observed in the absence of myelin suggests that injury and inflammation in MS can both proceed in the absence of a local myelin target. Theoretically, it also means that by studying the retina these other processes could potentially be better understood absent the sometimes overwhelming presence of myelin injury.

Given the high frequency of visual dysfunction in MS, it is not at all surprising that scientists have undertaken pathological investigations of the visual system. The most common and well-recognized clinical syndrome involving the visual system in MS is optic neuritis (ON). Although the episode is classically thought to initiate and focus injury in the retrobulbar optic nerve, the cell that suffers functional impairment resides in the retina. In ON, the absence of retinal findings defines one of the clinical aphorisms most commonly associated with the disease ("The patient sees nothing and the doctor sees nothing.") Unsurprisingly, there have been no recorded cases of pathology during acute optic neuritis. Optic nerve head swelling is seen in a minority of cases but associated retinal abnormalities are unusual and would lead a clinician to question the diagnosis.

On the other hand, tissue pathology has been far better characterized in MS and demonstrates unequivocally that injury to the anterior visual pathways is near universal in the disease. In fact, involvement of the visual pathway was reputed to be one of the defining pathological characteristics of the disease for early neuropathologists [2] including Charcot. In the 1930s Lisch described visual pathway demyelination in 12/12 MS pathology samples studied (only six of which came from patients who had a history of ON) [3]. In the middle part of the last century, Gartner described retinal and optic nerve atrophy in ten MS cases and documented the significant inner retinal injury seen in the disease [4]. He described demyelinating plaques in 100% of the optic nerves of patients with MS. All but one of these patients had significant nerve atrophy and the exception was noted to have a marked increase in reactive glial cells replacing the normal axonal constituents of the nerve. It was also noted that retinal atrophy was irregular but was concentrated in the papillomacular bundle. Ganglion cell loss was described as significant, including marked loss of perifoveal ganglion cells and atrophic shrunken appearance to the surviving ganglion cells. Furthermore, perivascular lymphocytes and increased glial populations and fibroblasts were described as well as thickened appearance to some blood vessels. In some cases, this gliosis was extensive with fibrosis that deformed the architecture of the retina and proximal optic nerve [4].

Toussaint conclusively demonstrated that demyelinating injury to the anterior visual pathway could be found in virtually all patients with MS in a larger series of 32 cases [5]. This was the first investigation to include some clinical characterization of source for the tissue sample and there was surprisingly little correlation between the degree of demyelination seen pathologically and the amount of visual loss that the patient experienced during life [5]. Subsequent studies have also confirmed the uniformity of optic nerve atrophy and demyelination on pathology in subjects with MS at end of life [6, 7].

Further small series confirmed the preference for injury of the papillomacular bundle [7] and suggested that the clinical periphlebitis described by Tar Braak and Rucker was in fact constituted by inflammatory infiltrate and was similar to perivascular lymphocyte cuffing seen in the brain [8–12]. An elegant modern study demonstrated size selective injury involving smaller retinal ganglion cells by studying their projections in the lateral geniculate nucleus. This provided a context for understanding the injury of the papillomacular bundle (which is predominantly constituted by the smaller parvocellular retinal ganglion cells that have both smaller axons and dendritic arbors). The authors demonstrated that even among parvocellular RGCs, smaller cells were more prone to injury and loss [13]. This study also documented that optic nerve atrophy extended into the tract and that optic nerve volume loss was at least in part the consequence of axonal loss. [13]

The largest and most definitive pathological description of retinal injury in MS included 132 eyes from 82 subjects with the disease (and 10 embedded reference subjects) [1]. Cases were examined in a standardized fashion with evaluators blind to the underlying diagnosis to reduce the influence of potential bias. Disease duration ranged from four months to more than five decades. Retinal injury was detected in all subtypes at all time points of the disease, but the degree of injury was variable. The study conclusively demonstrated that ganglion cells and their axons are lost in the large majority of retinas and optic nerves of patients with multiple sclerosis. Although difficult to study in the retinal nerve fiber layer itself, neurofilament staining (which labels axons) demonstrated significant loss of axons of the optic nerve, and this appeared to be partially dependent on the age of the patient and length of time that the patient had suffered from MS [1]. The series highlighted that retinal injury can be detected earlier in the course of disease by showing that patients documented to have relapsing remitting multiple sclerosis and acute fulminant disease at the time of death exhibited ganglion cell loss and loss of axons as well (Figure 14.1). Overall, 80% of subjects demonstrated qualitative cell loss in the retina and 71% demonstrated optic nerve atrophy [1]. Lastly, as an indication of the association between retinal cell loss and broader neurodegeneration in the rest of the CNS, brain volume was correlated with the degree of retinal atrophy identified in the series and there was trend detected between longer disease duration and qualitative assessment of retinal atrophy.

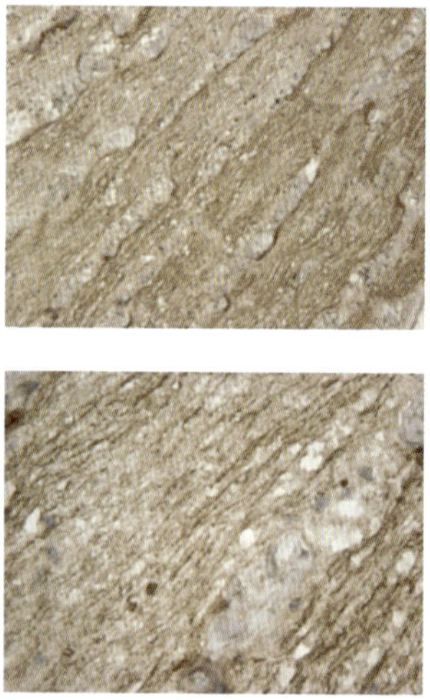

Figure 14.1 Axon loss in the optic nerve in multiple sclerosis. These images show significant reduction in normal axonal density in the optic nerves of patients with MS using a neurofilament stain (NF). Panel A shows loss of normal fiber bundles at 10x, whereas Panel B show loss of fibers themselves (40x) accompanied by an increased glial response.

Interestingly, significant inflammation was detected in the retinas of these subjects even though the samples were taken at the end of life. Many of the subjects had secondary progressive disease and the principle inflammatory response would be presumed to have abated. The study demonstrated further evidence of retinal inflammation in a subset of cases subjected to additional immunohistochemical assessment. This inflammation was characterized by the appearance of large numbers of cells expressing MHC Class II molecules (defining them as of immune lineage) throughout the retina, some of which were concentrated in the space around blood vessels (Figure 14.2). The rate of frank retinal periphlebitis was similar between the patients with progressive and relapsing MS. Foamy appearing cells that appeared to be of innate immune lineage were also seen, many of which were outside of the normal microglial network surrounding the inner nuclear layer of the retina (Figure 14.3). The finding of infiltrating and migrating native immune cells distributed throughout the retina means that some of the retinal layers seen using standard retinal imaging protocols may be constituted by cells that are not found in the healthy retina [1].

The retinal nerve fiber layer is defined at its inner edge by the internal limiting membrane and at its outer edge by the ganglion cell layer. Although the inner edge is a true biological interface, the outer edge is in large part conceptual. It is defined by the theoretical boundary between the cell soma of retinal ganglion cells and their axonal projections. The boundary appears sharp on optical coherence tomography images in part because of how OCT signal is produced – axonal microtubules reflect light differently when they are perpendicular to the light source.

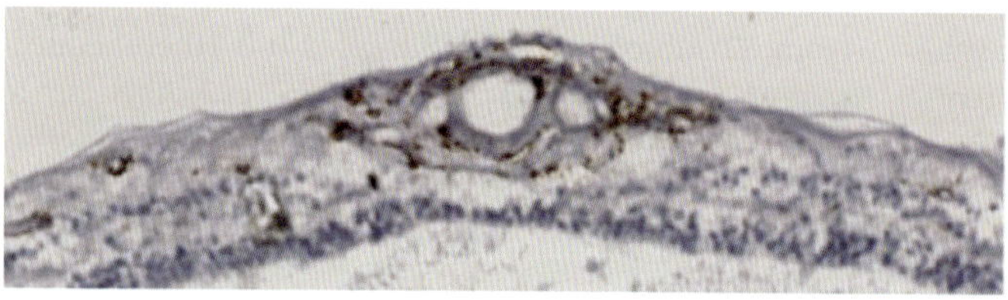

Figure 14.2: Immune activation in the retina in MS. HLA-DR staining showing MHC class II + cells in the inner retina, including in the retinal nerve fiber, ganglion cell, and inner nuclear/plexiform layers at 20x (Panel A) and inner nuclear layer at 40x (Panel B).

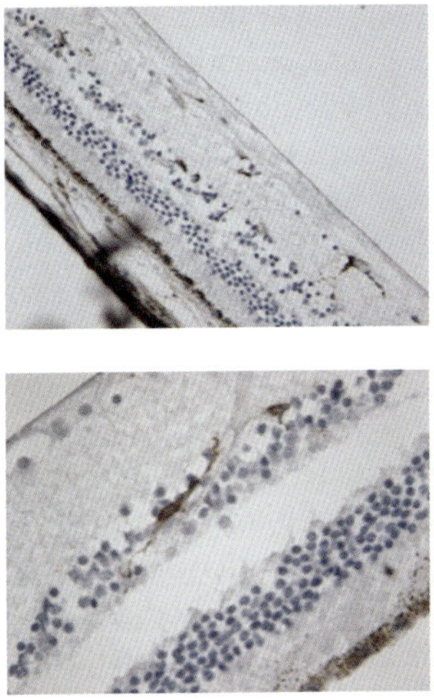

Figure 14.3 Reactive microglia in the retina in MS. Foamy reactive innate immune cells identified in the retina near optic nerve head in a subject with SPMS (HLA-DR Stain). These may constitute a reaction to degenerating neurons.

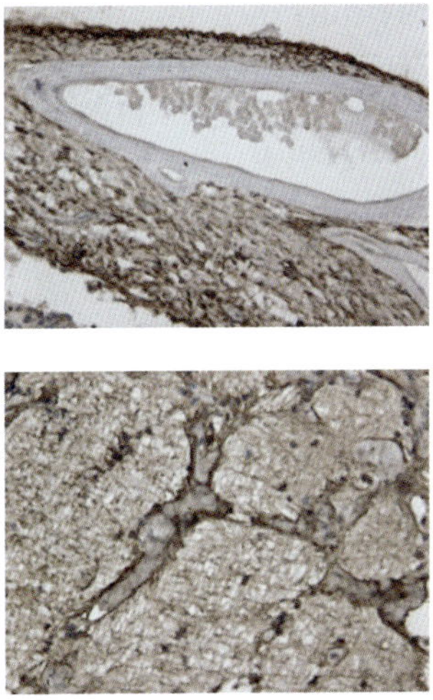

Figure 14.4 Immune cells in perivascular space. HLA-DR staining showing MHC class II positive immune cells adjacent to blood vessels in the nerve fiber layer of a subject with MS. Given the morphology, many of these cells appear to be lymphocytes.

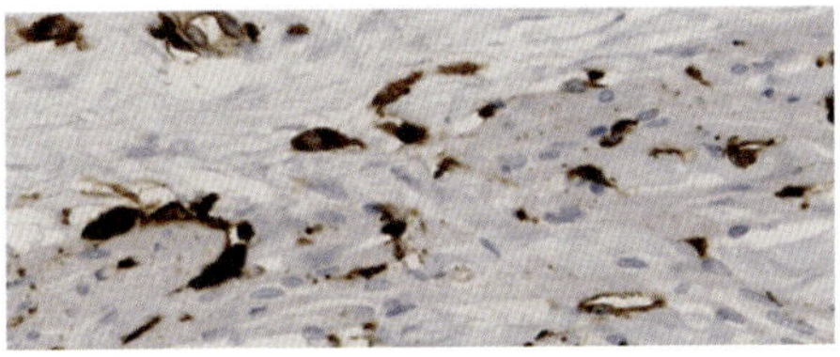

Figure 14.5 Gliotic scar in the retina and optic nerve. Perivenular gliosis near optic disc (Panel A) and within optic nerve (Panel B) in subject with SPMS (GFAP stain)

Between the ILM and the GCL inner boundary, the RNFL is constituted by RGC axons but also contains other cellular elements, including the inner retinal vascular branches of the central retinal artery and vein. The other constituents of the "RNFL" could include displaced amacrine cells, and Müller cell processes in the healthy state. (In fact, recent data suggests that up to half the cells of the GCL in the mouse may be amacrine cells rather than RGCs) [14]. In disease, infiltrating cells trapped anywhere between the ILM and GCL as well fibrosis/gliosis could also contribute volume to the RNFL[15]. In the pathology series 15% of patients had HLA-DR + cells found in the perivascular cuff (which would presumably be detected as RNFL) [Figure 14.4] [1], Outside of the peripapillary RNFL this would contaminate estimations of nerve fiber layer thickness of volume. However, this would only have limited impact on routine peripapillary RNFL thickness assessments because most perivascular sheathing has been identified to occur in the mid-periphery and not proximate to the optic disc [9, 11].

On the other hand, fibrosis especially at the optic nerve head was another frequently observed pathological phenomena seen in the pathology series [Figure 14.5]. This fibrosis was at times severe enough that appeared to lead to deformation of the normal architecture of the optic nerve head and could conceivably impact the shape of the cup and the volume of the RNFL [1, 4]. Additional, gliotic changes were detected using GFAP staining for astrocytes that showed reactive astrocytes next to vessels exhibiting blood retinal barrier disruption and located within the layer that constitutes RNFL [1].

Immune cells were not restricted to the RNFL in the study and HLA-DR positive cells with an activated appearance were found in deeper layers of the retina including the inner nuclear layer and inner plexiform layer [1]. Under normal circumstances microglial cells of the retina are tiled through the IPL and OPL surrounding the INL; however, in the state of activation they have the potential to migrate to sites of injury or inflammation [16].

One of the striking findings of the larger systematic evaluation of retinal samples from MS subjects was the identification of extensive injury involving the inner nuclear layer of the retina [1]. The population of neurons found in this layer (horizontal and bipolar cells) are not myelinated and, therefore, their loss suggests that there is either direct inflammatory mediated injury in the retina or that secondary trans-synaptic processes underlie cell loss in cells connected to a disrupted pathway.

In terms of the specificity of the findings this study had the added benefit that the evaluating pathologist was blinded to the underlying diagnosis (given embedded pathological controls). This served to reduce potential bias on the part of the evaluating pathologist in determining the frequency of the pathological features observed.

Neuronal ceroid lipofuscinosis

The neuronal ceroid lipofuscinoses are a set of inherited neurodegenerative diseases that exhibit significant progressive injury to the brain and retina. Considered together, they constitute the most common pediatric neurodegenerative disorders in humans with a cumulative prevalence of 1 per 10,000. Clinically, the diseases are characterized by developmental regression, visual disturbances, stimulus-induced myoclonus, seizures, and early death. The diseases typically manifest in the first decade of life – and the most common forms present with visual dysfunction – although later onset forms have been identified [17]. On ophthalmologic examination, most patients with NCL demonstrate significant optic atrophy and at least 70% have significant visual impairment at the time of death. Visual findings are particularly prominent in patients with infantile (CLN1) and juvenile (CLN3) onset NCL, where the injury is early and frequently profound. By contrast some of the other NCL subtypes, such as late infantile NCL (also known as CLN2), manifest visual symptoms and presumably retinal injury later in the disease. Most of the other NCL subtypes have also been described to have significant retinal injury – but are less common and the spectrum of disease has been less well described [17].

On brain imaging, NCL patients exhibit extensive confluent subcortical white matter injury along with severe brain atrophy and thalamic T2 hypointensities. The pathological characteristic feature of all these diseases is the intracellular accumulation of lipid- and protein-derived pigments called ceroid. Ceroid and lipofuscin are typically distinguished in that lipofuscin is lipopigment that accumulates as part of normal senescence but ceroid is lipopigment that accumulates as a consequence of a disease state. Both lipopigments and ceroid have the tendency to be endogenously autofluorescent, meaning that light of an appropriate frequency will elicit the release of photons with lower energy (i.e., a longer wavelength) [18]. In many instances, these autofluorescent materials are sensitive to a wide spectrum of stimulating light and, given their varied molecular structure, also emit a broad spectrum of photons in response.

The diagnosis of NCL is established through the identification of Periodic Acid Schiff and Luxol fast blue positive autoflourescent material in the brain and retina [17]. In these tissues, as well as in the muscle, subcutaneous fat, and skin, electron microscopy exhibits curvilinear bodies, fingerprint bodies, and Granular osmophilic deposits. Today, molecular diagnosis is the gold standard for confirming disease and establishing disease subtype. Given tissue accessibility and low morbidity of biopsy specimens, skin samples are typically the tissue of choice for disease identification and subtype confirmation can now frequently be confirmed via genetic testing.

Unfortunately, by the time of autopsy the disease has reached its end stage so that damage to neuronal and retinal populations is widespread. By some accounts, there is predominant injury to smaller cortical cells early, and injury in the retina and damage proceeds from the photoreceptor layers outwards. Clinical studies demonstrate retinal atrophy and pigmentary retinopathy that precede the development of nerve fiber layer loss of disc atrophy, suggesting the spread of disease to the inner retina [19, 20]. Histopathology from retinas on autopsy in Batten's disease (now known as NCL type 3) showed total loss of photoreceptors, including both rods and cones and extending into the outer plexiform layer. Pigmentary changes were less uniform and the degree of injury to the ganglion cell layer were also less consistent [20]. Electron microscopy also demonstrated curvilinear and fingerprint bodies in the ganglion cells of NCL subjects.

In almost all described histopathology cases of NCL type 3 (Batten's disease) there is accumulation of autofluorescent pigment in both retinal ganglion cells and cells of the inner nuclear layer. This distinguishes NCL from other ophthalmologic diseases with lipofuscin such as age-related macular degeneration in which lipofuscin accumulation is predominantly seen in the retinal pigment epithelium at the outer edge of the retina. Furthermore, lipopigment is not always found in cells that are degenerating – suggesting that lipofuscin/ceroid accumulation is not a necessary prerequisite for cell death [17, 20]. It should be noted, however, that only one autopsy case of NCL has been evaluated in the age of modern immunohistochemistry and that additional analyses and evaluations would be appropriate especially given the variety of genetic mutations described to date – even within a single disease causing gene. Furthermore, given the timing of tissue acquisition neither the precise evolution of tissue injury nor the cell types that are most susceptible to tissue injury is clear. Indeed, in CLN5, for example, there is not reported to be the "spread" of injury from the outer retina to the inner retina as described for CLN3 [17]. Furthermore, the number of retinas that have been pathologically described in the literature is small and a full characterization of the nature and extent of retinal injury remains to be performed.

Alzheimer's disease

Alzheimer's disease (AD) is the most common dementing illness of the elderly and accounts for more than half of dementia cases with pathological confirmation at autopsy. AD is pathologically characterized by neuron loss in specific areas of the brain as well as the presence of intraneuronal inclusions of hyperphosphorylated tau in vulnerable cell populations (known as neurofibrillary tangles) and plaques of amyloid beta (neuritic plaques). These amyloid plaques constitute the other pathological hallmark of AD and are composed of sheets of beta-amyloid peptides (these peptides in turn are 36–43 amino acids in length and are principally described by the peptide length detected).

Patients with AD have been reported to manifest visual dysfunction [21, 22], although the extent of these visual deficits has been difficult to characterize because of patients concomitant alterations in memory and behavior. There have been consistent reports documenting that patients with AD demonstrate significant inner retinal atrophy, including descriptions of disc pallor and nerve fiber loss documented with fundus photos and OCT [23–27]. Although most of the OCT studies were done on older technology the general impression has been that thinning predominantly involves the arcuate bundles rather than the papillomacular bundle. However, these studies have generally lacked pathological confirmation of diagnosis (and predated the use of amyloid PET-based imaging) and the total numbers of patients studied has been small.

A seminal paper in the field compared ten AD subjects with ten age-matched controls and described moderate levels of axonal degeneration in the optic nerves of subjects with AD. The investigators reported relatively selective loss of larger diameter axons in AD subjects (although very small axons of 0.5–1 micron diameter appeared to potentially be lost as well). Reactive gliosis was described in both the retina and the optic nerve [28]. The authors described particular diminution of the thickness of the nerve fiber layer. However, they specifically describe an absence of both intraneuronal tau and amyloid beta (as assessed by Thioflavin S staining) [29–31]. Ultrastructural assessments in a related set of samples reported a vacuolated frothy appearance to RGC cytoplasm. Using additional stains the investigators determined that in one case 20% of RGCs appeared to be actively degenerating [29]. Although the bulk of the literature in this area has suggested that inner retinal atrophy is detectable in AD, at least one well-documented series was unable to demonstrate any loss of RGCs or axonal loss in the retina [32].

The presence of amyloid beta fibrils in the retinae of AD patients is controversial and unclear. Most investigators have been unable to find amyloid deposits in the retinae of patients with AD. Age-related accumulation of amyloid beta has been described in the normal human and mouse retina [33], but only one group has reported the capacity to detect human retinal amyloid deposition in AD subjects [34, 35]. Others have found no evidence for either amyloid plaques or hyperphosphorylated tau in the AD retina [36].

In animal models of AD (mice genetically manipulated to recapitulate one or some of the major genetic defects associated with nonsporadic AD) pathological descriptions have suggested that Abeta deposition can be detected in the inner retina around blood vessels, and that this may be associated with ganglion cell loss and thinning of the retinal nerve fiber [34, 37]. This observation requires further replication and analysis.

Friedreich's ataxia

Friedreich's ataxia (FA) is an autosomal recessive neurodegenerative disease caused by excessive GAA repeats in intron 1 of the frataxin gene on chromosome 9. This leads to increased susceptibility to oxidative stress and mitochondrial dysfunction induced by aberrant iron influx. The disease is characterized by progressive leg weakness with ataxia and gait disturbance as well as loss of deep tendon reflexes and dysarthria. Up to 30% of patients with FA have been noted to manifest significant optic neuropathy [38, 39]. In addition, much less frequently patients exhibit progressive pigmentary retinopathy that appears similar to standard retinitis pigmentosa, and a different subset of patients has been reported to have more fuliminant and dramatic visual decline [38]. Although nearly all patients have evidence of injury to the anterior visual pathway, including thinning of nerve fiber, very few have significant visual symptoms. To date, there are no reported cases of pathological evaluation of the retina in patients with FA [38, 39].

Parkinson's disease and synucleinopathies

Idiopathic Parkinson's disease (IPD) is the second most common neurodegenerative disease in the industrialized world and is pathologically manifested by injury to dopaminergic cells of the central nervous system – most characteristically in the substantia nigra pars compacta of the midbrain. However, injury to the dopaminergic system is widespread in the disease and includes areas of the brainstem and cerebral hemispheres.

Induction of Parkinsonism in mice with the administration of 1-methyl-4-phenyl– 1,2,3,6-tetrahydropyridine (MPTP) produces a model of disease by selectively targeting dopaminergic function in the central nervous system. Use of MPTP causes a reversible but dose-dependent reduction in tyrosine hydroxylase in amacrine cells. In the absence of tyrosine hydroxylase, neurons cannot convert L-Tyrosine into L-DOPA (which is itself a necessary precursor for dopamine production) [40]. Decreases in retinal dopaminergic amacrine function might be predicted to result in failure of center surround antagonism in ganglion cells. Patients with IPD are known to have deficits detectable on flash electroretinograms and pattern electroretinograms – especially manifested in tests done with a high spatial frequency – as would be predicted by injury to amacrine cells. However, TH immunostaining in human subjects with IPD has been reported to be normal. Furthermore, intracellular aggregations of alpha-synuclein have been reported to be absent in the retina [41].

Despite interest in the field, and the recognition of visual functional deficits believed to be retinal in origin in subjects with IPD, there are no published descriptions of retinal histopathology in patients with IPD [36, 41]. A single pathological series including three patients has been the subject of two papers in patients with another major synucleinopathy – dementia with Lewy bodies. This analysis reported the identification of pale intracellular inclusions in the outer plexiform layer and cytoskeletal disorganization with enlarged rod inner segments. These inclusions were not synuclein, but their molecular structure was not identified [42].

Huntington's disease

Huntington's disease (HD) is a relentlessly progressive monogenic autosomal dominant hereditary neurodegenerative disease caused by expanded trinucleotide repeats in the gene encoding the protein huntingtin (Htt) on chromosome 4. The expanded CAG repeat gives rise to an excessively long polyglutamine region in mutant Htt. Disease onset is most typically in middle age and characterized by defects in motor function and psychiatric disturbances followed by the ultimate development of dementia and death. Principal injury occurs to the indirect pathway of the striatum including the caudate nucleus. A study of retinal function in living HD patients showed higher thresholds to blue light following adaptation to yellow light, suggesting deficient neural processing in the retina compared to both normal controls as well as with patients with Tourette's syndrome and schizophrenia [43].

Murine and drosophila models of HD exhibit clear evidence of retinal degeneration as part of the disease phenotype. The R6/1 mouse model expresses exon 1 of the HD gene with 115 CAG repeats driven by the human HD promoter. Similarly, the R6/2 model expresses the same exon but with 150 repeats (and thereby has accelerated and more severe disease). The R6/1 model shows cone dysfunction and injury starting around the same age as other manifestations of disease in the brain. Ultimately, these mice showed complete loss of cone opsin and transducin. The more severe R6/2 model demonstrates significant injury on light and electron microscopy affecting the entire retina, especially concentrated in the center [44]. The drosophila model of HD also has evidence of photoreceptor neuron degeneration [45]. Only a single subject with HD appears to have ever undergone detailed ophthalmic pathological analysis. The investigators failed to find any clear retinal injury, but examination of the photoreceptor layer, which is affected in the drosophila model, was limited by technical difficulties because it peeled off the retina during processing [45].

Spinocerebellar ataxia type VII

Spincerebellar ataxia type VII is an autosomal dominant progressive neurological syndrome characterized by gait ataxia, dysarthria, ophthalmoplegia, dysphagia pyramidal impairment, and visual loss. It is caused by a variable but expanded CAG (polyglutamine) repeat near the N-terminal end of the Ataxin-7 gene. As with other polyglutamine repeat disorders, the disease manifests genetic anticipation with repeat length inversely proportional to age of disease onset. Most patients ultimately progress to complete blindness. It has been reported that impairment of yellow–blue color vision may precede the onset of the disease by many years and may be one of the earliest signs of disease [46].

Descriptions of pathological injury in SCA-VII are sparse. However, one series described detailed retinal histopathology from five members of a single family and described severe inner and outer retinal abnormalities, including near complete loss of photoreceptors and ganglion cells. In addition, there was RPE degeneration and abnormal presence of pigment detected into the retina [46].

Toxic and metabolic states

Vitamin B12 deficiency is manifest by loss of both central nervous system and peripheral nervous system myelin (in addition to macrocytosis of erythrocytes). In the retina, B12 deficiency is characterized by loss of retinal ganglion cells in the macula and thinning of the temporal RNFL. There are no human cases of retinal pathology in subjects with documented B12 deficiency. On pathology, loss of axons, particularly in the temporal retina and retinal ganglion cells, is readily manifest in monkeys with induced cobalamin deficiency [47]. Other animal models of B12 deficiency are afoveate and the retina has not been studied.

In general, patients with nutritional deficiencies have appeared to follow the same pattern with predominant injury to the papillomacular bundle. Isolated cases of subjects with nutritional (tobacco) amblyopia have undergone retinal pathological evaluation and demonstrate profound loss of retinal ganglion cells and their axons of the temporal nerve fiber and replacement of normal RNFL with dense collagenous tissue, fibroblasts and glial cells [48, 49]. Methanol toxicity is associated with a more precipitous decline in vision but with the same pattern of injury – absent the gliosis [50]. Given the rarity of such fulminant cases in the industrialized world, additional pathological descriptions to confirm these findings are unlikely. However, the degree to which ganglion cell loss was accompanied by fibrotic response is an important caveat when considering retinal imaging findings.

Aging

In studying neurodegenerative disease, aging is both an important parameter for understanding the progression of the underlying disease and a confounder. There are changes in tissue architecture, cellular appearance, and tissue volume with normal aging. However, these diseases often manifest atrophy and cellular changes that reflect accelerated aging. It is, therefore, important to consider carefully the impact of aging on any pathological retinal specimen evaluated – especially as these samples in neurological disease almost uniformly are assessed at the end of life when pathological injury is most profound.

The total number of retinal neurons declines with age including loss of photoreceptors and retinal ganglion cells [51, 52]. Ubiquitin and alpha synuclein were both observed with high frequency in subjects older than age 80 and were principally found in the inner nuclear layer [53]. Tau as a cytoskeletal protein with high affinity for microtubules is found in highest concentration in the terminal end of developing axons and is involved in determining axon polarity and is required for normal axon development. It is, therefore, not surprising that unphosphorlyated tau can be found in the human retina. In one study, diffuse staining for unphosphorylated tau was observed in the inner plexiform layer of the retina in all subjects, including many with diseases having no relation to neurodegeneration; however, phosphorylated tau was not detected. Unphosphorylated tau was also observed to a lesser extent in photoreceptors [53].

Summary

In total, retinal pathology is a common feature of neurodegenerative diseases of the central nervous system. However, the pathological mechanisms underlying this injury remain elusive given the absence of conclusive histopathological evaluations in a wide variety of patients – with a few exceptions. Additional pathological evaluations in these diseases will help with understanding findings from the burgeoning field of retinal imaging and visual electrophysiology in the neurology clinic. Further studies in patients and animal models of disease, especially when done with correlative imaging, will help advance the field significantly and resolve lingering controversies.

References

1. Green, AJ. Mcquaid S, Hauser SL, et al Ocular pathology in multiple sclerosis: retinal atrophy and inflammation irrespective of disease duration. *Brain* 2010; **133** (Pt 6): 1591–1601.
2. Oppenheim H. Zur pathologie der disseminirten sklerose. *Berliner Klinische Wochenschrift* 1887; **48**:904–7.
3. Lisch K. Die Veranderung der peripheren schbahn bei Mulipler Sklerose Arch f. *Augehn* 1933;**107**:380.
4. Gartner S. Optic neuropathy in multiple sclerosis; optic neuritis. *AMA Arch Ophthalmol* December 1953;**50**(6):718–26.
5. Toussaint D, Périer O, Verstappen A, Bervoets S. Clinicopathological study of the visual pathways, eyes, and cerebral hemispheres in 32 cases of disseminated sclerosis. *J Clin Neuroophthalmol* September 1983;**3** (3):211–20.
6. Kerrison JB, Flynn T, Green WR. Retinal pathologic changes in multiple sclerosis. *Retina* 1994;**14**(5): 445–51.
7. Mogensen PH. Histopathology of anterior parts of the optic pathway in patients with multiple sclerose. *Acta Ophthalmol (Copenh)* April 1990;**68**(2):218–20.
8. ter Braak JWG, van Herwaarden A. Ophthalmo encephalomyelitis. *Klin Monatsbl Augenheilkd* 1933;**91**: 316–43.
9. Rucker CW. Sheathing of the retinal veins in multiple sclerosis. *Review of pertinent literature. Mayo Clin Proc* 1972;**47**:335–40.
10. Toussaint D. Perivenous sheathing in multiple sclerosis. *Bull Soc Belge Ophtalmol.* November 1983;**208** Pt 1:369–74.
11. Sanders MD. Retinal arteritis, retinal vasculitis and autoimmune retinal vasculitis. *Eye* 1987;**1**:441–65
12. Arnold AC, Pepose JS, Hepler RS, Foos RY. Retinal periphlebitis and retinitis in multiple sclerosis. *I. Pathologic characteristics. Ophthalmology* 1984; **91**:255–62.
13. Evangelou N, Konz D, Esiri MM, et al. Size-selective neuronal changes in the anterior optic pathways suggest a differential susceptibility to injury in multiple sclerosis. *Brain* 2001;**124**:1813–20.
14. Schlamp CL, Montgomery AD, Mac Nair CE, et al. Evaluation of the percentage of ganglion cells in the ganglion cell layer of the rodent retina. *Mol Vis* June 27, 2013;**19**:1387–96.
15. Wang L, Cioffi GA, Cull G, Dong J, Fortune B. Immunohistologic evidence for retinal glial cell changes in human glaucoma. *Invest Ophthalmol Vis Sci* April 2002;**43**(4):1088–94.
16. Liu S, Li ZW, Weinreb RN, Xu G, et al. Tracking retinal microgliosis in models of retinal ganglion cell damage. *Invest Ophthalmol Vis Sci* September 2012;**53** (10):6254–62.
17. Anderson GW, Goebel HH, Simonati A. Human pathology in NCL. *Biochim Biophys Acta* November 2013;**1832**(11):1807–26.
18. Seehafer SS, Pearce DA. You say lipofuscin, we say ceroid: defining autofluorescent storage material. *Neurobiol Aging* April 2006;**27**(4):576–88.
19. Bensaoula T, Shibuya H, Katz ML, Smith JE, Johnson GS, John SK, Milam AH. Histopathologic and immunocytochemical analysis of the retina and ocular tissues in Batten disease. *Ophthalmology* September 2000;**107**(9):1746–53.
20. Goebel HH, Fix JD, Zeman W. The fine structure of the retina in neuronal ceroid-lipofuscinosis. *Am J Ophthalmol* January 1974;**77**(1):25–39.
21. Cogan DG. Visual disturbances with focal progressive dementing disease. *Am J Ophthalmol* July 15, 1985;**100** (1): 68–72.
22. Tzekov R, Mullan M. Vision function abnormalities in Alzheimer disease. *Surv Ophthalmol* October 22, 2013. pii: S0039-6257(13) 00237-3.
23. Hedges TR 3rd, Perez Galves R, Speigelman D, et al. Retinal nerve fiber layer abnormalities in Alzheimer's disease. *Acta Ophthalmol Scand* June 1996;**74**(3):271–5.
24. Tsai CS, Ritch R, Schwartz B, Lee SS, et al. Optic nerve head and nerve fiber layer in Alzheimer's disease. *Arch Ophthalmol* February 1991;**109**(2):199–204.
25. Lu Y, Li Z, Zhang X, Ming B, et al. Retinal nerve fiber layer structure abnormalities in early Alzheimer's disease: evidence in optical coherence tomography. *Neurosci Lett* August 9, 2010 Aug 9;**480**(1):69–72.
26. Kesler A, Vakhapova V, Korczyn AD, et al. Retinal thickness in patients with mild cognitive impairment and Alzheimer's disease. *Clin Neurol Neurosurg* September 2011;**113**(7):523–6.
27. Berisha F, Feke GT, Trempe CL, et al. Retinal abnormalities in early Alzheimer's disease. *Invest Ophthalmol Vis Sci* May 2007;**48**(5):2285–9.

28. Hinton DR, Sadun AA, Blanks JC, Miller CA. Optic-nerve degeneration in Alzheimer's disease. *N Engl J Med* August 21, 1986;**315**(8):485–7.

29. Blanks JC, Torigoe Y, Hinton DR, Blanks RH. Retinal degeneration in the macula of patients with Alzheimer's disease. *Ann N Y Acad Sci* 1991;**640**:44–6.

30. Blanks JC, Torigoe Y, Hinton DR, Blanks RH. Retinal pathology in Alzheimer's disease. I. Ganglion cell loss in foveal/parafoveal retina. *Neurobiol Aging* May-June 1996;**17**(3):377–84.

31. Blanks JC, Schmidt SY, Torigoe Y, et al. Retinal pathology in Alzheimer's disease. II. Regional neuron loss and glial changes in GCL. *Neurobiol Aging.* May-June 1996;**17**(3):385–95.

32. Curcio CA, Drucker DN. Retinal ganglion cells in Alzheimer's disease and aging. *Ann Neurol* March 1993;**33**(3):248–57.

33. Hoh Kam J, Lenassi E, Jeffery G. Viewing ageing eyes: diverse sites of amyloid Beta accumulation in the ageing mouse retina and the up-regulation of macrophages. *PLoS One* October 1, 2010;**5**(10).

34. Koronyo-Hamaoui M, Koronyo Y, Ljubimov AV, et al. Identification of amyloid plaques in retinas from Alzheimer's patients and noninvasive in vivo optical imaging of retinal plaques in a mouse model. *Neuroimage* January 2011; **54** Suppl 1: S204–17.

35. Koronyo Y, Salumbides BC, Black KL, Koronyo-Hamaoui M. Alzheimer's disease in the retina: imaging retinal aβ plaques for early diagnosis and therapy assessment. *Neurodegener Dis* 2012;**10**(1–4):285–93.

36. Ho CY, Troncoso JC, Knox D, et al. Beta-amyloid, phospho-tau and alpha-synuclein deposits similar to those in the brain are not identified in the eyes of Alzheimer's and Parkinson's disease patients. *Brain Pathol* January 2014;**24**(1):25–32.

37. Alexandrov PN, Pogue A, Bhattacharjee S, Lukiw WJ. Retinal amyloid peptides and complement factor H in transgenic models of Alzheimer's disease. *Neuroreport* August 24, 2011;**22**(12):623–7

38. Fortuna F, Barboni P, Liguori R, et al. Visual system involvement in patients with Friedreich's ataxia. *Brain* January 2009;**132**(Pt 1):116–23.

39. Noval S, Contreras I, Sanz-Gallego I, et al. Ophthalmic features of Friedreich ataxia. *Eye (Lond)* February 2012;**26**(2):315–20.

40. Tatton WG, Kwan MM, Verrier MC, et al. MPTP produces reversible disappearance of tyrosine hydroxylase-containing retinal amacrine cells. *Brain Res* September 10, 1990;**527**(1):21–31.

41. Archibald NK, Clarke MP, Mosimann UP, Burn DJ. The retina in Parkinson's disease. *Brain* May 2009;**132** (Pt 5):1128–45.

42. Maurage CA, Ruchoux MM, de Vos R, et al. Retinal involvement in dementia with Lewy bodies: a clue to hallucinations? *Ann Neurol* October 2003;**54**(4):542–7.

43. Paulus W, Schwarz G, Werner A, et al. Impairment of retinal increment thresholds in Huntington's disease. *Ann Neurol* October 1993;**34**(4):574–8

44. Petrasch-Parwez E, Saft C, Schlichting A, et al. Is the retina affected in Huntington disease? *Acta Neuropathol* November 2005;**110**(5):523–5.

45. Jackson GR, Salecker I, Dong X, et al Polyglutamine-expanded human huntingtin transgenes induce degeneration of Drosophila photoreceptor neurons. *Neuron* September 1998;**21**(3):633–42.

46. Martin JJ, Van Regemorter N, Krols L, et al. On an autosomal dominant form of retinal-cerebellar degeneration: an autopsy study of five patients in one family. *Acta Neuropathol* 1994;**88**(4):277–86.

47. Agamanolis DP, Chester EM, Victor M, et al. Neuropathology of experimental vitamin B12 deficiency in monkeys. *Neurology* October 1976;**26** (10):905–14.

48. Smiddy WE, Green WR. Nutritional amblyopia. *A histopathologic study with retrospective clinical correlation.* Graefes Arch Clin Exp Ophthalmol 1987;**225** (5):321–4.

49. Victor M, Dreyfus PM. Tobacco-alcohol amblyopia. *Further comments on its pathology. Arch Ophthalmol.* November 1965;**74**(5):649–57.

50. Sharpe JA, Hostovsky M, Bilbao JM, Rewcastle NB. Methanol optic neuropathy: a histopathological study. *Neurology* October 1982;**32**(10):1093–100.

51. Curcio CA. Photoreceptor topography in ageing and age-related maculopathy. *Eye(Lond)* June 2001;**15** (Pt 3):376–83.

52. Pitts DG. The effects of aging on selected visual functions: dark adaptation, visual acuity, stereopsis and brightness contrast. In: Sekuler R, Kline DW, Dismukes K, editors. *Aging and Human Visual Function.* New York: 1982; p. 131–159.

53. Leger F, Fernagut PO, Canron MH, et al. Protein aggregation in the aging retina. *J Neuropathol Exp Neurol* January 2011;**70**(1):63–8.

Chapter 15

Retinal inflammation in multiple sclerosis revealed by optical coherence tomography and ophthalmoscopy

Elena H. Martinez-Lapiscina, Bernardo Sanchez-Dalmau, and Pablo Villoslada

Retinal abnormalities associated with multiple sclerosis (MS) are receiving increasing interest. The most significant are retinal vasculitis (periphlebitis) and pars planitis. Retinal vasculitis represents a group of diseases characterized by inflammation affecting the retinal vasculature. They represent a group of uncommon disorders that may occur as an isolated disease or more commonly in association with other ocular diseases or a variety of systemic diseases, including MS. Table 15.1 lists the different conditions that can be associated with retinal vasculitis. However, some other findings include presence of edema in different layers of the retina associated with different processes.

Retinal periphlebitis

Retinal periphlebitis is an inflammatory disorder of the retina characterized by focal or diffuse perivascular inflammatory infiltrates around retinal vessels. The pathology may be located anywhere on the retina, the peripheral retina being the most commonly affected site. Retinal periphlebitis affects retinal veins with normal retinal arteries and is asymptomatic. It is characterized by retinal venous sheathing (Rucker´s sign), especially on sites of arterio-venous crossover and focal perivenous exudation and hemorrhage (Figure 15.1A-B).

Retinal periphlebitis can be present in two forms. The first one is active periphlebitis, with venous sheathing, which may be focal or diffuse, and perivenous exudation and hemorrhage. The second is inactive periphlebitis, with vascular sclerosis and retinal pigmentary changes around the vein. The diagnosis of retinal periphlebitis is based on the retinal findings by ophthalmoscopy. Since retinal periphlebitis is most frequently found around veins of the retinal periphery, which cannot be reached by OCT, it is highly recommended to assess it using pupil dilatation and indirect or slit-lamp ophthalmoscopy. However, retinal periphlebitis is frequently undiagnosed in the clinical setting. Although some authors have tried to improve diagnosis by using retinal angiography in order to confirm the presence of retinal vessel leakage (typical of active retinal periphlebitis), angiography does not increase the identification of retinal periphlebitis [1]. The ultra-wide-field retinal imaging devices that provide a high-resolution image of up to 200 degrees of the retina in a single capture may help to identify retinal periphlebitis, allowing also a wide field fluorescein angiography (Figure 15.1C).

Most patients with retinal vascular sheathing have no visual complaints referable to the condition, but some patients develop recurrent episodes that may eventually become associated with severe retinal disease that ultimately results in retinal ischemia, retinal detachment, or other retinal dysfunction with consequent permanent visual loss.

The etiological process underlying retinal periphlebitis remains unclear. Retinal periphlebitis affects multiple veins with different evolution times and often results in relapses. This course is typical of immune-mediated disorders. Additionally, the presence of perivascular inflammatory infiltrate with mononuclear cells composed of lymphocytes, plasmacytes, and monocytes [2, 3] also argues in favor of an immune-mediated disorder. Moreover, retinal periphlebitis is associated with auto-immune disorders such as sarcoidosis [4], Behçet's disease [5], lupus erythematous [6], and mainly with MS [1, 2, 7–9].

Optical Coherence Tomography in Neurological Disease, ed. Peter A. Calabresi, Laura J. Balcer, and Elliot M. Frohman. Published by Cambridge University Press.

Table 15.1

Infectious disorders	Bacterial: tuberculosis, syphilis, Lyme disease, Whipple's disease, brucellosis, cat scratch disease, endophthalmitis, post-streptococcal syndrome, Mediterranean spotted fever, Rocky Mountain spotted fever Viral: human T cell lymphoma virus type 1, cytomegalovirus, herpes simplex virus, varicella zoster virus, Epstein-Barr virus, Rift Valley fever virus, hepatitis, acquired immunodeficiency syndrome, West Nile virus infection, dengue fever virus Parasitic: Toxoplasmosis
Neurologic disorders	Multiple sclerosis Microangiopathy of the brain, retina, and cochlea (Susac's syndrome)
Malignancy	Paraneoplastic syndromes Ocular lymphoma Acute leukemia
Systemic inflammatory diseases	Behçet's disease, sarcoidosis, systemic lupus erythematosus, Wegener's granulomatosis, polyarteritis nodosa, Churg-Strauss syndrome, relapsing polychondritis, rheumatoid arthritis, HLA-B27-associated uveitis, Crohn's disease, postvaccination, dermatomyositis, Takayasu's disease, Buerger's disease, polymyositis
Primary Ocular disorder	Frosted branch angiitis, Idiopathic retinal vasculitis, aneurysms, and neuroretinitis (IRVAN), acute multifocal hemorrhagic retinal vasculitis, idiopathic recurrent branch retinal arterial occlusion, pars planitis, birdshot chorioretinopathy.

Retinal periphlebitis in multiple sclerosis

Retinal periphlebitis can be found in 6–36% of patients with MS [1, 7–11]. These differences in prevalence rates may be explained by several factors related to MS subtype (relapsing-remitting or progressive forms), disease duration, time of monitoring of MS patients, and use of immunomodulatory therapy, as well as the instruments used for retinal ascertaining periphlebitis (direct ophthalmoscopy with or without mydriasis or ultra-wide-field retinal imaging devices).

Retinal periphlebitis in patients with MS may cause blurred vision [10] or a very mild decrease in visual acuity [9], but most frequently this condition is asymptomatic. Retinal periphlebitis most often affects the peripheral retina without relevant damage to the macula responsible for the most detailed central vision. This may explain why retinal periphlebitis associated with MS is rarely accompanied by clinical abnormalities. However, it is still unknown whether retinal periphlebitis may induce local damage in the retinal tissue. We have analyzed the effect of retinal periphlebitis in a given quadrant (temporal, nasal, superior, or inferior) and the corresponding retinal nerve fiber layer (RNFL) thickness in that quadrant [1]. The presence of retinal periphlebitis in a given quadrant was not associated with a significantly thinner RNFL in the corresponding quadrant [1]. However, the small sample size and the relatively low incidence rate of retinal periphlebitis during the study period may precluded our ability to establish a significant association. Moreover, retinal periphlebitis might damage retinal layers other than the RNFL.

Although the clinical impact of the retinal periphlebitis on visual function in MS patients might not be relevant, its pathogenic significance or its use as a biomarker is raising the interest in this finding. The perivascular inflammatory infiltrate with lymphocytes and monocytes [2, 3] is nearly indistinguishable from the histopathological signature of perivenular cuffs of inflammation within the central nervous system (CNS) of patients with MS, particularly in the cerebral white matter. Thus, the pathological substrate of both disorders is similar. This raises two questions. The first one is a theoretical issue. Myelin is the putative principal target of immune activation in MS, and the retina lacks myelin. However, the retina is a common site of inflammation in MS [2]. Therefore, it will be important to evaluate whether the immune response in MS patients with retinal periphlebitis differs from that of patients without it. The second question is a practical issue. The similarities in the pathological processes associated with MS and periphlebitis raise the possibility that retinal inflammation parallels the

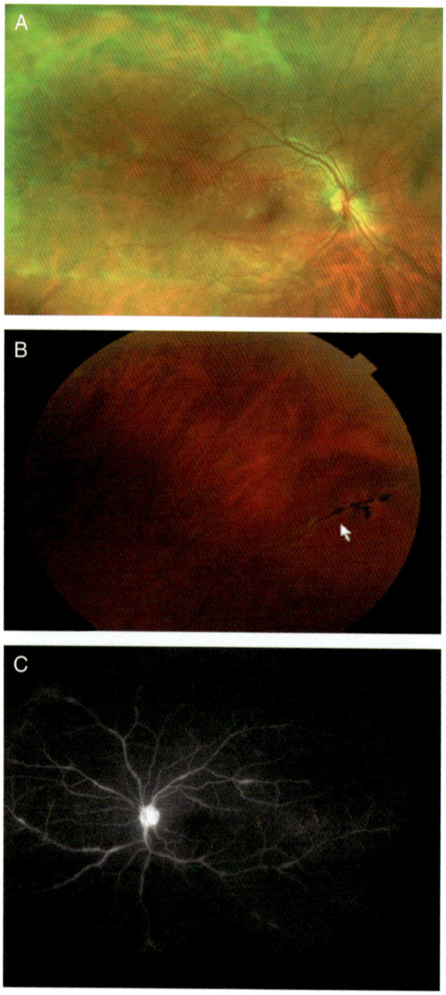

Figure 15.1 Retinal periphlebitis: (A) wide field retinography showing active retinal periphlebitis associated with MS; (B) non-active retinal periphlebitis, with pigmentary changes around the vein; (C) wide field fluorescein angiography in a case of diffuse periphlebitis.

inflammatory activity in the CNS in patients with MS as a part of the overall brain inflammatory activity. We have shown previously that patients with retinal periphlebitis had a 54% increased risk of new relapses [OR=1.52 95% IC (1.36–1.64)] in comparison with those without retinal inflammation [1]. Retinal periphlebitis is associated with both imaging and molecular biomarkers of disease activity, since it has been reported that MS patients with retinal periphlebitis have a higher gadolinium-enhancing lesion load [1, 9] and higher values of IgG index and intrathecal IgG synthesis [9] compared with patients without it. Consequently, retinal periphlebitis may become a suitable biomarker of inflammatory activity in MS.

Besides inflammation, MS causes neurodegeneration, which determines disease severity and impacts quality of life. Identifying appropriate biomarkers of axonal damage that can be easily assessed at the bedside is a key point for the development of neuroprotective therapies. Inflammation and neurodegeneration are directly correlated in MS [12]. Thus, retinal periphlebitis may be regarded also as biomarker of neurodegenerative damage in MS. We have recently shown that patients with retinal periphlebitis had a trend toward a higher EDSS score at baseline and accelerated disability progression after one year of follow-up when compared to patients without retinal inflammation [13]. Moreover, these patients had higher lesion volume and reduced T1 normalized brain parenchymal volume and normalized gray matter volume than patients without it. In comparison with MS patients without retinal inflammation, patients with retinal periphlebitis had also a thinner RNFL and smaller macular volumes, both surrogate retinal imaging markers of axonal damage [13].

In conclusion, retinal periphlebitis is associated with both the inflammatory and neurodegenerative processes in MS in terms of clinical parameters (relapses and disability), surrogate markers of inflammation (gadolinium-enhancing lesions, increased CSF IgG index, and intrathecal IgG synthesis rate), and features characteristic of neurodegeneration (lesion load, brain atrophy, and reduced RNFL thickness, and MV) (Table 15.2).

Edema of retinal layers in multiple sclerosis

The development of spectral-domain (SD) OCT devices has allowed studying in great detail the retina of patients with MS. The possibility of segmenting the different layers of the retina provides the opportunity for quantifying differences in layer thickness and identifying subtle abnormalities related with the inflammatory process associated with MS. Based on these enhanced capabilites, recent reports have described the presence of retinal edema, which can be localized to the inner nuclear layer, within the RNFL or in a pattern consistent with macular edema (e.g., as associated with fingolimod therapy) [15].

1. Microcystic Macular edema

Microcystic macular edema (MMO) refers to the presence of multiple retinal microcysts, preferentially involving the inner nuclear layer of retina, which can be revealed with SD-OCT [14] (Figure 15.2).

Table 15.2 Association between retinal periphlebitis and inflammatory and neurodegenerative parameters in multiple sclerosis

Parameters	Reference	Conclusion
Relapses	Sepulcre et al. Neurology 2007;68(7):544–49	RP is a risk factor of new Relapses over 2-years follow-up OR = 1.52 95% CI (1.36–1.64) p = 0.002
MRI gadolinium-enhancing lesions	Sepulcre et al. Neurology 2007;68(7):544–49	Patients with RP had larger gadolinium-enhancing lesion volume than patients without RP at baseline p = 0.003
	Stamenkoviæ M et al. Vojnosanit Pregl 2011;68(7):544–9	Patients with RP had gadolinium-enhancing lesions more commonly than patients without RP at baseline p = 0.012
CSF IgG index and intrathecal IgG synthesis	Stamenkoviæ M et al. Vojnosanit Pregl 2011;68(7):544–9	Patients with RP had increased values of IgG Index (1.39 ±0.42) and intrathecal IgG synthesis (26 ±20.3) than patients without RP [IgG Index:0.82 ±0.49 Intrathecal IgG synthesis: 9.6 ±13] p <0.001
Disability	Sepulcre et al. Neurology 2007;68(7):544–49	RP is not associated with disability progression over two-year follow-up.
	Ortiz Pérez S et al. Neurology 2013;81 (10):877-81	Patients with RP had a nonsignificant increased EDSS score at baseline [2.38 95%IC (1.44–3.32)] and EDSS progression after one-year follow-up [0.34 95%IC(0–0.75)] compared to patients without RP: EDSS score at baseline [1.87 95%IC (1.61–2.12)] and EDSS progression [0.17 95%IC(0–0.29)]
MRI total lesion volume	Ortiz Pérez S et al. Neurology 2013;81 (10):877-81	Patients with RP had higher lesion volume at baseline [19.0 95%IC (9.3–28.8)] compared to patients without RP [8.6 95%IC (6.0–11.3)] p = 0.038
MRI brain atrophy	Ortiz Pérez S et al. Neurology 2013;81 (10):877-81	Patients with RP had lower normalized brain parenchymal volume [1481 95% IC (1410–1552)]compared to patients without RP [1550 95%IC (1530–1569)] p = 0.059 Patients with RP had lower normalized gray matter volume [772 95%IC (733–811)] compared to patients without RP [806 95%IC (796–817)] p = 0.085
OCT RNFL thickness	Ortiz Pérez S et al. Neurology 2013;81 (10):877-81	Patients with RP had thinner RNFL [79.2 95%IC (68.2–90.2)] compared to patients without RP [92.6 95%IC (89.6–95.5)] p = 0.018
OCT macular volume	Ortiz Pérez S et al. Neurology 2013;81 (10):877-81	Patients with RP had a nonsignificant smaller MV [8.43 95%IC (8.07–8.80)] compared to patients without RP [8.55 95%IC (8.45–8.64)] p = 0.563

RP: Retinal periphlebitis; MRI: Magnetic resonance imaging; CSF: cerebrospinal fluid; EDSS: Expanded disability status scale; OCT: optical coherence tomography; RNFL: Retinal nerve fiber layer; MV: Macular volume.

This retinal abnormality was first identified as a complication of uveitis in MS patients [16]. However, recent studies have shown that MMO can be found in about 0.5–6% of patients with MS without uveitis or in those treated with fingolimod, as well as in a variety of other diseases that affect the visual pathways [13, 17–19]. Eyes with MMO had higher impaired visual acuity than eyes without MMO [17, 18].

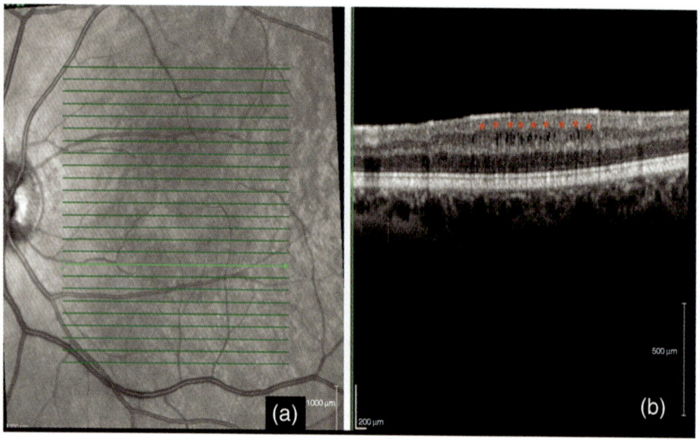

Figure 15.2 Microcystic macular edema associated with multiple sclerosis. A) OCT (Spectralis®) of the macula: the green arrow indicates the position of the OCT scans; B) Microcystic macular edema associated with Multiple Sclerosis: MMO is seen as small, round, and empty spaces in the inner nuclear layer: the red stars indicate the inner plexiform – retinal ganglion cell complex just above the cysts.

Visual complaints are more frequently found in patients with MMO than in those with retinal periphlebitis. However, eyes with MMO have thinner RNFL than eyes without it and MMO occurs more commonly in eyes with prior optic neuritis [17, 18]. Further, visual acuity remained significantly more abnormal among patients with MMO than those patients without MMO, even after adjustment for potential confounders such as age, sex, disease duration, and prior optic neuritis [17, 18]. The pathogenic mechanism underlying MMO in MS is not clear and different mechanisms may contribute to MMO such us Müller cell dysfunction [19], and blood-retinal barrier disruption and retinal inflammation [17, 18].

Clinically, MMO can be monitored by SD-OCT and this has led to the suggestion that MMO could be used as a suitable biomarker of MS disease activity in a subset of patients. MMO was associated with disease severity in an MS population investigated using cross-sectional analyses [13, 17, 18], whereas such an association was not identified when the patients were followed with a longitudinal strategy [17]. MMO is detected only among a small proportion of patients with MS (3–6%) and this low incidence may limit its value as a biomarker of disease activity. This hurdle can be overcome considering the following hypothesis postulated by Saidha and colleagues [17]. The increased thickness of the inner nuclear layer demonstrated by SD-OCT in MS patients may be a minor form of MMO. Retinal inflammation may cause thickening of the inner nuclear layer in the absence of visible MMO [17]. These authors showed that inner nuclear layer thickness was associated with both inflammatory activity in terms of relapses and gadolinium-enhancing lesions and new T2 lesions, and with neurodegenerative activity in terms of disability progression over two years of follow-up [17].

MMO has been identified in 26% patients with neuromyelitis optica [20]. The pathogenic mechanisms explaining MMO in patients with neuromyelitis optica are not completely understood, but they may be similar to those related to MS. MMO in patients with neuromyelitis optica is associated with higher visual disability and more severe retinal axonal damage regardless of prior optic neuritis episodes. Therefore, the presence of MMO may be a marker of poor visual outcome among patients with neuromyelitis optica [20].

2. RNFL edema due to interferon treatment

Ikebe and collegues described the first case of retinal hemorrhages and cotton-wool spots following interferon-alfa or -beta treatment in 1990 [21]. Since then, ophthalmological complications due to interferon administration have been reported especially among patients with hepatitis [22], but also among patients with MS [23–25]. The main fundoscopic sign of retinopathy due to interferon is cotton-wool spots (soft retinal exudates) [22]. SD-OCT has identified this finding as focal retinal nerve fiber layer edema with subsequent focal retinal thickening over the follow-up [26] (Figure 15.3). Cotton-wool spots represent retinal swellings resulting from focal occlusion of retinal arterioles that caused ischemic damage of the retinal nerve fiber layer. Cotton-wool spots are a common finding in patients with hypertension and diabetes mellitus, two well-recognized causes of ischemic microvascular damage by atherosclerosis. Interferon

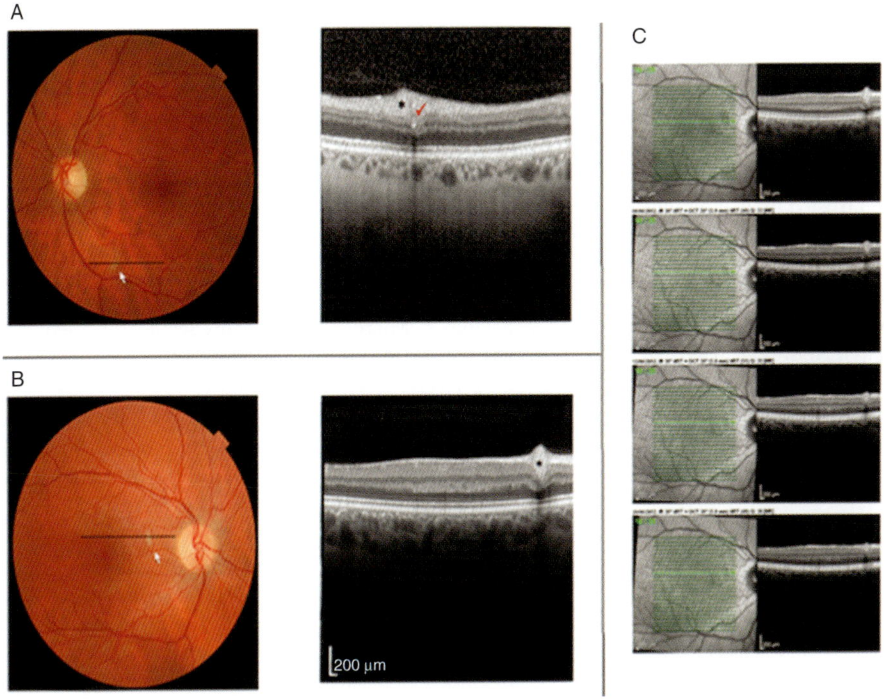

Figure 15.3 RNFL edema associated with interferon-beta treatment in MS. (A) OCT (Spectralis®): the black line indicates the position of the OCT scans. The white arrow points the RNFL edema as a grayish lesion in the funduscopic image. (B) The black star indicates the RNFL edema in OCT. Observe the RNFL thickening next to the focal edema. (C) SD-OCT monitoring of RNFL defect performed monthly over four-month follow-up. Notice the progressive resolution of the RNFL thickening.

can induce the production of autoantibodies leading to a local inflammatory infiltrate with deposition of cytokines, immune complexes, and leucocytes that finally occludes small retinal vessels leading to a focal retinal microinfarct [27–30]. RNFL defects due to interferon treatment may result as immune-mediated microvascular damage but the specific pathogenic mechanism of damage is not completely understood. Visual acuity impairment is the most common complaint found among patients with cotton-wool spots [22]. Improvement of visual complaints, fundoscopic exam, and SD-OCT abnormalities has been reported after interferon discontinuation [24] and also in patients that continue with this therapy [23]. However, the patient described by Sommer and colleagues suffered from new bilateral cotton-wool spots over the follow-up period, which finally disappeared after interferon disruption [23]. There is not enough evidence to determine whether treatment should be permanently discontinued or not. This interferon-associated retinopathy is a dynamic process, so if interferon is not discontinued, SD-OCT offers the possibility of a strict ophthalmologic monitoring even in absence of visual symptomatology. More importantly, SD-OCT evaluates not only the OCT correlate of these retinal soft exudates but also the subsequent RNFL thickening that might be relevant for MS patients.

References

1. Sepulcre J, Murie-Fernandez M, Salinas-Alaman A, Garcia-Layana A, Bejarano B, Villoslada P. Diagnostic accuracy of retinal abnormalities in predicting disease activity in MS. *Neurology* May 1, 2007;**68**(18):1488–94.
2. Green AJ, McQuaid S, Hauser SL, Allen IV, Lyness R. Ocular pathology in multiple sclerosis: retinal atrophy and inflammation irrespective of disease duration. *Brain* June 2010;**133**(Pt 6):1591–601.
3. Engell T. Neurological disease activity in multiple sclerosis patients with periphlebitis retinae. *Acta Neurologica Scandinavica* February 1986;**73**(2):168–72.
4. Herbort CP, Rao NA, Mochizuki M. International criteria for the diagnosis of ocular sarcoidosis: results of the first International Workshop On Ocular Sarcoidosis (IWOS). *Ocular Immunology and Inflammation* May–June 2009;**17**(3):160–9.

5. Mili-Boussen I, Letaief I, Zbiba W, Trabelsi O, Ben Younes N, Abid J, et al. [Retinal vasculitis. Epidemiological, clinical and etiological features]. *Journal Francais d'Ophtalmologie* October 2010;**33** (8):529–37. Les vascularites retiniennes: profils epidemiologiques, cliniques et etiologiques.
6. Quillen DA, Stathopoulos NA, Blankenship GW, Ferriss JA. Lupus associated frosted branch periphlebitis and exudative maculopathy. *Retina* (Philadelphia, Pa) 1997;**17**(5):449–51.
7. Rio J, Colin A, Salvador F, Tintore M, Viguera ML, Montalban J, et al. [Retinal periphlebitis in multiple sclerosis. *A prospective study].* Neurologia *(Barcelona, Spain).* October 1993;**8**(8):252–5.
8. Tola MR, Granieri E, Casetta I, Monari P, Scorrano R, Mazzeo V, et al. Retinal periphlebitis in multiple sclerosis: a marker of disease activity? *European Neurology* 1993;**33**(2):93–6.
9. Stamenkovic M, Obradovic D. Retinal periphlebitis in patients with multiple sclerosis. *Vojnosanitetski Pregled Military* – medical and pharmaceutical review July 2011;**68**(7):544–9.
10. Schmidt S, Wessels L, Augustin A, Klockgether T. Patients with multiple sclerosis and concomitant uveitis/periphlebitis retinae are not distinct from those without intraocular inflammation. *Journal of the Neurological Sciences* June 15, 2001;**187**(1–2):49–53.
11. Quentin CD, Altenhoff M, Schipper HI, Vogel M. [Retinal periphlebitis and multiple sclerosis. Incidence, cerebrospinal fluid and results of visual evoked potentials]. *Fortschritte der Ophthalmologie : Zeitschrift der Deutschen Ophthalmologischen Gesellschaft* 1990;**87** (4):359–61.
12. Barkhof F, Calabresi PA, Miller DH, Reingold SC. Imaging outcomes for neuroprotection and repair in multiple sclerosis trials. *Nature reviews Neurology* May 2009;**5**(5):256–66.
13. Ortiz-Perez S M-LE, Gabilondo I, Fraga-Pumar E, Martínez-Heras E, Saiz A, Sánchez-Dalmau B, *Villoslada P. Retinal periphlebitis is associated with multiple sclerosis severity. Neurology* 2013;**81**(10):877–81.
14. Mackenzie S, Schmermer C, Charnley A, Sim D, Vikas T, Dumskyj M, et al. SDOCT imaging to identify macular pathology in patients diagnosed with diabetic maculopathy by a digital photographic retinal screening programme. *PloS One* 2011;**6**(5):e14811.
15. Kappos L, Radue EW, O'Connor P, Polman C, Hohlfeld R, Calabresi P, et al. A placebo-controlled trial of oral fingolimod in relapsing multiple sclerosis. *The New England Journal of Medicine.* February 4, 2010;**362**(5):387–401.
16. Malinowski SM, Pulido JS, Folk JC. Long-term visual outcome and complications associated with pars planitis. *Ophthalmology* June 1993;**100**(6):818–24.
17. Saidha S, Sotirchos ES, Ibrahim MA, Crainiceanu CM, Gelfand JM, Sepah YJ, et al. Microcystic macular edema, thickness of the inner nuclear layer of the retina, and disease characteristics in multiple sclerosis: a retrospective study. *Lancet Neurol* November 2012;**11**(11):963–72.
18. Gelfand JM, Nolan R, Schwartz DM, Graves J, Green AJ. Microcystic macular edema in multiple sclerosis is associated with disease severity. *Brain.* June 2012;**135** (Pt 6):1786–93.
19. Balk LJ, Killestein J, Polman CH, Uitdehaag BM, Petzold A. Microcystic macular edema confirmed, but not specific for multiple sclerosis. *Brain* December 2012 Dec;**135**(Pt 12):e226; author reply e7.
20. Sotirchos ES, Saidha S, Byraiah G, Mealy MA, Ibrahim MA, Sepah YJ, et al. In vivo identification of morphologic retinal abnormalities in neuromyelitis optica. *Neurology* April 9, 2013 Apr 9;**80** (15):1406–14.
21. Ikebe T, Nakatsuka K, Goto M, Sakai Y, Kageyama S. *A case of retinopathy induced by intravenous administration of interferon.* Folia Ophthalmol Jpn *(Ganka-Kiyo).* 1990;**41**:6.
22. Fragoso YD, Paggiaro MS, Mastromauro R, Jacondino Gda S, Wilson HM. Literature systematic review on the ophthalmological side effects of interferons. *Arquivos Brasileiros de Oftalmologia.* July–August 2011;**74** (4):306–10.
23. Sommer S, Sablon JC, Zaoui M, Rozot P, Hosni A. [Interferon beta-1 b retinopathy during a treatment for multiple sclerosis]. *Journal Francais d'Ophtalmologie.* May 2001;**24**(5):509–12.
24. Mallada-Frechin J, Abellan-Miralles I, Alfaro-Beltra ML, Medrano V, Munoz-Gil MB, Fernandez-Izquierdo S, et al. [Retinopathy secondary to treatment with Interferon beta-1a in a patient with multiple sclerosis]. *Revista de Neurologia.* April 16–30, 2005;**40**(8):482–4.
25. Hara K, Tanito M, Ohira A. Retinal nerve fibre layer defects associated with cotton-wool spots in patients with interferon retinopathy. *Acta Ophthalmologica.* March 2012;**90**(2):e158–60.
26. Ioannides A, Georgakarakos ND, Elaroud I, Andreou P. Isolated cotton-wool spots of unknown etiology: management and sequential spectral domain optical coherence tomography documentation. *Clinical Ophthalmology* (Auckland, NZ). 2011;**5**:1431–3.
27. Taylor JL, Grossberg SE. The effects of interferon-alpha on the production and action of other cytokines. *Seminars in Oncology.* Febrary 1998;**25**(1 Suppl 1): 23–9.
28. Sugano S, Suzuki T, Watanabe M, Ohe K, Ishii K, Okajima T. Retinal complications and plasma C5a

levels during interferon alpha therapy for chronic hepatitis C. *The American Journal of Gastroenterology*. December 1998;**93**(12):2441–4. PubMed PMID: 9860406. Epub 1998/12/22. eng.

29. Lohmann CP, Kroher G, Bogenrieder T, Spiegel D, Preuner J. Severe loss of vision during adjuvant interferon alfa-2 b treatment for malignant melanoma. *Lancet*. April 17, 1999;**353**(9161):1326.

30. Guyer DR, Tiedeman J, Yannuzzi LA, Slakter JS, Parke D, Kelley J, et al. Interferon-associated retinopathy. *Archives of Ophthalmology*. March 1993;**111**(3):350–6.

Chapter 16

Optical coherence tomography and optic nerve magnetic resonance imaging in demyelinating diseases

Robert T. Naismith

Introduction

Studies of optical coherence tomography (OCT) and optic nerve magnetic resonance imaging (MRI) provide opportunities to cross-validate very distinct tools to assess visual pathway integrity. MRI of visual pathways provides distinct advantages for testing quantitative sequences and relating these to other measures of clinical function, structure, and physiology. These techniques are not in competition, as they can offer complementary information. Selection of one or both techniques would depend upon the investigative question, the timing of study, and other design features, and the advantages and disadvantages of each imaging method as it relates to a particular patient population. Indeed, OCT has clear advantages in acquisition time, equipment expense, operator expertise, and patient convenience. One major advantage for MR sequences is that, once validated on visual systems, they can then be implemented within other regions of the central nervous system directly hidden from view by OCT (e.g., spinal cord, brain).

Optic nerve imaging and the clinical-radiologic paradox

The optic nerve has major relevance in multiple sclerosis (MS) as a prime site for clinical and subclinical inflammatory demyelinating events that result in axon injury and disability. Optic "nerve" is a misnomer, because the structure is a direct "tract" of the central nervous system and has myelin derived from oligodendrocytes. While the propensity for the optic nerve to become involved in MS is clear, the rationale for the predominance of optic nerve involvement in MS is not. Perhaps the proclivity is conferred by a combination of vascular and immunologic features, which result in a particular vulnerability for attack [1]. Because MS white-matter plaques are often centered upon blood vessels, the dual arterial supply, high metabolic demands of the retina, and prominent venous drainage may contribute to potential for blood brain barrier breakdown within the optic nerve. The posterior visual pathways are also frequently affected in MS due to close proximity of optic radiations to the ventricles, a prime location for the classic periventricular plaque.

Regulatory agencies that approve disease-modifying therapies are most interested in surrogate measures with high clinical relevance toward disability and patient reported outcomes. Because imaging events are much more frequent than relapses and disability, MRI has been transformational for evaluating new therapeutics over a reasonable time frame for phase I and phase II studies. MRI metrics in corroboration with standard clinical endpoints (i.e., relapses, sustained disability progression) have been of major importance in phase III trials of MS therapeutics. Because the visual pathways represent a well-circumscribed structural system that is frequently involved in MS and have clinical outcome measures that relate to quality of life, and with little redundancy or confounding purpose, the optic nerve MRI serves as a model system for investigating how imaging techniques correspond with clinical dysfunction. The relation of imaging to a clinically meaningful event and quality of life is paramount for regulatory agencies to consider approval of new MS medications. This relation has been elusive for MRI sequences in clinical practice but, based on optic nerve imaging, it can be improved upon with more specialized sequences.

Optical Coherence Tomography in Neurological Disease, ed. Peter A. Calabresi, Laura J. Balcer, and Elliot M. Frohman. Published by Cambridge University Press.

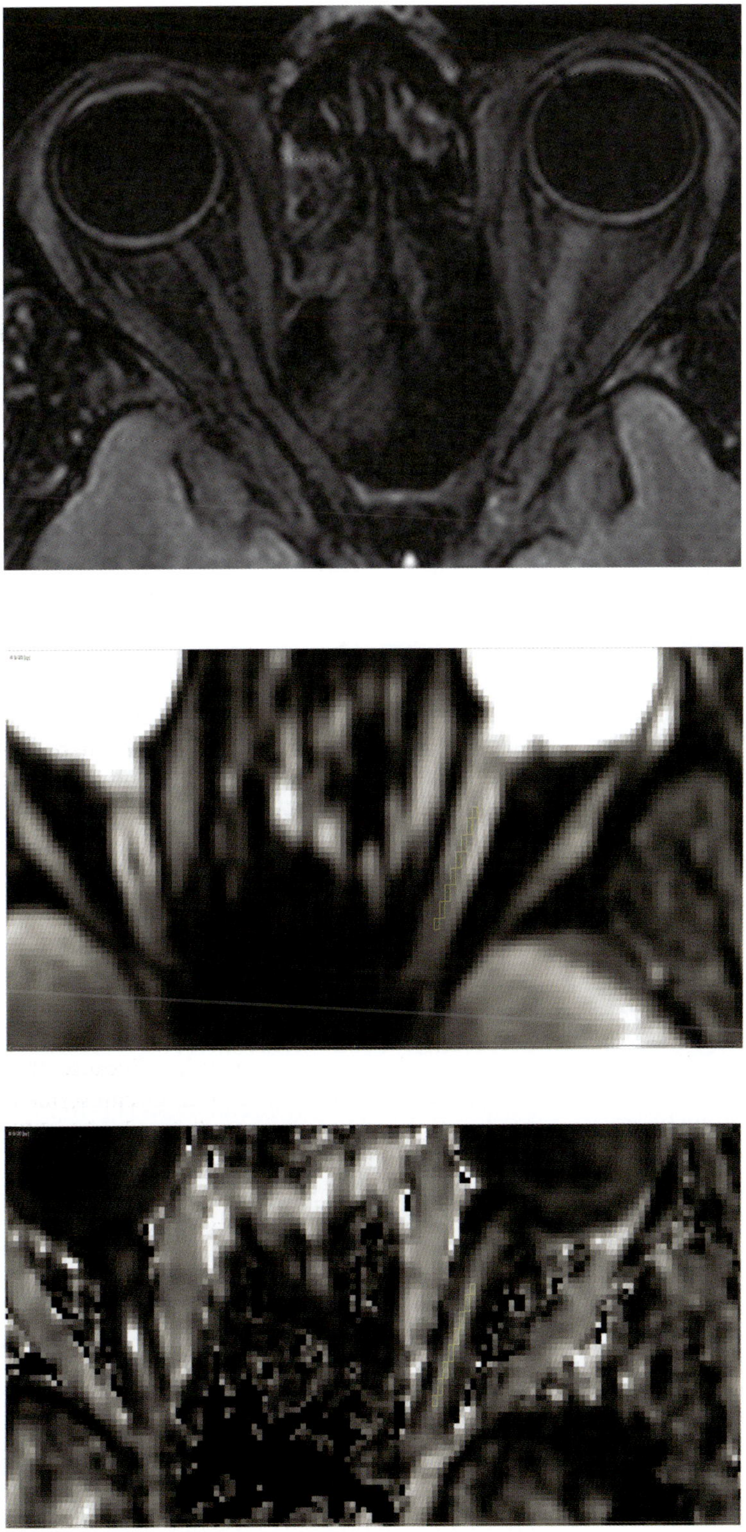

Figure 16.1 Axial optic nerve slice representing T2-weighted and diffusion-weighted sequences. (A) Optic nerve FLAIR MRI demonstrates increased T2 signal and swelling within the left nerve. (B) B0 image used for generating region of interest (yellow) consisting of 22 voxels within the nerve center. (C) Fractional anisotropy map demonstrating high directionality of the optic nerve on the left (right optic nerve cut by plane of slice).

Optic nerve MRI has high sensitivity and specificity for diagnosing optic neuritis and evaluating for other etiologies in clinical practice. The addition of optic nerve MRI to select clinical trials utilizing OCT and other visual outcomes can help support a treatment effect, if all measures are beneficially affected in a positive manner [2, 3]. Specialized MR sequences may have potential to evaluate acute axon injury, susceptibility to axonal loss, the composition of inflammatory infiltrates, and the potential for remyelination and efficacy of neural repair (Figure 6).

Challenges of optic nerve MRI

Optic nerve measures 3–4 mm in diameter in a healthy subject, less in someone with long-standing MS due to atrophy. High spatial resolution is a requisite for deriving reliable imaging measures of the optic nerve. The optic nerve is surrounded by different imaging interfaces, such as cerebral spinal fluid, orbital fat, air within sinuses, and bone. These different tissue interfaces create potential for imaging artifacts to negatively impact scan quality. Additionally, optic nerve imaging is impacted by eye or head movement, both of which can degrade image quality. Even arterial pulsations may negatively impact high-resolution quantitative techniques. The fast acquisition times and immediate processing of OCT does have an advantage for patient optimization and high-quality scans.

Optic nerve imaging in clinical practice is utilized frequently and with a high degree of success. However, investigational techniques require high-resolution and high signal-to-noise ratio (SNR), two qualities that require time and increase the chances for excessive movement. As the resolution increases, so must the scanning time and propensity to movement and other potential artifacts.

Optic nerve MRI in clinical practice

Standard optic nerve imaging includes high-resolution sequences in axial, sagittal, and coronal views. T2-weighted short tau inversion recovery (STIR) sequence is utilized to assess the presence of abnormal T2 hyperintense signal within the nerve, can provide information about whether the nerve is swollen or atrophic, and can assess for other impinging or infiltrating structures on the optic nerve [4]. A fat-suppressed T1-weighted sequence after administration of Gadolinium contrast can assess for the presence of blood–brain barrier breakdown, frequently seen in the acute setting of optic neuritis [5, 6].

T1-weighted sequences after administration of gadolinium reveals optic nerve enhancement with a sensitivity of 66–94%, typically lasting 1–2 months [7]. While optic nerves with more extensive enhancement had worse vision acutely, the association of final clinical outcome to enhancement length and presence of enhancement in the intracanicular portion of the optic nerve has conflicted among investigations [7–10]. Owing to the high sensitivity for contrast enhancement in the setting of acute optic neuritis, the absence of enhancement should at least make one consider an alternate diagnosis, such as ischemic optic neuropathy [11].

T2-weighted signal abnormalities can be observed in both the acute and chronic setting of optic neuritis. The length of chronic optic nerve hyperintensity has been demonstrated to correlate with thinning of the retinal nerve fiber layer (RNFL) by OCT [12]. However, MRI hyperintense lesion length did not appear to correlate with clinical outcomes. The decision to treat optic neuritis with anti-inflammatory glucocorticoids should be made on clinical and individual patient circumstances, as intravenous methylprednisolone did appear to shrink the resultant length of MRI hyperintense T2-signal within the optic nerve [13].

Optic nerve volumes

Volumetric measures of the CNS can serve as a surrogate of axonal loss and perhaps demyelination. Unfortunately, tissue volume measures also involve a number of confounding pathologic processes such as edema, cellular infiltration, and gliosis [14–16]. The time course of optic nerve volume changes has relevance for interpreting studies of OCT with regard to timing. Due to the inflammation and edema, the optic nerve can have prominent swelling during the acute period, with a mean 20% expansion over control nerve, and remain swollen for up to 60 days [17]. One year after optic neuritis, the nerve becomes atrophic by 14% compared to control.

While the more severely swollen optic nerves had worse baseline visual function, neither the amount of swelling nor the amount of atrophy predicted clinical visual outcomes at one year. Similar to what was observed with intravenous methylprednisolone and chronic T2-weighted lesion length, glucocorticoids did not appear to impact the degree of optic nerve atrophy when administered in the acute setting [18]. This implies that anti-inflammatory agents have little effect on axonal injury, even when administered within days of optic neuritis clinical onset [19]. This also illustrates how the visual pathway can provide important information about MS pathogenesis and treatment effect (or lack thereof).

Optic nerve diffusion tensor imaging

Diffusion tensor imaging (DTI) is a quantitative technique that can assess tissue directionality and integrity. Because the visual system is a tightly packed, structured tract of axons and myelin, DTI can be utilized to define the location and trajectory of the visual pathways. Diffusion imaging is based upon the Brownian motion of protons, which will diffuse along the trajectory of the axon. Mean diffusion will increase when there is loss of tissue.

DTI is acquired in six or more directions, and the largest direction of diffusion within a voxel is called the *principal eigenvector*. The principal eigenvector is referred to as lambda-1. By convention, eigenvectors perpendicular to lambda –1 include lambda-2 and lambda-3. From these eigenvectors, one can derive several interrelated DTI parameters to summarize and describe the diffusion within a specified voxel. Lambda-1, or the principal eigenvector, is sometimes referred to as axial diffusivity and has been proposed to be a surrogate for axonal injury during acute inflammation [20–23]. Radial diffusivity is the mean of the two perpendicular diffusivities (lambda-2 plus lambda-3 divided by 2) and has been proposed as a marker of both demyelination and tissue integrity [24–27]. DTI summary parameters include mean diffusivity (lambda1 + lambda2 + lambda 3/3) and fractional anisotropy, a scalar value of a directional ellipsoid between zero to one. Axial diffusivity and fractional anisotropy both imply a principal direction in their measure.

In remote optic neuritis, radial diffusivity and fractional anisotropy of the optic nerve have established strong correlations with RNFL by OCT, high- and low-contrast vision, and visual-evoked potentials (Figure 16.2) [26, 28–31]. Similarly, FA and radial diffusivity of the optic radiations have been demonstrated to correlate with RNFL, multifocal VEPs, and visual acuity [31–33]. These studies help to cross-validate OCT and DTI because they hold high concordance among all outcome measures despite assessing two different areas of the optic nerve, with vastly different techniques and methodologies.

In contrast to remote optic neuritis studies previously discussed, acute optic neuritis must be interpreted through a different set of DTI parameters, underscoring the importance of clinical correlation and a temporal evaluation. After acute optic neuritis, axial diffusivity has been found to be depressed for one to three months, followed by a period of apparent "normalization" around six months, and finally elevation of axial diffusivity after one year [34, 35, http://journals.plos.org/plosone/article?id=10.1371/journal.pone.0083825]. The precise etiology for this decrease is not clear, but an explanation can include axonal swelling and beading as a result from mitochondrial dysfunction, cytotoxic edema, and aggregation of intracellular proteins with increased intracellular

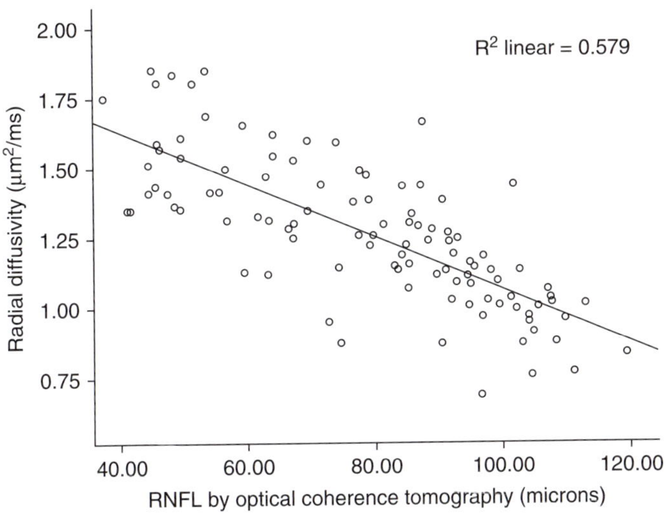

Figure 16.2 Correlation of optic nerve radial diffusivity with retinal nerve fiber layer thickness. Retinal nerve fiber layer thickness has a striking correlation with radial diffusivity within the optic nerve. The correlation cross-validates the techniques for assessing tissue integrity within the anterior visual pathway when also considering the robust relationship to clinical outcomes for each methodology. Radial diffusivity measures included 1–2 mm of the optic nerve, a location contiguous but separated in space from the RNFL.
(Reproduced with permission from Naismith et al, Neurology, 2009)

viscosity and impaired fast transport through microtubules. This initial depression in axial diffusivity has been found to correspond to long-term outcomes of RNFL by OCT, high- and low-contrast sensitivities, and visual evoked potentials at 6 and 12 months. The other DTI parameters, mean and radial diffusivities, and fractional anisotropy, do not appear to convey this acute alteration. Three months after optic neuritis onset, radial diffusivity begins to increase and reaches a plateau between 6 to 12 months. This increase in radial diffusivity has also been shown to correspond to RNFL and visual function parameters. The increases in axial and radial diffusivities between three and six months might be explained by axonal drop-out and loss of tissue integrity, both of which would result in an increased total diffusivity within the affected voxel. The MS lesions thus have a variety of pathologies which can change over time.

Optic nerve magnetization transfer imaging

Magnetization transfer imaging (MTI) is a quantitative technique proposed for the assessment of tissue macromolecules such as myelin. The technique uses an off-resonance radiofrequency pulse to saturate macromolecular protons rather that the standard pulse that saturates protons within the liquid pool. This hydrogen saturation is transient as the energy is transferred from the immobile macromolecular hydrogen pool to the free-water hydrogen pool, thus decreasing the free water signal in a predictable manner. By evaluating the ratio (MTR) of the saturated and the unsaturated sequences, one can obtain an indirect measure of macromolecular concentration and, thus, myelin [36]. MTR is beginning to be utilized to assess therapies designed to preserve myelin or enhance remyelination in MS.

On a cross-sectional basis in remote optic neuritis, optic nerve MTR has correlated with RNFL thickness and macular volumes by OCT, and visual evoked potential latency and amplitude [37, 38]. In longitudinal studies, MTR does not appear to be substantially impacted in acute optic neuritis [39, 40]. Rather, MTR appears to decrease between 3 and 6 months after optic neuritis clinical onset and, at that time, has been found to correlate with 12-month RNFL by OCT, high- and low-contrast visual acuity, and multifocal VEP. Subsequent to 6 months, MTR can appear to increase and improve for some patients, remain stable, or continue to drop through 12 months. The trend towards increasing MTR after 6 months has been hypothesized to represent remyelination post inflammation, and these post-6 month changes have been found to correspond to less volume loss in 12 month RNFL compared with those whose MTR continued to have a late decline [40].

Conclusions

Optic nerve MRI opens new opportunities to test novel imaging techniques and provide critical structural and metabolic information about the central nervous system in demyelinating diseases. One of the major goals of MR imaging is to develop a sequence with pathologic specificity to axon injury, myelin loss, and inflammation. Incorporation of OCT and VEPs with imaging helps to validate the degree to which the MRI technique discerns axonal and myelin pathologies. While the perfect technique for accomplishing this specificity has not been definitively established, optic nerve imaging has most certainly brought the MS field closer to this realization. Similarly, OCT in MS seeks to meet some of these needs to study inflammation and neurodegeneration.

References

1 Schmidt S. Candidate autoantigens in multiple sclerosis. *Multiple Sclerosis* 1999; **5**: 147–60.

2 Sühs K-W, Hein K, Sättler MB, *et al.* A randomized, double-blind, phase 2 study of erythropoietin in optic neuritis. *Annals of Neurology* 2012; **72**: 199–210.

3 Connick P, Kolappan M, Crawley C, et al. Autologous mesenchymal stem cells for the treatment of secondary progressive multiple sclerosis: an open-label phase 2a proof-of-concept study. *The Lancet Neurology* 2012; **11**: 150–6.

4 Miller DH, MacManus DG, Bartlett PA, Kapoor R, Morrissey SP, Moseley IF. Detection of optic nerve lesions in optic neuritis using frequency-selective fat-saturation sequences. *Neuroradiology* 1993; **35**: 156–8.

5 Guy J, Mao J, Bidgood Jr WD, Mancuso A, Quisling RG. Enhancement and demyelination of the intraorbital optic nerve: Fat suppression magnetic resonance imaging. *Ophthalmology* 1992; **99**: 713–9.

6 Guy J, Mancuso A, Quisling RG, Beck R, Moster M. Gadolinium-DTPA-enhanced magnetic resonance imaging in optic neuropathies. *Ophthalmology* 1990; **97**: 592–9.

7 Kupersmith MJ, Alban T, Zeiffer B, Lefton D. Contrast-enhanced MRI in acute optic neuritis: Relationship to visual performance. *Brain* 2002; **125**: 812–22.

8 Dunker S, Wiegand W. Prognostic value of magnetic resonance imaging in monosymptomatic optic neuritis. *Ophthalmology* 1996; **103**: 1768–73.

9 Miller DH, Newton MR, Van der Poel JC, et al. Magnetic resonance imaging of the optic nerve in optic neuritis. *Neurology* 1988; **38**: 175–9.

10 Hickman SJ, Toosy AT, Miszkiel KA, *et al.* Visual recovery following acute optic neuritis. *J Neurol* 2004; **251**: 996–1005.

11 Rizzo Iii JF, Andreoli CM, Rabinov JD. Use of magnetic resonance imaging to differentiate optic neuritis and nonarteritic anterior ischemic optic neuropathy. *Ophthalmology* 2002; **109**: 1679–84.

12 Kallenbach K, Simonsen H, Sander B, Wanscher B, Larsson H, Larsen M, Frederiksen JL. Retinal nerve fiber layer thickness is associated with lesion length in acute optic neuritis. *Neurology* 2010; **74**: 252–8.

13 Kapoor R, Miller DH, Jones SJ, et al. Effects of intravenous methylprednisolone on outcome in MRI-based prognostic subgroups in acute optic neuritis. *Neurology* 1998; **50**: 230–7.

14 Frisén L, Quigley HA. Visual acuity in optic atrophy: A quantitative clinicopathological analysis. *Graefe's Arch Clin Exp Ophthalmol* 1984; **222**: 71–4.

15 Hickman SJ, Brex PA, Brierley CMH, et al. Detection of optic nerve atrophy following a single episode of -unilateral optic neuritis by MRI using a fat-saturated short-echo fast FLAIR sequence. *Neuroradiology* 2001; **43**: 123–8.

16 Hickman SJ, Brierley CM, Brex PA, MacManus DG, Scolding NJ, Compston DA, Miller DH. Continuing optic nerve atrophy following optic neuritis: A serial MRI study. *Multiple Sclerosis* 2002; **8**: 339–42.

17 Hickman SJ, Toosy AT, Jones SJ, et al. A serial MRI study following optic nerve mean area in acute optic neuritis. *Brain* 2004; **127**: 2498–505.

18 Hickman SJ, Kapoor R, Jones SJ, Altmann DR, Plant GT, Miller DH. Corticosteroids do not prevent optic nerve atrophy following optic neuritis. *Journal of Neurology, Neurosurgery & Psychiatry* 2003; **74**: 1139–41.

19 Beck RW, Cleary PA, Anderson MM, et al. A Randomized, Controlled Trial of Corticosteroids in the Treatment of Acute Optic Neuritis. *New England Journal of Medicine* 1992; **326**: 581–8.

20 Budde MD, Kim JH, Liang HF, Russell JH, Cross AH, Song SK. Axonal injury detected by in vivo diffusion tensor imaging correlates with neurological disability in a mouse model of multiple sclerosis. *NMR Biomed* 2008; **21**: 589–97.

21 Budde MD, Xie M, Cross AH, Song S-K. Axial Diffusivity Is the Primary Correlate of Axonal Injury in the Experimental Autoimmune Encephalomyelitis Spinal Cord: A Quantitative Pixelwise Analysis. *The Journal of Neuroscience* 2009; **29**: 2805–13.

22 Song SK, Sun SW, Ju WK, Lin SJ, Cross AH, Neufeld AH. Diffusion tensor imaging detects and differentiates axon and myelin degeneration in mouse optic nerve after retinal ischemia. *Neuroimage* 2003; **20**: 1714–22.

23 Naismith RT, Xu J, Tutlam NT, Lancia S, Trinkaus K, Song S-K, Cross AH. Diffusion tensor imaging in acute optic neuropathies: Predictor of clinical outcomes. *Arch Neurol* 2011: archneurol.2011.243.

24 Song S-K, Sun S-W, Ramsbottom MJ, Chang C, Russell J, Cross AH. Dysmyelination revealed through MRI as increased radial (but unchanged axial) diffusion of water. *Neuroimage* 2002; **17**: 1429–36.

25 Song S-K, Yoshino J, Le TQ, Lin S-J, Sun S-W, Cross AH, Armstrong RC. Demyelination increases radial diffusivity in corpus callosum of mouse brain. *Neuroimage* 2005; **26**: 132–40.

26 Naismith RT, Xu J, Tutlam NT, Trinkaus K, Cross AH, Song S-K. Radial diffusivity in remote optic neuritis discriminates visual outcomes. *Neurology* 2010; **74**: 1702–10.

27 Naismith RT, Xu J, Tutlam NT, et al. Increased diffusivity in acute multiple sclerosis lesions predicts risk of black hole. *Neurology* 2010; **74**: 1694–701.

28 Kolbe SC, Marriott M, van der Walt A, et al. Diffusion tensor imaging correlates of visual impairment in multiple sclerosis and chronic optic neuritis. *Investigative Ophthalmology & Visual Science* 2012; **53**: 825–32.

29 Smith SA, Williams ZR, Ratchford JN, et al. Diffusion tensor imaging of the optic nerve in multiple sclerosis: Association with retinal damage and visual disability. *American Journal of Neuroradiology* 2011; **32**: 1662–8.

30 Dasenbrock HH, Smith SA, Ozturk A, Farrell SK, Calabresi PA, Reich DS. Diffusion tensor imaging of the optic tracts in multiple sclerosis: Association with retinal thinning and visual disability. *Journal of Neuroimaging* 2011; **21**: e41-e9.

31 Li M, Li J, He H, et al. Directional diffusivity changes in the optic nerve and optic radiation in optic neuritis. *British Journal of Radiology* 2011; **84**: 304–14.

32 Reich DS, Smith SA, Gordon-Lipkin EM, et al. Damage to the optic radiation in multiple sclerosis is associated with retinal injury and visual disability. *Archives of Neurology* 2009; **66**: 998–1006.

33 Kolbe S, Bajraszewski C, Chapman C, et al. Diffusion tensor imaging of the optic radiations after optic neuritis. *Hum Brain Mapp* 2012; **33**: 2047–61.

34 Naismith RT, Xu J, Tutlam NT, et al. Disability in optic neuritis correlates with diffusion tensor-derived directional diffusivities. *Neurology* 2009; **72**: 589–94.

35 Naismith RT, Xu J, Tutlam NT, et al. Diffusion tensor imaging in acute optic neuropathies: Predictor of clinical outcomes. *Archives of Neurology* 2012; **69**: 65–71.

36 Inglese M, Ghezzi A, Bianchi S, et al. Irreversible disability and tissue loss in multiple sclerosis: A conventional and magnetization transfer magnetic resonance imaging study of the optic nerves. *Archives of Neurology* 2002; **59**: 250–5.

37 Trip S, Schlottmann P, Jones S, et al. Optic nerve magnetization transfer imaging and measures of axonal loss and demyelination in optic neuritis. *Multiple Sclerosis* 2007; **13**: 875–9.

38 Klistorner A, Chaganti J, Garrick R, Moffat K, Yiannikas C. Magnetisation transfer ratio in optic neuritis is associated with axonal loss, but not with demyelination. *Neuroimage* 2011; **56**: 21–6.

39 Hickman SJ, Toosy AT, Jones SJ, et al. Serial magnetization transfer imaging in acute optic neuritis. *Brain* 2004; **127**: 692–700.

40 Wang Y, van der Walt A, Paine M, et al. Optic Nerve Magnetisation Transfer Ratio after Acute Optic Neuritis Predicts Axonal and Visual Outcomes. *PLoS One* 2012; 7: e52291.

Chapter 17

Optical coherence tomography in neurologic clinical trials

Robert A. Bermel and Peter K. Kaiser

Introduction

Clinical trials of any new therapeutic agent depend on sensitive indices of disease activity or progression to detect benefit. Surrogate measures, which ideally are directly linked to the mechanism of disease, are not available for many neurological diseases. In multiple sclerosis (MS) clinical trials, MRI markers of inflammatory disease activity have been crucial to rapid acceleration in development of therapies that impact the inflammatory mechanisms of the disease, which manifest as new MRI lesions and relapses. The development of new imaging measures that quantify axonal loss or neurodeneration in MS would likely facilitate acceleration in the discovery and testing of new therapeutic options, especially for progressive MS. Optical coherence tomography (OCT) is currently being applied and evaluated in the context of neurologic clinical trials to fill that need.

Advantages to using OCT as an outcome measure

OCT is an appealing outcome measure to include in clinical trials, for multiple reasons. First, as the fields of multiple sclerosis and neurodegenerative disease move toward a goal of neuroprotection, having a measure of unmyelinated axonal integrity (as can be obtained from the peripapillary retinal nerve fiber layer [pRNFL]) is of great appeal. Second, OCT also offers the ability to specifically examine the preservation of first-order sensory neurons, at the macula, either by total macular volume or by quantifying the ganglion cell layer (GCL) thickness. Third, OCT links very intuitively to a sensitive clinical outcome within the same pathway, namely low-contrast letter acuity [1]. Finally, feasibility of OCT is extremely high, with widespread availability of the equipment in either ophthalmology or neurology departments of most academic medical centers, excellent reproducibility, and the advantage of rapid, painless testing without any significant medical risks [2–4].

Possible designs for trials

Trials in neurological disease may be designed with OCT as either a primary or key secondary outcome measure. Given the lack of an established precedent and ineligibility for imaging measures to serve as the primary outcome measure of phase III trials to support definitive regulatory approval, the current focus is on phase II trial designs. Some examples of trial designs which might be designed with OCT as primary or key secondary outcome measure include an acute neuroprotection design, in acute optic neuritis, and a chronic neuroprotection design, in secondary progressive MS (SPMS) (Figure 17.1).

Advantages of the acute neuroprotective study design include the relative large magnitude of pRNFL loss that occurs over a short period of time following optic neuritis, which averages 10–20 uM and is largely complete by six months after the attack [5]. Challenges for trials in acute optic neuritis include the narrow window of opportunity for action (making recruitment difficult) and also the difficulty calculating change in pRNFL when the baseline pRNFL in the affected eye may be increased due to pRNFL swelling. Requiring a narrow window (<14 days) from optic neuritis onset to randomization poses a challenge to enrollment but maximizes the chance of starting the drug during a theoretical window of opportunity for neuroprotection. Possible solutions to the recruitment issue involve inclusion of sites who have an established rapid referral network composed of optometrists, ophthalmologists,

Optical Coherence Tomography in Neurological Disease, ed. Peter A. Calabresi, Laura J. Balcer, and Elliot M. Frohman. Published by Cambridge University Press.

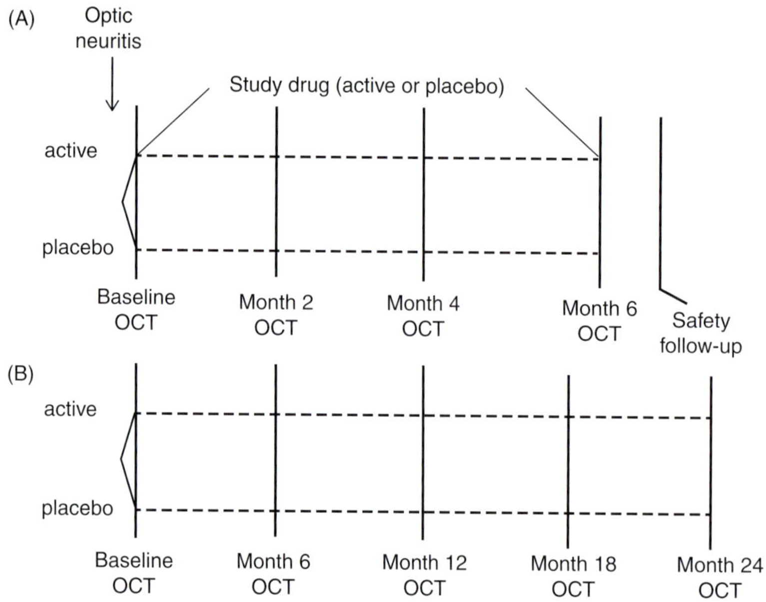

Figure 17.1 Commonly proposed multi-center study designs that utilize OCT as a key outcome measure for parallel-group, placebo-controlled multi-centered trials. (A) acute optic neuritis; (B) progressive MS.

and neuroophthalmologists, who may represent "first responders" for acute optic neuritis. To combat the problem of pRNFL swelling, the fellow (unaffected) eye can be utilized to statistically control for swelling of the pRNFL in the affected eye, an analysis which assumes that both eyes were equal without prior occurrence of optic neuritis in the fellow eye. This requires a prior history of optic neuritis be added to the exclusion criteria of the trial, with the associated potential of limiting the eligible population. Alternatively, parameters measured at the macula, such as the GCL thickness, are not increased due to swelling in acute optic neuritis and may be used as the outcome of interest in acute optic neuritis trials. Challenges for OCT-focused trials in SPMS include the required length of the trial (2–3 years, which is longer than is optimal for phase II trials) given the generally slow rate of decline of OCT measures in purely progressive MS [6].

Key variables of interest

For the purposes of neurological studies, both peripapillary and macular scans are obtained. Key variables of interest for OCT trials in neurological disease include the pRNFL, total macular volume (TMV), and the ganglion cell/inner plexiform layer (GCL/IPL) thickness (obtained at the macula). The primary reason for using these measures is that they are readily available using instrument-derived algorithms, although the scan patterns, availability, and derivation of these measures vary across technologies and manufacturers. Other variables of potential interest include the macular RNFL, and subsets of the pRNFL measured in individual quadrants or specific regions such as the papillomacular bundle. Utilization of the latter set of measures in multi-center clinical trials has not been extensively explored. At present, no multi-center clinical trial has conducted an OCT analysis using third-party or platform-agnostic retinal segmentation and quantification algorithms. Thus, instrument-specific algorithms are currently relied upon, which introduces inherent incompatibilities when combining data across platforms. Retinal segmentation algorithms that can analyze data from different OCT scanner platforms are being developed. A set of common data elements (CDE) is provided by the U.S. National Institute for Neurological Disorders and Stroke (NINDS), to guide the collection of core OCT variables in MS clinical trials [7]. The CDE provide example source documents and key component variables for the two most commonly utilized spectral-domain OCT platforms in neurological trials (Zeiss Cirrus and Heidelberg Spectralis). Beyond this, there is no standard data dictionary agreed upon for use when integrating OCT into clinical trials.

Technical and practical issues

One of the factors that makes implementation of any imaging modality in multi-center clinical trials a challenge is the issue of different technologies, different manufacturers, and upgrades or changes to the equipment or software during the course of a trial. The MS clinical trials community has experience with these issues from years of using MRI in multi-center trials [8]. Technical issues with MRI have been dealt with by restricting the technologies accepted for use by sites in the trial (by manufacturer, magnetic field strength, etc.), restricting the outcomes and pulse sequences utilized (advanced MRI outcomes have been slow to move into multi-center trials for this reason), placing restrictions on equipment or software upgrades during the trial, and employing a central reading center to ensure quality control and uniform implementation of procedures. There are analogous solutions that are utilized in trials driven by OCT, and the community's prior experience with MRI somewhat eases the adoption of some of these solutions for OCT.

Deciding which technologies to allow in a trial always requires a compromise between uniformity of data (highest if only a single technology or manufacturer is included) and feasibility (more sites can be easily included if there are fewer restrictions). For OCT, time-domain OCT (TD-OCT) is being rapidly supplanted in the neurological community by spectral-domain OCT (SD-OCT), which is now widely available. Even within SD-OCT however, there are multiple manufacturers, each of which has its own unique implementation of the variables of interest. Strategies to deal with the inclusion of partially incompatible platforms include restricting certain analyses to a subset of patients scanned on a single platform, or transforming the data in a validated way to improve compatibility across platforms. Such a transformation has been described for total macular volume, which is calculated differently by the Spectralis (restricted to the ETDRS circle) than by the Cirrus (calculated for the entire 6 × 6 × 2 mm acquired macular cube).[9]

Combining pRNFL data from Cirrus and Heidelberg devices in the context of a multi-center clinical trial is supported by one validation study [9], as long as any individual patient within the trial is scanned consistently on the same platform (ideally the same exact instrument) throughout the entire trial. In that study, overall agreement for pRNFL between SD-OCT platforms Cirrus and Spectralis was high, suggesting the two platforms could be utilized in parallel in the context of a multi-center clinical trial, analogous to different sites using different MRI platforms. The same was not true of TD-OCT (Zeiss Stratus) values, which differ significantly from corresponding SD-OCT-measured values for pRNFL. The ability to combine the data across SD-OCT platforms is one of the primary advantages to utilizing pRNFL as a key outcome measure in large multi-center clinical trials. For trials which restrict OCT acquisition to one platform, other platform-specific algorithm-derived measures such as GCL/IPL provided by the Cirrus or papillomacular bundle thickness provided by Spectralis may also prove to be useful outcome measures.

Specific acquisition protocols are delineated at the outset of the trial, and if instruments from multiple manufacturers are being utilized in the trial, the acquisition protocol and manual of operations (MOOP) are designed to provide data that are as analogous as is possible across manufacturers.

A general requirement to reduce variability is that any one patient be scanned on the same instrument for all study visits. The "repeat scan" (co-registration of scan pattern based on fundus photograph) feature available on most SD-OCT scanners can be employed to maximize reproducibility of placement of the pRNFL circle. Changes to equipment or software during the course of a trial are discouraged.

Sample sizes for trials using OCT

For any clinical trial, the sample size and power of the trial is dependent largely on the anticipated effect size of the treatment of interest and the variability of the measurement. For trials employing OCT as an outcome measure, this can be understood as percent preservation of the OCT variable of interest (such as pRNFL) compared to the natural history, placebo-treated state, or active comparator depending on the trial design.

For trials in acute optic neuritis, the natural history of pRNFL loss following acute optic neuritis is well described, and detailed sample size calculations are published for a range of statistical techniques, anticipated effect sizes, and statistical power levels [10]. Common analyses rely on the fellow-eye-controlled change in pRNFL, as previously discussed. Although these sample sizes were derived using data from TD-OCT, the overall results are felt likely to be applicable to SD-OCT, though SD-OCT affords greater inter-scan reliability, likely lower variance, and therefore slightly smaller sample sizes when deployed in a clinical trial compared to TD-OCT [4]. Depending on the chosen power level, duration of follow-up, and anticipated treatment effect, between 40 and 100 participants are required per arm to demonstrate differences in pRNFL between groups [10].

For trials in progressive MS, sample size estimates are not well established. Quantifying the natural history of OCT in progressive MS requires longitudinal measurement over time, which is complicated by changing technology and the need for large cohorts given the heterogeneity of disease. The most robust estimates for rate of decline come from one study pooling TD-OCT data across three centers that examined 299 patients with at least two time points spread over ≥ 6 months' time, showing pRNFL thinning that averaged 2.9 uM over 2–3 years of follow-up [11]. This study excluded patients who experienced acute optic neuritis during the course of follow-up, but was composed mostly of patients with relapsing MS, with median disease duration of nine years. Most of the patients (87%) were on standard MS disease modifying therapies. In the absence of more robust published data on purely progressive MS, these are the most analogous natural history data on which to base sample size calculations for progressive MS trials. Although groups of patients with secondary progressive MS (SPMS) have thinner pRNFL than those with CIS or RRMS when evaluated in cross-sectional studies [12], this does not necessarily mean that the yearly rate of thinning is greater in SPMS. It is likely, based on the Talman study, that there is substantial inter-individual variability in the rate of pRNFL thinning. Patients with shorter disease duration and more active inflammatory characteristics such as new T2 or gadolinium-enhancing lesions appear to have more rapid neurodegeneration [6]. Clinical trials may, therefore. potentially be enriched by including patients with these characteristics. These enrichment tactics may be particularly useful if macular GCL/IPL is utilized as an outcome measure, as disease activity and shorter disease duration have been shown to correlate with rapidity of GCL/IPL thinning more so than pRNFL thinning [6].

Role of the OCT reading center

Given the complexities involved in the incorporation of OCT in multi-center clinical trials, use of an OCT reading center to provide expertise and facilitate the collection of study results could be justified as essential on a logistical basis alone. Oversight by an experienced OCT reading center also confers advantages that result in improved data quality and usability. Some of these advantages were highlighted in a recent report that examined the difference in the quality of TD-OCT data obtained in the context of a study planned without the use of an OCT reading center, with OCT obtained at individual sites without a structured protocol or central oversight compared to OCT data obtained in the context of a similar study except for centrally specified and coordinated OCT data collection [13]. Inclusion of the OCT reading center with preplanned OCT study protocol was associated with more usable data, fewer errors, and higher signal strengths [13].

Favorable study characteristics facilitated by an OCT reading center that likely improve data quality include implementation of a standard OCT protocol with well-defined quality standards, certification of OCT technicians, and real-time data transmission with quality assurance feedback to sites [14]. Figure 17.2 shows how an OCT reading center integrates with overall study architecture. Specific roles of the OCT reading center throughout the course of a trial are outlined in Table 17.1.

Differences between OCT-driven trials in ophthalmology and neurology

Because early experience with OCT in clinical trials was in the ophthalmology space, OCT instrument vendors and OCT reading centers may have substantial experience with ophthalmological clinical trials. Important differences exist, however, between trials conducted in ophthalmology and those in neurologic disease. Ophthalmology trials (especially those in retinal disorders) rely heavily on categorical or subjective grading of OCT scans to classify outcomes, whereas the focus in neurological trials to date is on quantitative data. Although there is less of a focus on categorical grading in neurological trials (and commonly instrument-generated quantitative data could be created for each scan at the site), it is still important for independent raters to look at each scan in a trial to assure accurate collection of the variables of interest, especially if multiple scans are obtained at each visit, as is common practice to maximize opportunity for quality control. Optimally, each scan is evaluated by two or more independent raters, and if there is disagreement between the two raters that exceeds a given

Table 17.1 Potential roles of an OCT reading center

Potential Roles of an OCT Reading Center:

1. Provide input into protocol development with respect to OCT
2. Draft instrument-specific manual of operations
3. Site and technologist training, qualification and certification
4. Handling, storage, archiving of source images
5. Quantitative data management using regulatory-compliant methods
6. On-study individual scan review and grading
7. Quality assurance with real-time feedback to sites
8. Study closeout, query resolution, OCT database lock

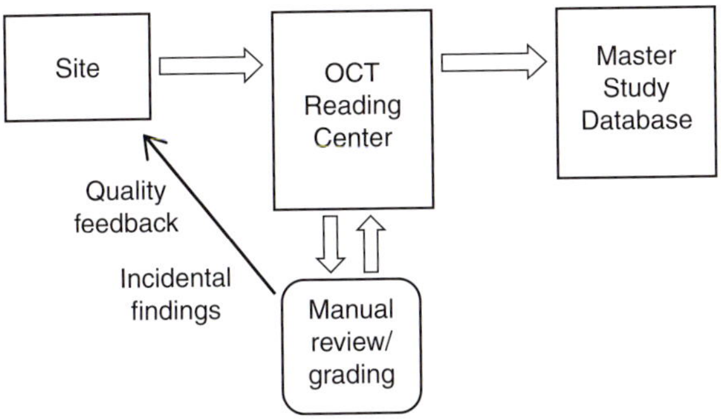

Figure 17.2 Interaction of the OCT reading center in the context of multisite clinical trials of neurological disease

threshold, then a third rater will examine the scan. Neurological trials always collect binocular data (even in monocular pathologies such as unilateral optic neuritis), whereas sometimes monocular data is utilized in ophthalmology trials. It is important to recognize that neurological patients may not have had a dilated ophthalmoscopic exam prior to trial entry; therefore, the possibility of incidental ophthalmological findings is greater in neurological trials, and a workflow must be built to effectively convey those findings back to the sites.

Examples of neurologic clinical trials utilizing OCT

The first large-scale trials to utilize OCT at all were the phase III trials of fingolimod, FREEDOMS I and FREEDOMS II. OCT was initially included in these trials as a key safety outcome, due to the potential for fingolimod to cause macular edema. In FREEDOMS I, OCT was employed by most sites as a safety screening test and to monitor on-study for macular edema, but scan protocol and analysis was conducted locally at the sites and not centrally coordinated or aggregated. Because of the time frame in which those trials were conducted, time-domain OCT was the available technology. No specific OCT protocol was mandated, rather this was left up to the treating ophthalmologist at the site. Quantitative OCT results from this trial were not systematically collected, are not available in aggregate, and would have marginal utility given the lack of standardized acquisition or analysis protocol. FREEDOMS II included oversight from the UC Davis OCT reading center, and baseline OCT results from that trial were recently reported [15]. In that multi-center trial cohort, pRNFL and TMV thinning was common at baseline, with 34% of the patients having a mean pRNFL value below the fifth percentile in at least one eye compared to a normative database.

The OCTAGON trial was a randomized double-blind parallel group trial of glatiramer acetate (GA) vs. placebo in acute optic neuritis, conducted at multiple sites in the United States. Change in peripapillary RNFL over six months (measured by time-domain OCT) was the primary outcome measure. The study is notable because it was the first planned acute optic neuritis study utilizing OCT outcomes. With a planned enrollment of 100 patients per arm, the study was designed to have 80% power to detect a difference of 5 uM in baseline to six-month RNFL between groups [16]. After enrollment occurred more slowly than planned, the trial was closed in late 2010, with 44 patients having enrolled in total. The OCTAGON study confirmed two anticipated issues with acute optic neuritis trials driven by OCT: difficult enrollment within an acute neuroprotective window of opportunity, and the confound of baseline pRNFL swelling (baseline pRNFL = 130.5 ±8.9 uM in the placebo arm) [16].

The first multi-center neuroprotective trial in acute optic neuritis to show benefit on OCT was a trial of erythropoietin versus placebo as add-on to intravenous methylprednisolone, enrolling at three centers in Germany between August 2006 and February 2011. Measured by TD-OCT, pRNFL decreased by a median of 7.5 μm in the erythropoietin group compared to a median of 16.0 μm in the placebo group by week 16 ($p = 0.0357$) [17]. Other outcomes including retrobulbar optic nerve diameter and VEP latency showed benefit of erythropoietin compared to placebo. The trial is also notable because they had to screen 97 participants to include 40, likely a factor of the stringent requirement of a seven-day window from optic neuritis onset to randomization. A follow-up study, Treatment of Optic Neuritis with Erythropoetin (TONE), is planned, randomizing between erythropoietin or placebo, with pRNFL measured using SD-OCT as the primary outcome measure, planning to enroll 100 participants with onset of first symptoms less than 10 days prior to randomization [18].

A single-center study conducted in Iran in 60 participants with visual symptoms eight days or less in duration showed a benefit of memantine versus placebo on preservation of pRNFL at three months (78.9 uM in placebo group vs. 91.3 uM in memantine group, $p = 0.01$), with no difference in full-field visual evoked potentials or full-contrast visual acuity found between treatment groups [19].

There are two notable large-scale multi-center trials currently planned or in process which are attempting to utilize OCT to support a neuroprotective effect of experimental therapy in progressive MS. The Secondary and Primary Progressive Ibudilast NeuroNext Trial in MS (SPRINT-MS) will randomize 250 patients with either primary or secondary progressive MS to receive either ibudilast or placebo [20]. The primary outcome of the trial is whole brain atrophy measured on MRI, though pRNFL on OCT is a key secondary outcome measure. All 19 sites in the trial are providing OCT data on all patients. Either Zeiss Cirrus or Heidelberg Spectralis OCT is being accepted by the central OCT reading center. The Multiple Sclerosis-Secondary Progressive Multi-Arm Randomisation Trial (MS-SMART) anticipates enrolling 440 participants randomized to amiloride, riluzole, ibudilast, or placebo and followed for two years. OCT is a tertiary/supportive outcome measure in MS-SMART [21].

Randomized placebo-controlled phase II clinical trials of multiple agents in acute optic neuritis are currently ongoing. A trial of phenytoin versus placebo is being conducted in the United Kingdom, and plans for enrollment of 90 total participants within 14 days of onset of visual loss, followed for six months, with final data collection planned in April 2014 [22]. The amiloride clinical trial in optic neuritis (ACTION) study estimates enrollment of 46 participants, with primary outcome being the difference in pRNFL at 6 months and 12 months, with data collection anticipated to be complete by September 2014 [23]. A multi-center trial of fingolimod in acute demyelinating optic neuritis (ADON), which aimed to recruit 126 total participants with a first episode of ADON andrandomize to fingolimod or placebo for 18 weeks, was planned but closed prior to completing enrollment [24]. A randomized study of BIIB033, an anti-LINGO monoclonal antibody, is being conducted in acute optic neuritis, with planned recruitment of 80 total participants. Nerve conduction velocity on full-field visual evoked potential is the primary outcome measure, although both pRNFL and GCL/IPL at week 24 are key secondary outcome measures [25].

Multiple other trials have incorporated OCT or utilized it as a secondary outcome measure. In a phase IIa open-label study of autologous mesenchymal stem cells in 10 patients with SPMS, there was no significant change in pRNFL on follow-up compared to baseline [26]. A phase II trial of riluzole in early MS employed TD-OCT as a secondary outcome measure found no significant difference between treatment arms in pRNFL over 36 months in 43 participants, consistent with the negative result on the primary outcome measure, percent brain volume change [27].

Conclusions

As the field of multiple sclerosis clinical trials enters into an era of testing treatments for neuroprotection, OCT will play a key role as an outcome measure given its feasibility and early track record in acute optic neuritis of showing proof of concept for neuroprotention in a short time frame.

References

1. Balcer LJ, Baier ML, Cohen JA, Kooijmans MF, Sandrock AW, Nano-Schiavi ML, et al. Contrast letter acuity as a visual component for the Multiple Sclerosis Functional Composite. *Neurology* 2003; **61**:1367–1373.

2. Frohman EM, Costello F, Stuve O, Calabresi P, Miller DH, Hickman SJ, et al. Modeling axonal degeneration within the anterior visual system: implications for demonstrating neuroprotection in multiple sclerosis. *Arch Neurol* 2008; **65**:26–35.
3. Cettomai D, Pulicken M, Gordon-Lipkin E, Salter A, Frohman TC, Conger A, et al. Reproducibility of optical coherence tomography in multiple sclerosis. *Arch Neurol* 2008; **65**:1218–1222.
4. Syc SB, Warner CV, Hiremath GS, Farrell SK, Ratchford JN, Conger A, et al. Reproducibility of high-resolution optical coherence tomography in multiple sclerosis. *Mult Scler* 2010; **16**:829–839.
5. Costello F, Coupland S, Hodge W, Lorello GR, Koroluk J, Pan YI, et al. Quantifying axonal loss after optic neuritis with optical coherence tomography. *Ann Neurol* 2006; **59**:963–969.
6. Ratchford JN, Saidha S, Sotirchos ES, Oh JA, Seigo MA, Eckstein C, et al. Active MS is associated with accelerated retinal ganglion cell/inner plexiform layer thinning. *Neurology* 2013; **80**:47–54.
7. Multiple Sclerosis Standards – NINDS Common Data Elements.; 2014.
8. Bermel RA, Fisher E, Cohen JA. The use of MR imaging as an outcome measure in multiple sclerosis clinical trials. *Neuroimaging Clin N Am* 2008; **18**:687–701, xi.
9. Warner CV, Syc SB, Stankiewicz AM, Hiremath G, Farrell SK, Crainiceanu CM, et al. The impact of utilizing different optical coherence tomography devices for clinical purposes and in multiple sclerosis trials. *PLoS One* 2011; **6**:e22947.
10. Henderson APD, Altmann DR, Trip AS, Kallis C, Jones SJ, Schlottmann PG, et al. A serial study of retinal changes following optic neuritis with sample size estimates for acute neuroprotection trials. *Brain* 2010; **133**:2592–2602.
11. Talman LS, Bisker ER, Sackel DJ, Long DA,Jr, Galetta KM, Ratchford JN, et al. Longitudinal study of vision and retinal nerve fiber layer thickness in multiple sclerosis. *Ann Neurol* 2010; **67**:749–760.
12. Costello F, Hodge W, Pan YI, Eggenberger E, Freedman MS. Using retinal architecture to help characterize multiple sclerosis patients. *Can J Ophthalmol* 2010; **45**:520–526.
13. Keltner JL, Cello KE, Balcer LJ, Calabresi PA, Markowitz CE, Werner JS. Stratus OCT Quality Control in Two Multi-Centre Multiple Sclerosis Clinical Trials. *Neuro-Ophthalmology* 2011; **35**:57–64.
14. Sakai RE, Feller DJ, Galetta KM, Galetta SL, Balcer LJ. Vision in multiple sclerosis: the story, structure-function correlations, and models for neuroprotection. *J Neuroophthalmol* 2011; **31**:362–373.
15. Winges KM, Werner JS, Harvey DJ, Cello KE, Durbin MK, Balcer LJ, et al. Baseline retinal nerve fiber layer thickness and macular volume quantified by OCT in the North American Phase 3 Fingolimod Trial for Relapsing-Remitting Multiple Sclerosis. *Journal of Neuro-Ophthalmology* 2013; **33**: 322–329 10.1097/WNO.0b013e31829c51f7.
16. OCTAGON trial. http://clinicaltrials.gov/ct2/show/results/NCT00856635; Accessed 12/2013.
17. Suhs KW, Hein K, Sattler MB, Gorlitz A, Ciupka C, Scholz K, et al. A randomized, double-blind, phase 2 study of erythropoietin in optic neuritis. *Ann Neurol* 2012; **72**:199–210.
18. Treatment of Optic Neuritis With Erythropoietin (TONE). http://clinicaltrials.gov/ct2/show/results/NCT00856635; Accessed 01/2014.
19. Esfahani MR, Harandi ZA, Movasat M, Nikdel M, Adelpour M, Momeni A, et al. Memantine for axonal loss of optic neuritis. *Graefes Arch Clin Exp Ophthalmol* 2012; **250**:863–869.
20. Safety, Tolerability and Activity Study of Ibudilast in Subjects With Progressive Multiple Sclerosis. http://clinicaltrials.gov/show/NCT01982942; Accessed 12/2013.
21. MS-SMART: Multiple Sclerosis-Secondary Progressive Multi-Arm Randomisation Trial. http://clinicaltrials.gov/show/NCT01910259; Accessed 01/2014.
22. Neuroprotection with phenytoin in optic neuritis. http://clinicaltrials.gov/show/NCT01451593; Accessed 12/2013.
23. Amiloride clinical trial in optic neuritis. http://www.clinicaltrials.gov/show/NCT01802489; Accessed 12/2013.
24. Fingolimod (FTY720) in Acute Demyelinating Optic Neuritis (ADON). http://www.clinicaltrials.gov/show/NCT01802489; Accessed 01/2014.
25. 215ON201 BIIB033 In Acute Optic Neuritis (AON) (RENEW). http://clinicaltrials.gov/show/NCT01721161; Accessed 01/2014.
26. Connick P, Kolappan M, Crawley C, Webber DJ, Patani R, Michell AW, et al. Autologous mesenchymal stem cells for the treatment of secondary progressive multiple sclerosis: an open-label phase 2a proof-of-concept study. *Lancet Neurol* 2012; **11**:150–156.
27. Waubant E. A phase II trial of neuroprotection with riluzole in early relapsing-remitting MS. *ECTRIMS* 2013, Copenhagen, Denmark. Late Breaking News Session 10/05/2013.

Chapter 18

Optical coherence tomography in a multi-center setting: quality control issues

Axel Petzold, Laura J. Balcer, Peter A. Calabresi, Fiona Costello, Elliot M. Frohman, Ari J. Green, Alexander Klistorner, Friedemann Paul, Sven Schippling, and Pablo Villoslada

Introduction

The many advantages of retinal OCT imaging described in this book do not come without attention to quality control (QC). Qualitatively poor OCT scans may cause loss of data or wrong data due to measurement artifacts [13, 4]. This remains of particular concern for *longitudinal data* in a multi-center setting typical for randomized controlled trials (RCT). Therefore, the authors of this chapter convened in 2012 with the aim to establish robust and transparent QC criteria for the use of retinal OCT in multiple sclerosis (MS) research and trials.

In this chapter we will first review the published evidence on the effect of poor-quality scans. Next, we will illustrate how substantial measurement artifacts can be introduced by breaking a few rules with an otherwise well-acquired OCT scan. This is followed by a detailed description of seven QC criteria which permit one to identify scans that should be rejected from analysis in a multi-center setting. For didactic reasons, this is followed by a number of examples seen in an OCT reading center. For brevity, this chapter predominantly deals with the peripapillary ring scan, but points relevant for macular volume scans will also be discussed. The chapter concludes with pragmatic advice on how to obtain high quality OCT scans.

The problem of poor-quality OCT scans

Recognized reasons for poor quality OCT scans are poor illumination, boundary line errors, or algorithm failures and imperfect centering of the ring-scan around the head of the optic nerve [4]. In some cases there will be obvious protocol violations such as scanning with the wrong protocol at the wrong retinal location. Any such scans should be recognized early and excluded if the error cannot be repaired. Still, there are more subtle pitfalls that can lead to inappropriate quantitative data if left unchecked.

Quantitative measurement artifacts due to QC issues

To illustrate the size of the problem, the annual loss of the peripapillary retinal nerve fiber layer (RNFL) in MS is about 1–2 μm per year. This is over 10 times the expected 0.1 μm observed in healthy subjects [12]. It is relevant to notice that the small quantity of localized changes caused by neurodegeneration may easily be masked by measurement artifacts. For example, a localized measurement artifact up to 40 μm can be the result of off-center placement of the measurement beam [2], but this will not readily be visible to an OCT reading center. Poor placement of the peripapillary ring-scan results in artifacts around the 3.4 μm range of the global average [5]. Poor signal is a problematic issue, and measurement artifacts in the 10 μm range can readily arise [1]. For this reason, OCT scans containing such measurement artifacts may contaminate the data and mask the detection of relevant retinal layer atrophy. We are the opinion that such artifactual OCT ought to be excluded from clinical studies or trials.

Optical Coherence Tomography in Neurological Disease, ed. Peter A. Calabresi, Laura J. Balcer, and Elliot M. Frohman. Published by Cambridge University Press.

Reliable QC assessment in a multi-center setting

A set of seven quality control (QC) criteria which address all of the above discussed issues was validated in a previous study [13]. These criteria could be reliably used with a substantial inter-rater agreement in a multi-center setting. For mnemonics reasons the set was called "OSCAR-IB," where each of the letters indicates one of seven QC criteria which have to be met [13].

The OSCAR-IB criteria

A summary of the seven OSCAR-IB criteria is shown in Table 18.1. Each of the seven criteria is discussed in more detail later in this chapter. For didactic reasons, representative examples that have been rejected in a reading center setting are presented for illustration.

O-criterion

For the first of the OSCAR-IB criteria, "obvious" (O), scans will be rejected for highly apparent issues, including severe lens opacities, vitreous hemorrhage, or poor focus of the lens. See Figure 18.1 for a typical real-life example of a poorly focused image. Rejection also occurred if there was a protocol violation such as deliberately not averaging several B-scans by turning off the ART mode. In our experience, the rejection rate based on this criterion is low, but the reasons remain unpredictable.

S-criterion

For the second of the OSCAR-IB criteria, signal strength (S), we had arbitrarily chosen a cut-off of 15 dB [13] based on our experience and published evidence suggesting that poor signal strength decreases the signal-to-noise ratio of RNFL measures (Figure 18.2) [14, 8]. However, scans with poor signal strength (defined as < 15 dB for the Heidelberg Spectralis and < 10 dB for the Cirrus) but relatively good contrast between layers allowing for proper image post-processing and segmentation do exist. In absence of a transparent way to judge signal strength other than dB, we recommend to aim for a signal of at least 15 dB for the Heidelberg Spectralis and 10 dB for the Cirrus (the cut-off may be different for different devices entering the ever-increasing OCT market), but allow for a reasonable margin of judgment in OCT scans that give a good inter-layer contrast despite a lower signal strength. In order words, the S-criterion should be used as a soft criterion.

C-criterion

The third of the OSCAR-IB criteria, correct centration of the ring scan (C), is a hard criterion (Figure 18.3). Even a small degree of displacement between peripapillary ring scans can lead to a measurement artifact above 3.4 μm [5]. It should be highlighted that any change of position between a baseline and follow-up scan should be rejected for this reason. Likewise, any large level of imperfect centering at baseline, which in the worst-case scenario may cut through the optic nerve head itself, should be rejected (Figure 18.4). To judge what a "large displacement" means, we proposed to use the Royal Air Force (RAF) logo as a guide and reject peripapillary ring scans that cross two of the RAF logo rings [13]. What might be permissible is a slight displacement that is taken into consideration at follow-up

Table 18.1 The OSCAR-IB quality-control criteria for retinal OCT scans. Table modified with permission from reference [13].

Item	criteria
O	Obvious problems (e.g., unfocused image, wrong scan protocol, etc.).
S	Is the OCT signal sufficient to give a sharp contrast between layers needed for layer segmentation? We recommend a signal > 10 for the Cirrus and > 15 for the Heidelberg Spectralis OCT., appropriate B–scan averaging (ART function activated).
C	Is the scan correctly centered?
A	Is there an algorithm failure?
R	Is there visible retinal pathology which may potentially impair the RNFL reading? (minor floaters casting a shadow are not relevant)
I	Is the fundus well illuminated?
B	Is the measurement beam placed centrally?

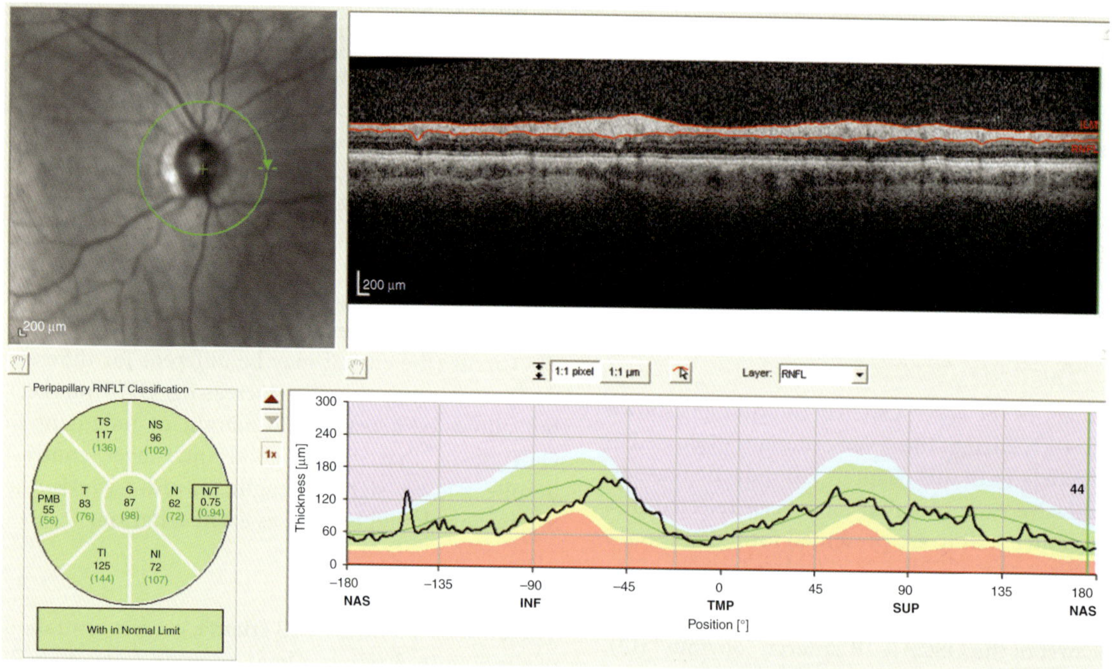

Figure 18.1 This OCT scan is poorly focused, as illustrated by the blurred cSLO image to the left. This scan was QC rejected according to the [O] criterion for this reason alone, but also conflicts with the [C] and [S] criteria.

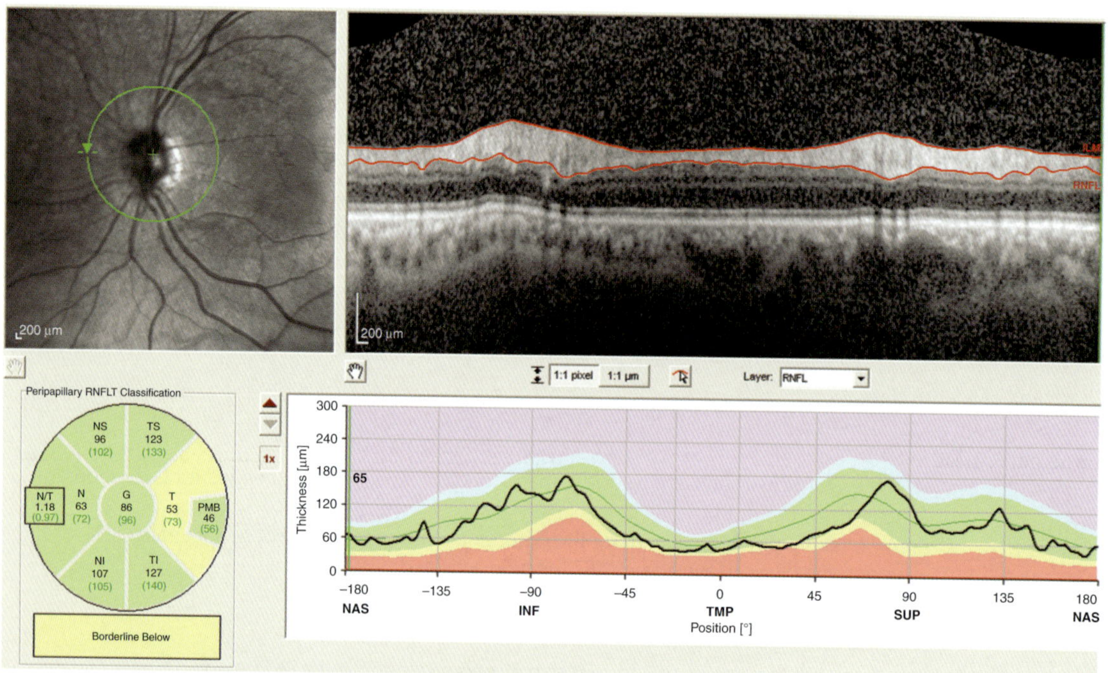

Figure 18.2 The poor signal strength in this image (5 dB) causes a grainy and very noisy image. In addition, the (C, B) criteria are violated. The contrast levels between retinal layers are so poor that image post-processing will become questionable. This scan was QC rejected.

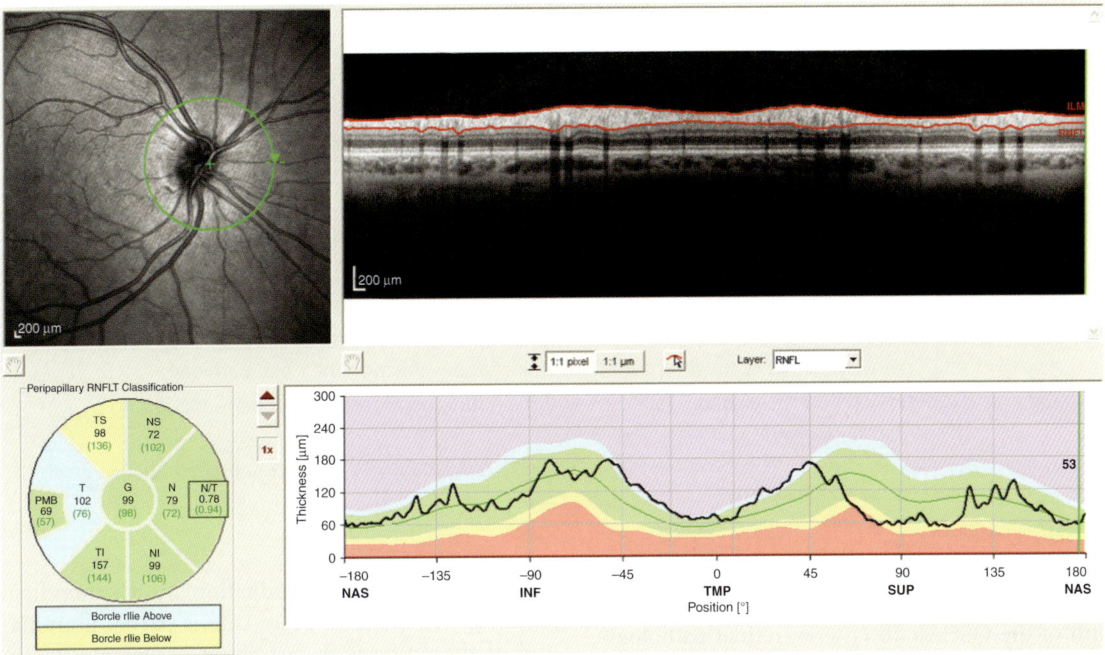

Figure 18.3 Poor centering of the peripapillary ring scan. The cSLO image to the left shows that the green circle is not placed centrally over the optic nerve head, but is shifted to the right. As a result, the thickness profile of the temporal quadrant (T, TMP, −45–45 degree position) appears to be artificially thickened. This scan was QC rejected.

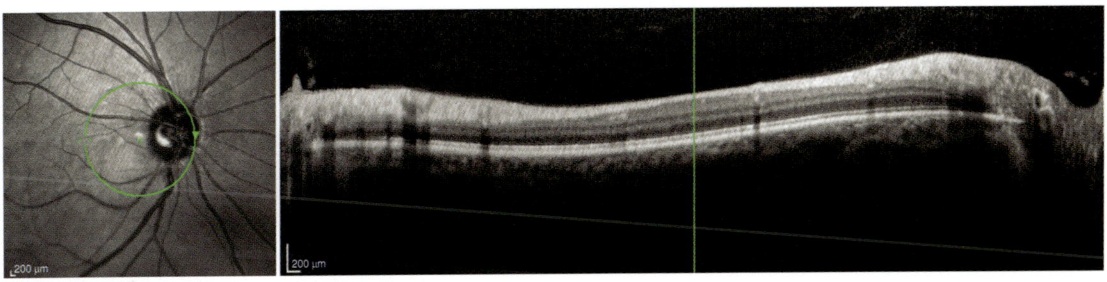

Figure 18.4 Another example of a poorly centered OCT technician ring scan submitted to a reading center in a multi-center setting. In this example, the nasal quadrant cuts through the cup of the optic disc. This scan was QC rejected.

scans by means of scan registration. Having some flexibility here is relevant because of the variable anatomy of the optic nerve head.

A-criterion

The fourth of the OSCAR-IB criteria, algorithm failures (A), also present a serious issue. Any localized algorithm failure invalidates data taken from the respective retinal region. Such scans will need to be rejected. Importantly, this can be corrected by the reading center and in contrast to the other criteria re-assessment of a patient may not be needed.

In selected cases, it may be possible to correct such errors by image post-processing techniques, including manual correction. This procedure is extremely time-consuming. A decision may be made on individual scans. While this criterion should be handled rather strictly on the baseline scan in order to ensure optimal settings for longitudinal studies, one may accept that a minor, manually correctable algorithm failure on a valuable follow-up scan should not necessarily lead to immediate rejection. An OCT technician should be aware of this fact, because manual correction of algorithm failures may be possible prior to uploading a scan to a reading center.

Table 18.2 Pathology of the retina to be considered by the OSCAR-IB criteria. Table reproduced with permission from reference [13].

Summary	Diseases
Structural	Drusen, Cysts, Detachment, Large discs, Small crowed discs, presence of myelinated axons, naevus, tumor, peripapillary atrophy, optic disc edema, more than six diopters of myopia or hyperopia
Vascular	AION & PION, NA-AION & NA-PION, GCA, CRO, CRBO, AVM, Cotton-wool spots, CVA affecting the optic pathways
Immune	paraneoplastic, MAR, NMO, CAR, SLE, uveitis, birdshot retinochoroiditis
Infectious	Viral, bacterial, fungus, HIV, Lyme disease, secondary syphilis
Hereditary	Leber's, DOA, albinism, cone dystrophy, retinitis pigmentosa
Iatrogenic	Retina surgery, photocoalgulation, solar retinopathy, central serous chorioretinopathy, Purtscher's retinopathy, optic nerve sheet fenestration, brain surgery affecting the optic pathways
Metabolic/ toxic	Diabetes, Vit A deficit, alcohol-, tobacco– and malnutrition-induced amblyopia, amiodarone, chloroquine, vigabatrin
Other	Glaucoma, macular degeneration, acute posterior multifocal placoid pigment epitheliopathy, acute macular neuroretinopathy

R-criterion

The fifth of the OSCAR-IB criteria, retinal pathology (R), unrelated to MS can independently influence RNFL measures (see Figure 18.5) and ought to be taken into account in studies focused on MS. A list of pathologies to be considered is presented in Table 18.2.

At present, a number of recent OCT studies have provided evidence that retinal pathology other than RNFL thinning exists in MS [11, 6, 10, 3], including microcystic macular edema (MME) predominantly affecting the inner nuclear layer (INL) of the retina. We, therefore, do not recommend rejecting OCT scans showing evidence of MME because this may be a clinically relevant finding in the disease.

I-criterion

The sixth of the OSCAR-IB criteria refers to poor illumination of scans (I). Poor or unequal illumination had been made one of the first QC criteria in other studies but remains difficult to judge on its own. In most cases poor illumination will also cause a loss of signal and related problems (see Figure 18.6). Therefore, a scan may be rejected on the basis of a combination of several OSCAR-IB criteria.

What remains difficult is how to judge poor illumination in isolation. To give one example, Figure 18.7 shows a shadow cast on the retina by a floater. Should this scan be rejected? We would not do so because the scan quality is such that all retinal layers can clearly be distinguished and the scan would not fail because of any of the other OSCAR-IB criteria.

In contrast, poor illumination by a suboptimal placement of the laser beam causes partial illumination of the retina with just about acceptable B-scan quality in some areas and very dark B-scans from poorly illuminated areas. Typically, the poorly illuminated areas are located at the border of the IR image. Clearly, in poorly illuminated areas the signal drops to such low levels that no image post-processing can be performed. In summary, a shadow caused by floaters, cataracts, long eye lashes, and the like should not be considered a general cause of exclusion for the I-criterion in cases where A- and B-scan quality is good.

B-criterion

The last of the OSCAR-IB criteria, the beam placement criterion (B), may not be intuitively obvious to everyone. To put it simply, it is important to keep the OCT scan in the live window horizontally orientated whenever possible.

Problems with the B-criterion arise when a scan is tilted in one direction at baseline and to the opposite direction at follow-up, because measurement errors in the range of 9–40 μm can be introduced [2]. The reason for this is illustrated in Figure 18.8. Therefore, scans with suboptimal beam placement as described, should be rejected.

In some cases the anatomy of the retina may make it difficult to achieve a perfectly horizontally aligned OCT. In this context, the QC rating of the follow-up scan will ensure that the same direction of tilting is

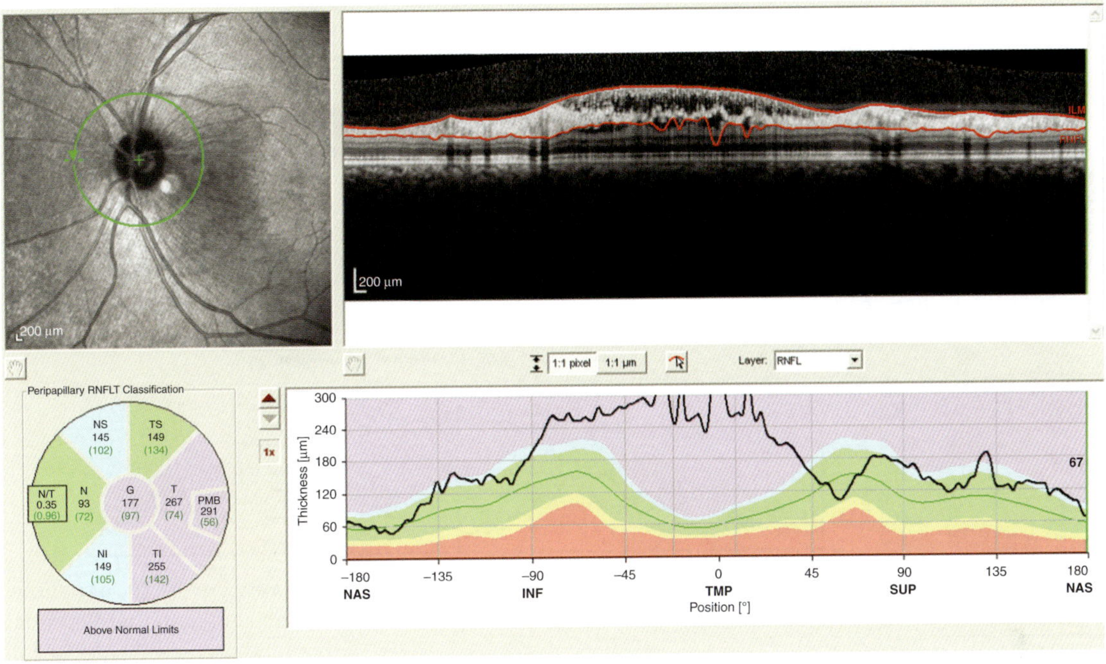

Figure 18.5 In this patient central serous edema extends to the area captured by the peripapillary ring scan. Consequently the temporal quadrant of the RNFL appears to be thickened artificially. This scan was QC rejected.

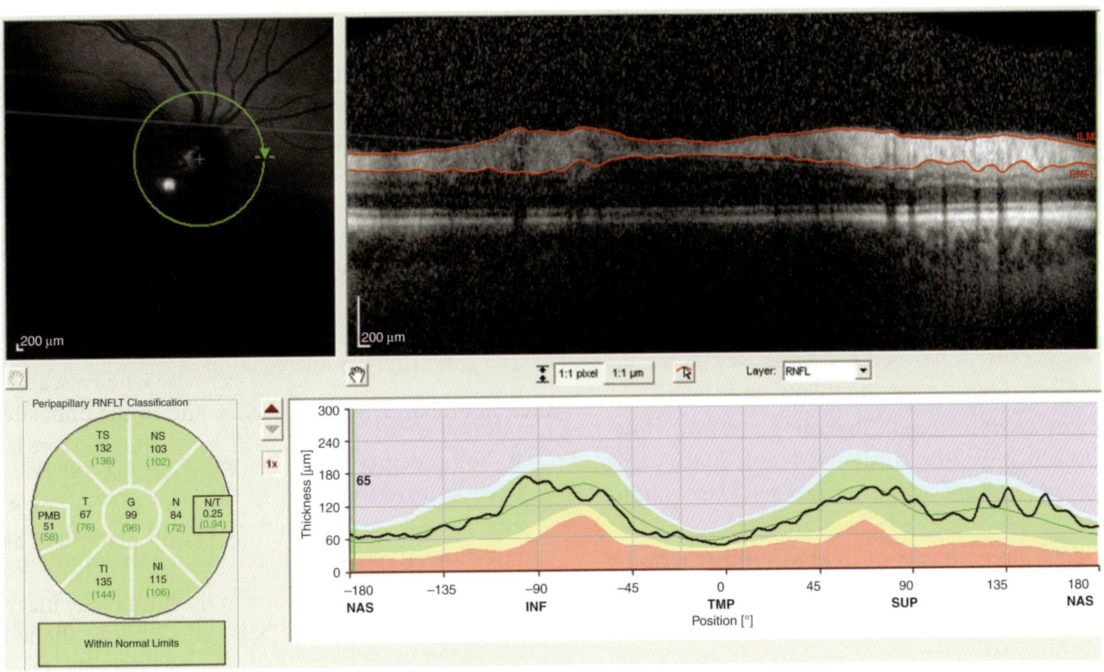

Figure 18.6 A poorly illuminated OCT scan, which also causes a low signal such that it is impossible to recognize any of the retinal layers but the RNFL in the temporal quadrant. The (B) criterion is also violated. This scan was QC rejected.

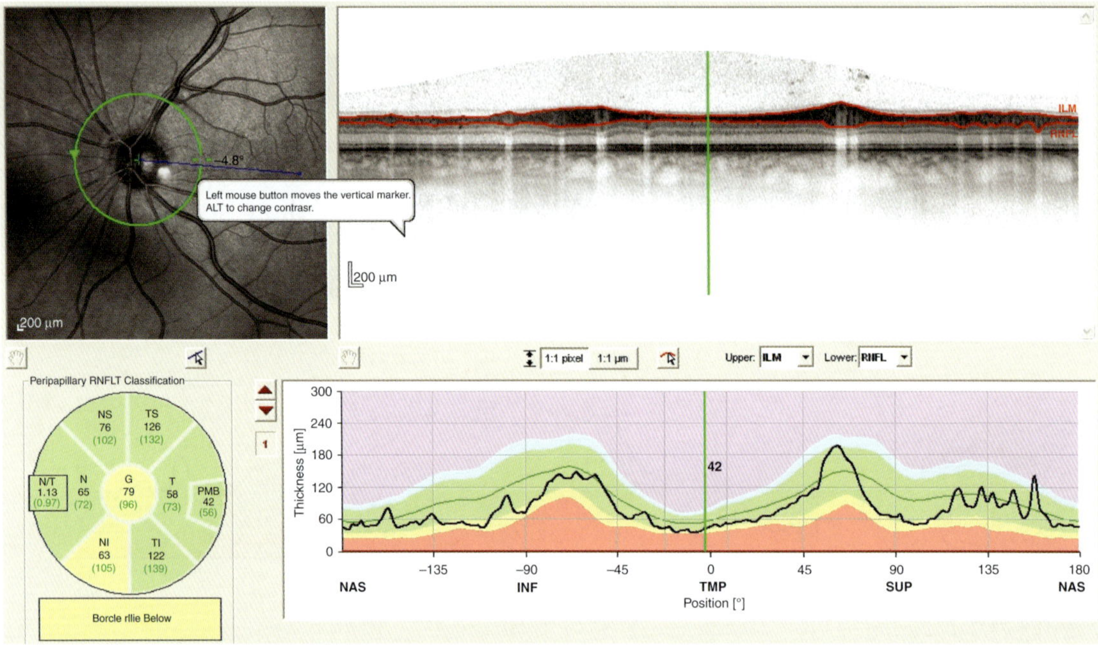

Figure 18.7 This OCT scans appears to be unequally illuminated. What happened here is that a floater casts a shadow in the lower-left part of the IR image. The scan does not violate any of the OSCAR-IB criteria. This scan was QC accepted.

repeated, thus ensuring consistency. The core of the B-criterion is that the direction of tilt causes a characteristic, reproducible, robust signal pattern in the outer plexiform (OPL) and outer nuclear layers (ONL, Figure 18.9). This sign allows tracing possible errors due to off-center beam placement.

We recommend the rejection of any scans that combine an obvious violation of the B-criterion with an associated change of retinal layer thickness values in the corresponding retinal area.

Macular volume scans

Validated QC criteria for macular volume scans do not exist at present. We propose that the same seven OSCAR–IB criteria be used the same way as for the peripapillary ring scan for the following reasons:

1. O: Any obvious reason including protocol violations which led to exclusion of a peripapillary ring scan very likely compromise macular volume scans as well.
2. S: Signal strength may be used as a soft criterion if image post-processing is possible such that reliable quantitative data can be obtained from relevant B-scans.
3. C: Poor centering of a macular scan is a clear reason for rejection because considerable measurement artifacts are introduced [9]. The possibility of post hoc repositioning of the EDTRS grid needs to be considered.
4. A: Algorithm failures are more frequent in areas with very thin retinal layers. Because the foveola itself does not contain any measurable degree of several retinal layers, algorithm failures in this region are common, but they should not lead to rejection if image post-processing remains possible for relevant B-scans.
5. R: Any retinal pathology other then MME affecting the macula should be discussed for rejection in MS research.
6. I: Poor and unequal illumination should be used as a soft criterion for rejection of macular scans if present in isolation of on a small number of less relevant (peripheral) B-scans.
7. B: Some degree of off-center beam placement is likely to occur in parts of the large area scanned and should not be used as a hard criterion for rejection if not combined with corresponding measurement artifacts on longitudinal scans. There is published evidence demonstrating that off-center beam placement affects retinal thickness measurements [7] as it did for peripapillary ring scans [2].

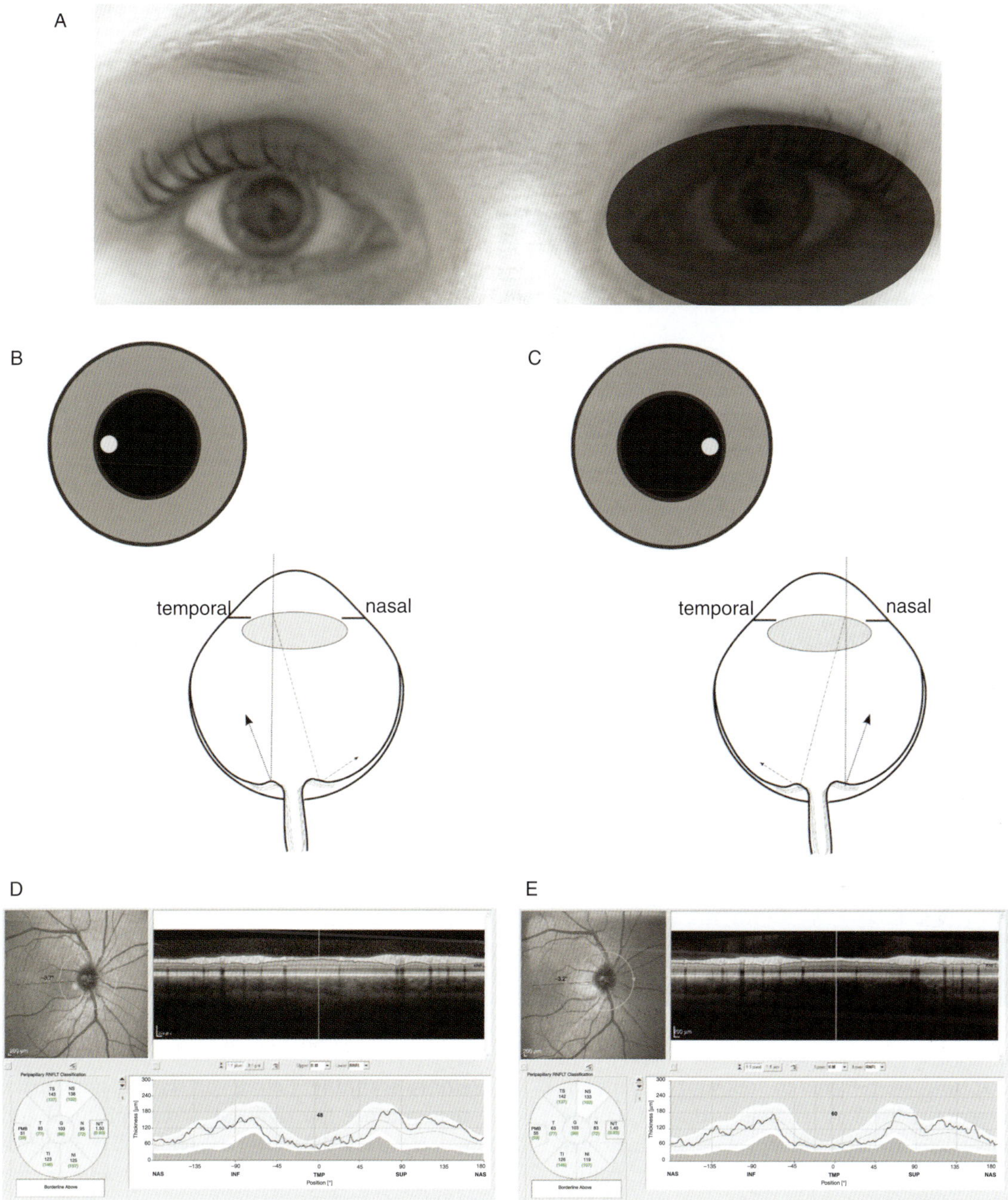

Figure 18.8 (A) The OCT measurement beam is focused on the dilated right eye of a healthy control subject. (B) temporal off-center placement of the measurement beam results in a shorter light path to the temporal part of the optic nerve head (dotted line) and a longer pathway from the nasal part of the optic nerve head (dotted-dashed line). The difference in path length results in a tilted appearance of the B-scan. (C) Nasal off-center placement of the measurement beam results in a mirror pattern. The resulting averaged OCT image is of good quality (ART 25, signal strength 35 dB) for both (D) temporal off-center placement and (E) nasal off-center placement. The quantification of the RNFL thickness by the algorithm is, however, clearly different (Global average OD with temporal off-center placement 106 μm and nasal off-center placement 103 μm). Figure reprinted with permission from reference [2].

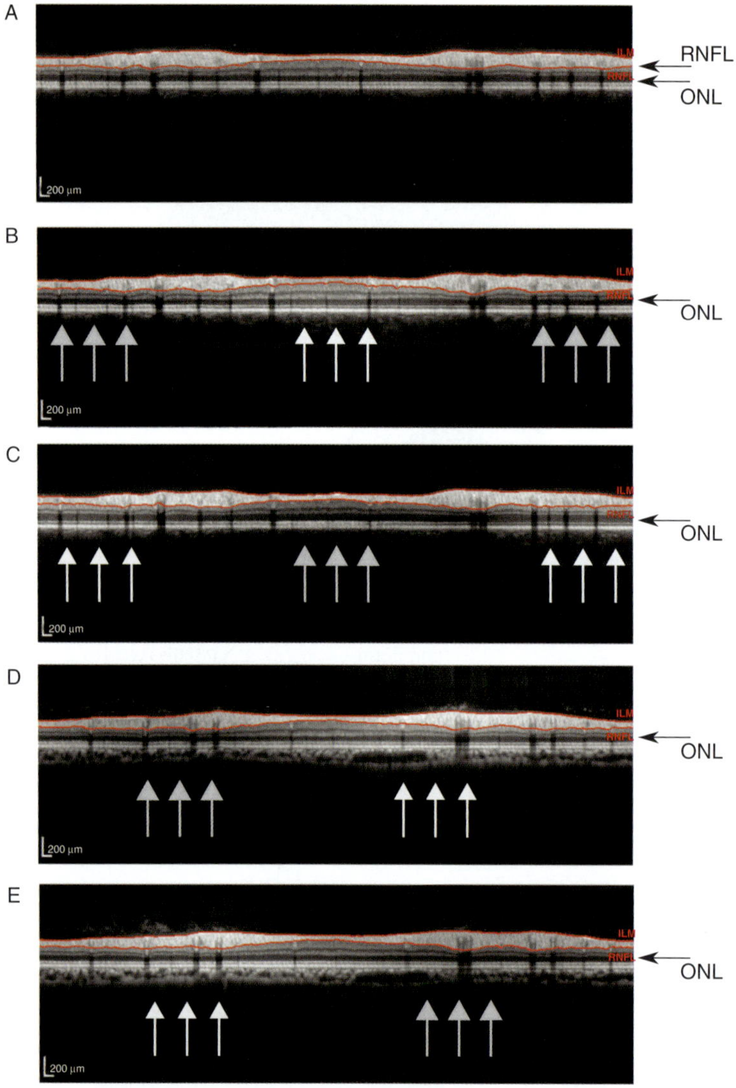

Figure 18.9 Inhomogeneous reflectivity of the outer part of the ONL indicates off-center placement of the OCT measurement beam. (A) The averaged summary scan obtained from the correctly, horizontally orientated live images of the reference scan. This images shows a homogeneous reflectivity of the outer ONL (black arrow). The automated segmentation identifies the borders of the RNFL (red/gray lines). Note, this is the image that is sent to the reading center and used for automated calculation of the RNFL thickness. (B) temporal off-center placement results in a inhomogeneous outer-ONL reflectivity. The ONL reflectivity is increased for the centrally elevated part in the live image (white arrows) and decreased in the periphery (gray arrows). (C) nasal off-center placement, (D) rostral off-center placement, (E) caudal off-center placement.

Several times we referred to "relevant B-scans" in this proposed QC list. The rationale is that QC failure of B-scans taken through the foveola or perimacular rim posed a proportional greater risk than QC failure of a B-scan taken at the extreme edges (Figure 18.10). Therefore, one may handle the QC criteria softer at the edge of a macular volume scan but remain rigorous in the center.

Practical advice for obtaining high-quality OCT scans

As a rule of thumb we advise to keep the mnemonics of the OSCAR-IB criteria in mind.

Prior to scanning Before you start imaging make sure that you use the right OCT scan protocol and obtain a clearly visible OCT image (O). If available activate automated B-scan averaging and/or the eye-tracking function.

While scanning During imaging, center your peripapillary ring scan and/or macular scan well (C); take care of good and equal illumination (I); keep the B-scan horizontally aligned in the live window to ensure central beam placement (B).

After scanning After scanning briefly revise your scans asking two questions. Is there any obvious algorithm failure (A)? Is there any retinal pathology visible that may lead to exclusion (R)?

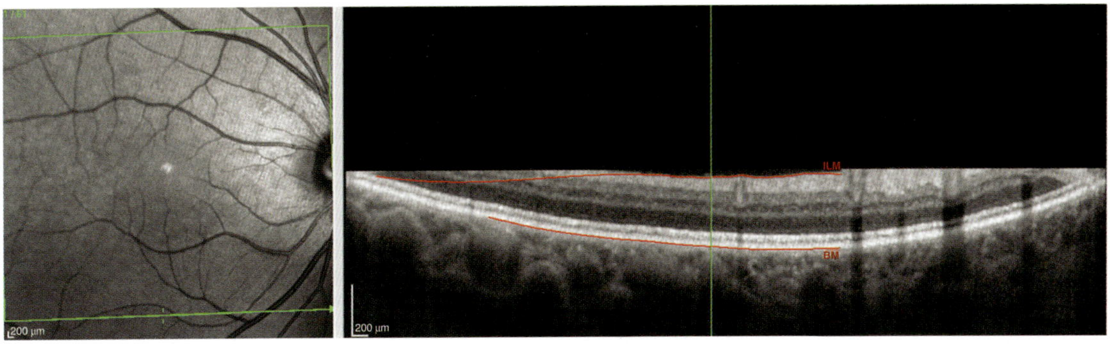

Figure 18.10 This OCT scan is cut on the edges. Potential rejection of such a scan taken at the very edge of the macular volume scan should be carefully considered if all other, more relevant, OCT B-scans of the entire volume are acceptable.

Conclusion

This chapter showed that transparent, reliable, and validated QC criteria are available for retinal OCT in MS research. It is advisable to take these criteria into account, particularly in a multi-center setting, in order to maximise the efficacy of this new and promising technology.

References

1 Madhusudhanan Balasubramanian, Christopher Bowd, Gianmarco Vizzeri, Robert N. Weinreb, and Linda M. Zangwill. "Effect of image quality on tissue thickness measurements obtained with spectral domain-optical coherence tomography." *Opt Express* **17** (2009), pp. 4019–4036.

2 Lisanne J. Balk, Willemien A E J. de Vries-Knoppert, and Axel Pet- zold. "A Simple sign for recognizing off-axis OCT measurement beam placement in the context of multicentre studies." *PLoS One* **7** (2012), e48222.

3 Lisanne J. Balk, Joep Killestein, Chris H. Polman, Bernard M J. Uit- dehaag, and Axel Petzold. "Microcystic macular edema confirmed, but not specific for multiple sclerosis." *Brain* **135** (2012), e226.

4 Amitha Domalpally, Ronald P Danis, Baoyan Zhang, Dawn Myers, and Christina N Kruse. "Quality issues in interpretation of optical coherence tomograms in macular diseases." *Retina* **29** (2009), pp. 775–781.

5 Michelle L Gabriele, Hiroshi Ishikawa, Gadi Wollstein, Richard A Bilonick, Kelly A Townsend, Larry Kagemann, Maciej Wojtkowski, Vivek J Srinivasan, James G Fujimoto, Jay S Duker, and Joel S Schuman. "Optical coherence tomography scan circle location and mean retinal nerve fiber layer measurement variability." *Invest Ophthalmol Vis Sci* **49** (2008), pp. 2315–2321.

6 Jeffrey M. Gelfand, Rachel Nolan, Daniel M. Schwartz, Jennifer Graves, and Ari J. Green. "Microcystic macular edema in multiple sclerosisis associated with disease severity." *Brain* (2012), pp. 1786–93.

7 Amirhossein Hariri, Sun Young Lee, Humberto Ruiz-Garcia, Muneeswar Gupta Nittala, Florian M. Heussen, and Srinivas R. Sadda. "Effect of angle of incidence on macular thickness and volume measurements obtained by spectral-domain optical coherence tomography." *Invest Ophthalmol Vis Sci* **53** (2012), pp. 5287–5291.

8 Christopher Kai-shun Leung, Carol Yim-lui Cheung, Dusheng Lin, Chi Pui Pang, Dennis S C Lam, and Robert N Weinreb. "Longitudinal variability of optic disc and retinal nerve fiber layer measurements." *Invest Ophthalmol Vis Sci* **49** (2008), pp. 4886–4892.

9 Jeong W. Pak, Ashwini Narkar, Sapna Gangaputra, Ronald Klein, Barbara E K.Klein, Stacy Meuer, Yijun Huang, and Ronald Danis. "Effect of optical coherence tomography scan decentration on macular center subfield thickness measurements." *Invest Ophthalmol Vis Sci* (2013).

10 Shiv Saidha, Elias S. Sotirchos, Mohamed A. Ibrahim, Ciprian M. Crainiceanu, Jeffrey M. Gelfand, Yasir J. Sepah, John N. Ratchford, Jiwon Oh, Michaela A. Seigo, Scott D. Newsome, Laura J. Balcer, Elliot M. Frohman, Ari J. Green, Quan D. Nguyen, and Peter A. Cal- abresi. "Microcystic macular edema, thickness of the inner nuclear layer of the retina, and disease characteristics in multiple sclerosis: a retrospective study." *Lancet Neurol* **11** (2012), pp. 963–972.

11 Shiv Saidha, Stephanie B. Syc, Mohamed A. Ibrahim, Christopher Eckstein, Christina V. Warner, Sheena K. Farrell, Jonathan D. Oak- ley, Mary K. Durbin, Scott A. Meyer, Laura J. Balcer, Elliot M. Frohman, Jason M. Rosenzweig, Scott D. Newsome, John N. Ratchford, Quan D. Nguyen, and Peter A. Calabresi. "Primary

retinal pathology in multiple sclerosis as detected by optical coherence tomography." *Brain* **134** (2011), pp. 518–533.

12 Lauren S Talman, Esther R Bisker, David J Sackel, David A Long, Kristin M Galetta, John N Ratchford, Deacon J Lile, Sheena K Far- rell, Michael J Loguidice, Gina Remington, Amy Conger, Teresa C Frohman, Dina A Jacobs, Clyde E Markowitz, Gary R Cutter, Gui- Shuang Ying, Yang Dai, Maureen G Maguire, Steven L Galetta, El- liot M Frohman, Peter A Calabresi, and Laura J Balcer. "Longitudinal study of vision and retinal nerve fiber layer thickness in multiple sclerosis." *Ann Neurol* **67** (2010), pp. 749–760.

13 Prejaas Tewarie, Lisanne Balk, Fiona Costello, Ari Green, Roland Martin, Sven Schippling, and Axel Petzold. "The OSCAR-IB Con– sensus Criteria for Retinal OCT Quality Assessment." *PLoS One* **7** (2012), e34823.

14 Gianmarco Vizzeri, Christopher Bowd, Felipe A. Medeiros, Robert N. Weinreb, and Linda M. Zangwill. "Effect of signal strength and improper alignment on the variability of stratus optical coherence tomography retinal nerve fiber layer thickness measurements." *Am J Ophthalmol* **148** (2009), 249–255.e1.

Chapter 19

Future technological advances in optical coherence tomography

Hiroshi Ishikawa and Joel Schuman

Since its commercial introduction in 1996, optical coherence tomography (OCT) has gone through numerous iterations of technological improvement. The most dramatic and important change was the transition from time-domain (TD) to commercially available spectral-domain (SD) OCT in 2006. SD-OCT eliminated the need for the physically moving reference mirror that dictated the scan speed, so that commercial SD-OCT devices achieved 40 times faster scanning compared to even the fastest TD-OCT systems. This enabled three-dimensional (3-D) sampling of the retinal tissue in vivo rather than the two-dimensional (2-D) scanning formerly performed. In addition to the faster scanning, SD-OCT also provided higher resolution (4–5 μm compared to 8–10 μm).

3-D scanning allowed visualization of retinal tissue in coronal sections in addition to the conventional sagittal and transverse (axial) sections. Coronal sectioning confirmed that the seemingly random reflections below the retina in TD-OCT sagittal or transverse images were the choroidal vasculature (Figure 19.1). Also, the OCT fundus image (summed coronal view of the 3-D OCT data) permitted us to pinpoint the sampling location within the 3-D cube OCT data relative to the structures that can be used as references (e.g., major retinal blood vessels, optic nerve head (ONH), etc.) (Figure 19.2). This change can be recognized as analogous to the transition in radiology from the simple x-ray to CT scanning.

The transition to SD-OCT also changed how the OCT technology was commercialized. With the apparent public domain nature of the SD-OCT technology, multiple companies jumped into the medical OCT market. Currently, there are at least nine companies manufacturing SD-OCT. This competition accelerates technological improvement and innovation in a very positive way, as well as driving prices down for consumers.

In this chapter, many new technological advancements in the ocular OCT imaging field are discussed. Some are still in purely experimental stages, but others are on the verge of clinical commercialization or even already on the market. All provide particular advantages in a variety of aspects of OCT imaging that are useful for both clinical and research purposes.

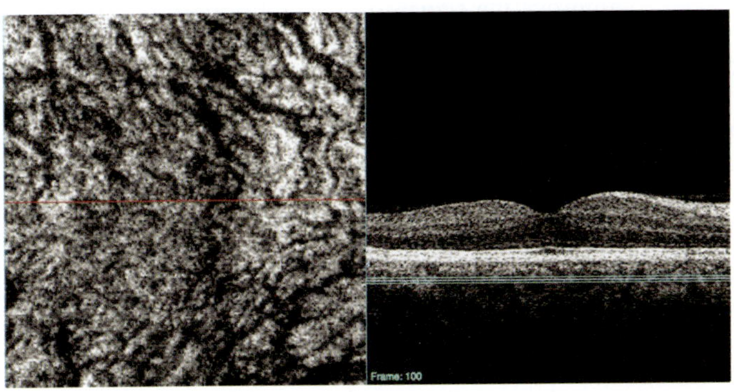

Figure 19.1 The coronal sectioning of 3-D SD-OCT data showed the seemingly random noise below the retina in cross-sectional images to be choroidal vasculature. (A) C-mode image of choroidal vasculature, which was generated by summing up the information within the slab of thickness indicated by the three horizontal light blue lines shown on the cross-sectional image (B).

Optical Coherence Tomography in Neurological Disease, ed. Peter A. Calabresi, Laura J. Balcer, and Elliot M. Frohman. Published by Cambridge University Press.

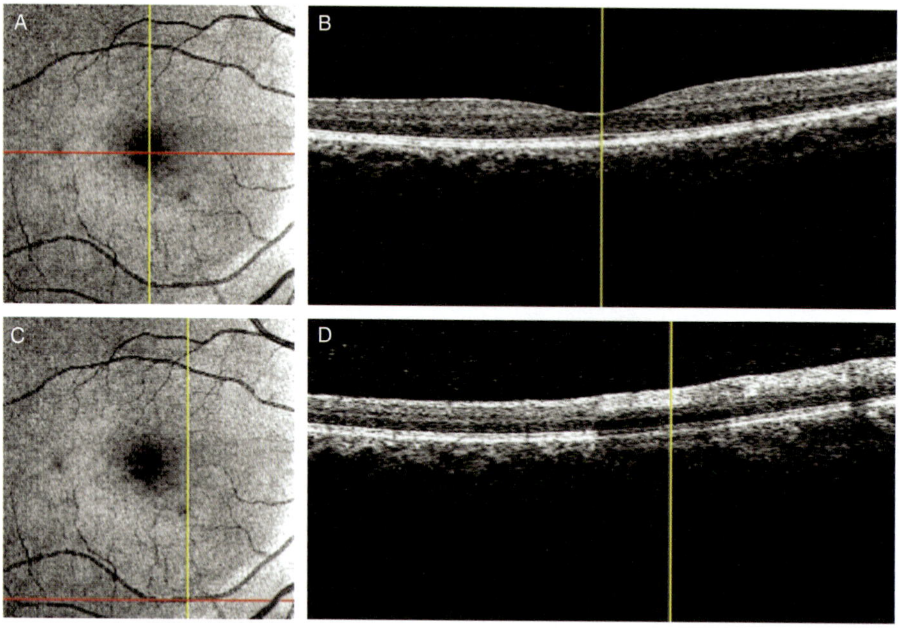

Figure 19.2. The optical coherence tomography (OCT) fundus image (summed coronal view of the 3-D OCT data), as shown in (A) and (C), permits pinpointing of the sampling location within the 3-D cube OCT data. Red lines on the fundus image indicate where the corresponding cross-sectional images on the right were sampled. The vertical yellow lines point the same location in the corresponding fundus and cross-sectional images. In (B), the vertical yellow line points out the position of the foveola, while in (D) it indicates the location of the blood vessel.

Eye-tracking system

Eye movement artifacts on OCT images have been one of the biggest problems that affect both qualitative and quantitative assessment from the very beginning. When SD-OCT was commercialized, we hoped that the faster scanning speed of SD-OCTs would have solved the eye movement artifact problem. Ironically, the faster speed was used to increase sampling density (from 768 samplings on six radial 2-D slices to 40,000 samplings on a 3-D cube covering 6 × 6 mm area for approximately the same scan time of 1.2 to 1.4 seconds) instead of decreasing scanning time, resulting in the same eye movement artifacts in SD-OCT exhibited with TD-OCT (Figure 19.3). On the other hand, it is easier to catch such artifacts on SD-OCT than TD-OCT because the 3-D scanning allows an en face view of the image. Also, eye movements including micro-saccades are so fast that even near instantaneous scanning might still demonstrate some eye movement artifacts, although the magnitude becomes small with extremely fast scanning. Therefore, it seems common sense to add eye tracking to OCT.

Eye-tracking OCT is not really a new technological advancement as of June 2014, because there are some commercial SD-OCT devices that already have this feature. They send two beams of light to the target eye simultaneously: one beam for tracking and the other beam for OCT scanning. With eye tracking, it not only resolves eye movement or blink artifacts occurring during scanning, but also enables repeated scanning at the same location. This allows signal averaging to improve the signal-to-noise ratio, resulting in greater image quality (Figure 19.4) [1–5]. It is also possible to register the scanning location to the previous scan so that scan-to-scan measurement variability can be minimized. This is particularly useful for longitudinal study to assess changes in a given subject [6].

The one practical drawback of eye-tracking OCT is its prolonged scanning time. The fast eye movement and blinking during scanning forces the machine to discard the frame just taken and simply repeat scanning at the same location until there is no detectable motion for that particular frame. This means that the overall scanning time is a function of the number of eye movement/blinking events during scanning. Unfortunately, as the number of

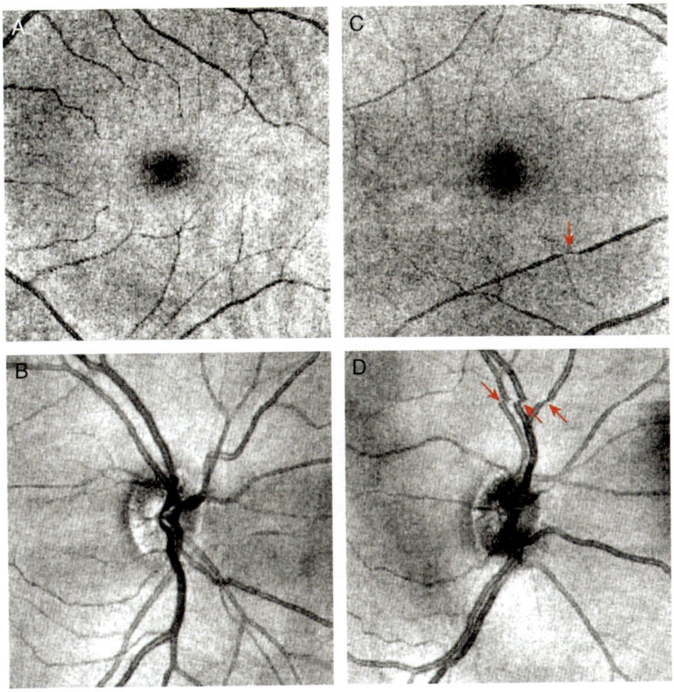

Figure 19.3. Eye motion artifacts during scanning. (A) and (C) present good scans, without eye motion artifacts or blinking, of macular region. (B) and (D) show scans with eye movement during the scans, as indicated by the red arrows. Eye motion artifacts can be observed as the discontinuity of the blood vessels on the fundus images and significantly affect the analysis results.

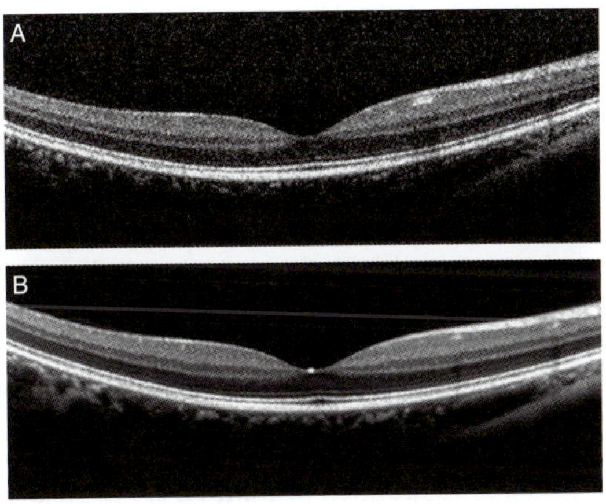

Figure 19.4 Cross-sectional images through the fovea from the same eye using OCT device with an eye-tracking system. (A) no frame averaging is applied. (B) 100 frames averaged. 100-frame averaged scan reveals stronger and clearer definition of the retinal layer structures with less speckle noise compared to a non-frame-averaged scan.

eye movement/blinking events increases with age and severity of vision impairment, the overall scan time may become sometimes intolerably long for such cases if a dense 3-D volume scan is needed. This also indicates that the scanning speed of the current SD-OCT is still not fast enough to capture “motion-free” 3-D OCT image.

Swept-source OCT

Swept-source (SS) OCT is similar to SD-OCT in the use of detected wavelength to determine reflection depth. In SS-OCT, an A-scan line is obtained by scanning with a starting frequency and then “sweeping” the frequency over a period of time to obtain the different spectral components of the detected signal, using a tunable laser source with a continuous “sweeping” mode. Instead of using a spectrometer to determine different spectral components, which is the speed bottle neck in SD-OCT, a single detector gathers all the information of the “sweep” [7]. The acquisition speed of SS-OCT is dictated by the tuning speed of the laser light source. It reaches 100,000 to 400,000 A-scans in one second, substantially increasing the scanning speed to 4 to 8 times faster than SD-OCT. SS-OCT has been reported to scan at MHz rates as well [8–10].

With the dramatically improved scanning speed, regular 200 × 200 A-scans covering a 6 × 6 mm area can be done within a fraction of a second, and therefore we are getting one step closer to motion-free 3-D OCT images even without an eye-tracking system. However, the faster speed is generally used for denser sampling so that the overall scanning time for a 3-D cube scan remains about one second. This is because the sampling density has not reached the optimal number for both qualitative and quantitative assessment yet. Even with potential eye movement artifacts, denser sampling gets higher priority in OCT imaging for both clinical and research purposes.

Tunable laser light sources dramatically improve the scanning speed; however, they also bring disadvantages. The major disadvantage is the lower axial resolution than SD-OCT (5.3 to 8 μm (SS-OCT) vs. 4 to 5 μm (SD-OCT)). [11] Ironically, the narrow bandwidth of the swept-source laser, which achieves faster scanning, decreases the axial resolution because resolution is proportional to the bandwidth. Therefore, a narrower-bandwidth light source results in worse axial resolution

On the other hand, SS-OCT does not exhibit some of the problems seen with SD-OCT. Unlike with SD-OCT, neither the sensitivity nor the resolution of SS-OCT diminishes with increasing distance from the "zero-delay." The zero-delay can be thought of as the point in space representing the beginning of each given A-scan, such that the farther a point is from the zero-delay, the deeper into the tissue the scan point is acquired.

Adaptive optics optical coherence tomography

OCT technology is known to provide great axial resolution (4 to 5 μm with SD-OCT). However, the transverse, or lateral, resolution is still limited to the range of 15 to 20 μm. This asymmetric proportion of the resolution in different dimensions hinders its visualization clarity in the coronal plane. For example, inner and outer borders of the photoreceptor layer together with the inner/outer segment junction can be recognized in axial slices, while the photoreceptor mosaic cannot ordinarily be visualized except in high A-scan density coronal slices. [12,13]

Adaptive optics (AO) was originally developed and used in astronomical telescopes in order to improve the resolution of astronomical imaging and remove the effects of atmospheric distortion. [14] It is now incorporated into OCT devices to correct ocular aberrations. AO systems measure the distortion in the wave shape of the reflected signal and compensate for them with a deformable mirror. In this way, AO fixes the ocular aberrations caused by wavefront distortions when the signal passes through the eye and, therefore, is able to markedly improve transverse resolution. Combined with OCT, it provides detailed visualization of individual retinal cells and generates 3-D images of photoreceptors in vivo. Since AO-OCT has better focus on the retina and more efficient collection of backscattered light by reducing the diffraction effect, it enhances image contrast and quality as well as transverse resolution. With a pupil diameter of > 6 mm, a transverse resolution of 2–3 μm can be achieved, which enables visualization of individual rods and cones as well as individual nerve fiber bundles [15,16].

Doppler OCT

Assessment of retinal vasculature and blood flow is an important clinical observation for evaluating various pathological conditions and understanding pathophysiology. Conventionally, fluorescein angiography (FA) and indocyanine green angiography (ICGA) have been used to observe the retinal blood vessel morphology, and Doppler ultrasound has been used for blood flow measurement. However, FA and ICGA imaging are invasive due to the requirement of dye injection [17, 18], and Doppler ultrasound can target only one or two vessels at a time and its measurement is largely operator dependent.

Doppler OCT (D-OCT) was developed for observation of both the vasculature morphology and blood flow measurement in a noninvasive fashion. The principle behind D-OCT is similar to the Doppler ultrasound. It is based on the frequency shift caused by the moving blood cells. When the incident light signal is scattered or reflected back from moving particles, a shift in frequency will be observed due to the Doppler effect. The shift in the central frequency of the reflected light can be detected as the phase change between sequential A-scans [19].

With the ability to detect the frequency shifts or phase changes, D-OCT allows imaging blood vessels in vivo with high resolution and sensitivity and offers valuable information regarding the blood flow direction and velocity, as well as detailed structural investigation of the vasculature [20–28]. With sophisticated image-processing techniques, quantitative flow investigation of retinal perfusion is now possible with commercially available OCT devices, though it still remains challenging. The most important contribution of D-OCT is to provide 3-D tissue retinal microvascular information in a noncontact and noninvasive fashion compared to FA and ICGA; however, D-OCT cannot identify leakage of fluid from vessels. D-OCT uses Doppler to generate image contrast without the use of dye through a technique called *optical coherence angiography* (OCA) and, therefore, enables segmentation and display of vasculature. Enabling the 3-D visualization of the vasculature, especially retinal and choroidal vasculature, provides an alternative means for diagnosis and management of many retinal pathologies related to vasculature damage [29, 30].

Polarization-sensitive OCT

Conventional OCT visualizes different tissues (mainly various retinal layers) based on the differences in their optical indices of refraction. However, the intensity-based contrasts can be less optimal for distinguishing certain adjacent tissues (e.g., boundary between ganglion cell and inner plexiform layers), especially under pathological conditions. There are other types of optical properties that the conventional OCT is not detecting, such as absorption, fluorescence, luminescence, and polarization. Polarization sensitive (PS) OCT can assess birefringence and depolarization of target tissues with depth information.

Fibrous tissues (e.g., nerve fiber bundles) that consist of long parallel fibrils surrounded by tissues with different refractive indices exhibit birefringence. Multiple scattering at large particles or scattering at nonspherical particles causes depolarization of incoming light. PS-OCT visualizes tissue specific contrast by detecting these optical properties. Initially, PS-OCT was only implemented in TD-OCT but now is adapted to SD-OCT and able to provide a contrast-enhanced OCT image with better sensitivity in real time [31–35].

Retinal tissues show both good birefringence and depolarization effects, so they can be good targets for PS-OCT. Scanning laser polarimetry (SLP or GDx) has been used for glaucoma assessment by measuring the retardation amount of the laser light (RNFL birefringence) that is supposed to linearly correlate with RNFL thickness [36–41]. Several studies suggest that RNFL birefringence changes may precede RNFL thickness changes that can be measured using conventional OCT [42–45]. The biggest limitation of SLP is that it measures tissue retardation as a whole. In other words, the RNFL measurements are confounded by other birefringent tissues in the eye (e.g., cornea, vitreous, sclera, etc.).

Since PS-OCT allows a depth-resolved optical probe of birefringence, RNFL birefringence can be separately measured from other confounding structures with birefringence properties. RPE exhibits depolarization, so it can also be a good target for PS-OCT, especially in eyes with pathologies involving RPE (e.g., macular degeneration, pigment epithelial detachments, pseudo vitelliform dystrophy, etc.) [46]. With potentially more accurate and detailed assessment of birefringent tissues using PS-OCT, we may be able to detect minute changes in the integrity of nerve fiber bundles at much earlier stages than currently possible.

High penetration OCT

One of the limitations of conventional OCT is its relatively short penetration depth. Although the scanning window covers ~2mm in the axial direction, OCT signals quickly become attenuated below the RPE. In the ONH area, visibility of lamina cribrosa depends on the thickness of the pre-lamina tissue. Additionally, SD-OCT exhibits gradual image dynamic range loss along the depth. In other words, images look sharp on the top but blurry on the bottom. This is an inherent problem stemming from the SD-OCT principle. In cases in which the region of interest is a deep tissue (e.g., choroid, lamina cribrosa), the so-called enhanced depth imaging (EDI) technique can be applied, in which the dynamic range deterioration can be reversed (blurry top and sharp bottom) [47–63]. However, there are other ways to overcome this limitation, such as by using a longer wavelength light source (so-called high penetration (HP) OCT).

Conventional OCT devices use infrared light with center wavelengths around 830 nm as the light source because signals around 830 nm are widely available and are well transmitted by water, the main content of the vitreous [64]. However, signals with wavelengths of 830 nm have limited reflected signal strength beyond the RPE and, therefore, limit the ability to visualize the deeper structures. Instead of using 830 nm, HP-OCT seeks an alternative local minimum on the spectrum of the water absorption, which is located around 1,050 nm, and uses it as the light source. Besides minimal absorption by the water, signals with wavelength around 1,050 nm exhibit less scattering in the choroid and less attenuation in the RPE. Therefore, signals can penetrate beyond the RPE and enable the visualization of tissue structure of choroid and sclera with better image quality and contrast [65–67]. This approach is different from EDI in using a longer wavelength light source.

HP-OCT has been employed in several studies to evaluate the high-penetration effects and clinical benefits [67–76]. HP-OCT is able to provide information posterior to the retina, like choroid, choroidal vasculature, and sclera, to observe choroid or sub-RPE damage or morphological changes caused by various pathologies, such as the development of choroidal neovascularization (CNV) beneath the RPE induced by age-related macular degeneration (AMD) and polypoidal choroidal vasculopathy (PCV) [67, 72], and to evaluate choroidal thickness with better reproducibility. Some statistically significant differences in choroidal thickness or morphological changes of the ocular tissues between healthy and pathological cases have been reported [73, 75, 76]. Furthermore, combining the OCA technology with an HP-OCT engine, high-penetration optical coherence angiography (HP-OCA), enables vascular imaging of the deep posterior eye in a noninvasive manner. A recent study showed that HP-OCA revealed depth-resolved abnormal vasculature in exudative macular disease and the en face HP-OCA images showed high similarity with FA and ICGA images. This suggests that HP-OCA may be clinically useful in noninvasive 3-D angiography [74].

Joint aperture OCT

As we have seen so far, improving the scanning speed has been one major focus of OCT technology advancements. However, it is known that higher speeds may degrade image quality due to shorter exposure time. One of the key components that dictate overall image quality is sensitivity, the minimum detectable fraction of back reflected light. Naturally, under the same illumination condition (light source power in OCT domain), shorter exposure lowers sensitivity. One way to overcome this law of physics is a new approach called joint aperture (JA) OCT.

JA-OCT is an angle-resolved OCT method, in which illumination from an active channel is simultaneously probed by several passive channels. In other words, JA-OCT combines multiple imaging channels that are targeting the same subject from different angles that are strategically placed. JA-OCT increases the collection efficiency and effective sensitivity of the OCT system without increasing the light source power on the sample, hence no further exposure or safety risk. Additionally, JA-OCT provides angular scattering information about the sample in a single acquisition, so the OCT imaging speed is not reduced. Therefore, JA-OCT is especially suitable for ultrahigh-speed in vivo imaging [77]. Based on the angle diversity concept, JA-OCT is able to generate a high-quality image with reduced speckle noise without sacrificing imaging speed by organizing multiple channels in an asymmetric configuration and varying beam sizes. With multiple channels, JA-OCT provides angular scattering information about the sample in a single acquisition, which may be useful for automatic tissue identification detection [78].

Klein et al. demonstrated that, scanning with JA-OCT, the acquisition time for human retina with 2,112 × 258 axial scans for each channel is 0.46 seconds [77]. The acquired data showed significantly reduced speckle noise, increased collection efficiency, higher signal-to-noise ratio (SNR), reduction of specular and parasitic reflections, and better visualization of retinal layers. With all these advantages, JA-OCT successfully compensates the dim signal level problem of ultrahigh-speed OCT devices, and provides high-quality images with substantially reduced speckle noise at megahertz imaging speed. JA-OCT may be able to provide more ocular tissue structural information, originally hidden because of limited image acquisition speed and image quality. Furthermore, JA-OCT also offers new perspectives for OCT functional imaging: increased channels may allow for reconstruction of the true Doppler vector and the angular scattering characteristics may make tissue identification feasible.

Conclusions

OCT is a rapidly evolving technology. The advances described in this section represent only a small number of the many areas in which OCT is continuing to develop. As lasers improve and prices drop, other new OCT iterations will appear, such as is possible in laboratories today with vertical cavity lasers permitting OCT imaging of the entire length of the eye in a single A-scan. The excitement and possibilities in OCT development are palpable.

References

1. Sander, B., M. Larsen, L. Thrane, et al., Enhanced optical coherence tomography imaging by multiple scan averaging. *Br J Ophthalmol* 2005; **89**(2): 207–12.
2. Sakamoto, A., M. Hangai, and N. Yoshimura, Spectral-domain optical coherence tomography with multiple B-scan averaging for enhanced imaging of retinal diseases. *Ophthalmology*, 2008;**115**(6): 1071–1078 e7.

3. Pappuru, R.R., C. Briceno, Y. Ouyang, et al., Clinical significance of B-scan averaging with SD-OCT. *Ophthalmic Surg Lasers Imaging*, 2012;**43**(1): 63–8.
4. Jorgensen, T.M., J. Thomadsen, U. Christensen, et al., Enhancing the signal-to-noise ratio in ophthalmic optical coherence tomography by image registration–method and clinical examples. *J Biomed Opt*, 2007;**12**(4): p. 041208.
5. Wu, W., O. Tan, R.R. Pappuru, et al., Assessment of frame-averaging algorithms in OCT image analysis. *Ophthalmic Surg Lasers Imaging Retina*, 2013;**44**(2): 168–75.
6. Chin, E.K., R.W. Sedeek, Y. Li, et al., Reproducibility of macular thickness measurement among five OCT instruments: effects of image resolution, image registration, and eye tracking. *Ophthalmic Surg Lasers Imaging*, 2012; **43**(2) 97–108.
7. Drexler, W. and J.G. Fujimoto, *Optical Coherence Tomography: Technology and Applications*. 2008. New York:Springer.
8. Blatter, C., T. Klein, B. Grajciar, et al., Ultrahigh-speed non-invasive widefield angiography. *J Biomed Opt*, 2012. **17**(7): 070505.
9. Goda, K., A. Fard, O. Malik, et al., High-throughput optical coherence tomography at 800 nm. *Opt Express*, 2012. **20**(18): 19612–7.
10. Klein, T., W. Wieser, C.M. Eigenwillig, et al., Megahertz OCT for ultrawide-field retinal imaging with a 1050 nm Fourier domain mode-locked laser. *Opt Express*, 2011. **19**(4): 3044–62.
11. Potsaid, B., B. Baumann, D. Huang, et al., Ultrahigh speed 1050nm swept source/Fourier domain OCT retinal and anterior segment imaging at 100,000 to 400,000 axial scans per second. *Opt Express*, 2010. **18**(19): 20029–48.
12. Zawadzki, R.J., S.S. Choi, S.M. Jones, et al., Adaptive optics-optical coherence tomography: optimizing visualization of microscopic retinal structures in three dimensions. *J Opt Soc Am A Opt Image Sci Vis*, 2007. **24**(5): 1373–83.
13. Zawadzki, R.J., S.S. Choi, A.R. Fuller, et al., Cellular resolution volumetric in vivo retinal imaging with adaptive optics-optical coherence tomography. *Opt Express*, 2009. **17**(5): 4084–94.
14. Ragazzoni, R., E. Marchetti, and G. Valente, Adaptive-optics corrections available for the whole sky. *Nature*, 2000. **403**(6765): 54–6.
15. Miller, D.T., O.P. Kocaoglu, Q. Wang, et al., Adaptive optics and the eye (super resolution OCT). *Eye (Lond)*, 2011. **25**(3): 321–30.
16. Kocaoglu, O.P., S. Lee, R.S. Jonnal, et al., Imaging cone photoreceptors in three dimensions and in time using ultrahigh resolution optical coherence tomography with adaptive optics. *Biomed Opt Express*, 2011. **2**(4): 748–63.
17. Yannuzzi, L.A., K.T. Rohrer, L.J. Tindel, et al., Fluorescein angiography complication survey. *Ophthalmology*, 1986. **93**(5): 611–7.
18. Hope-Ross, M., L.A. Yannuzzi, E.S. Gragoudas, et al., Adverse reactions due to indocyanine green. *Ophthalmology*, 1994. **101**(3): 529–33.
19. Drexler, W. and J.G. Fujimoto, State-of-the-art retinal optical coherence tomography. *Prog Retin Eye Res*, 2008. **27**(1):45–88.
20. Wehbe, H., M. Ruggeri, S. Jiao, et al., Automatic retinal blood flow calculation using spectral domain optical coherence tomography. *Opt Express*, 2007. **15**(23): 15193–206.
21. Makita, S., T. Fabritius, and Y. Yasuno, Quantitative retinal-blood flow measurement with three-dimensional vessel geometry determination using ultrahigh-resolution Doppler optical coherence angiography. *Opt Lett*, 2008. **33**(8): 836–8.
22. Wang, Y., B.A. Bower, J.A. Izatt, et al., Retinal blood flow measurement by circumpapillary Fourier domain Doppler optical coherence tomography. *J Biomed Opt*, 2008. **13**(6): 064003.
23. Szkulmowska, A., M. Szkulmowski, D. Szlag, et al., Three-dimensional quantitative imaging of retinal and choroidal blood flow velocity using joint Spectral and Time domain Optical Coherence Tomography. *Opt Express*, 2009. **17**(13): 10584–98.
24. Makita, S., Y. Hong, M. Yamanari, et al., Optical coherence angiography. *Opt Express*, 2006. **14**(17): 7821–40.
25. An, L. and R.K. Wang, In vivo volumetric imaging of vascular perfusion within human retina and choroids with optical micro-angiography. *Opt Express*, 2008. **16**(15): 11438–52.
26. Kim, D.Y., J. Fingler, J.S. Werner, et al., In vivo volumetric imaging of human retinal circulation with phase-variance optical coherence tomography. *Biomed Opt Express*, 2011. **2**(6): 1504–13.
27. Makita, S., F. Jaillon, M. Yamanari, et al., Comprehensive in vivo micro-vascular imaging of the human eye by dual-beam-scan Doppler optical coherence angiography. *Opt Express*, 2011. **19**(2): 1271–83.
28. Miura, M., S. Makita, T. Iwasaki, et al., Three-dimensional visualization of ocular vascular pathology by optical coherence angiography in vivo. *Invest Ophthalmol Vis Sci*, 2011. **52**(5): 2689–95.
29. Hwang, J.C., R. Konduru, X. Zhang, et al., Relationship among visual field, blood flow, and neural structure measurements in glaucoma. *Invest Ophthalmol Vis Sci*, 2012. **53**(6): 3020–6.

30. Adhi, M. and J.S. Duker, Optical coherence tomography–current and future applications. *Curr Opin Ophthalmol*, 2013. **24**(3): 213–21.
31. Pircher, M., E. Goetzinger, R. Leitgeb, et al., *Transversal phase resolved polarization sensitive optical coherence tomography. Phys Med Biol*, 2004. **49**(7): 1257–63.
32. Pircher, M., E. Gotzinger, R. Leitgeb, et al., Imaging of polarization properties of human retina in vivo with phase resolved transversal PS-OCT. *Opt Express*, 2004. **12**(24): 5940–51.
33. Gotzinger, E., M. Pircher, and C.K. Hitzenberger, High speed spectral domain polarization sensitive optical coherence tomography of the human retina. *Opt Express*, 2005. **13**(25): 10217–29.
34. Zotter, S., M. Pircher, E. Gotzinger, et al., Measuring retinal nerve fiber layer birefringence, retardation, and thickness using wide-field, high-speed polarization sensitive spectral domain OCT. *Invest Ophthalmol Vis Sci*, 2013. **54**(1): 72–84.
35. Gotzinger, E., M. Pircher, B. Baumann, et al., Three-dimensional polarization sensitive OCT imaging and interactive display of the human retina. *Opt Express*, 2009. **17**(5): 4151–65.
36. Windisch, B.K., P.J. Harasymowycz, J.L. See, et al., Comparison between confocal scanning laser tomography, scanning laser polarimetry and optical coherence tomography on the ability to detect localised retinal nerve fibre layer defects in glaucoma patients. *Br J Ophthalmol*, 2009. **93**(2): 225–30.
37. Ferreras, A., L.E. Pablo, A.B. Pajarin, et al., Scanning laser polarimetry: logistic regression analysis for perimetric glaucoma diagnosis. *Eye (Lond)*, 2009. **23**(3): 593–600.
38. Yamanari, M., M. Miura, S. Makita, et al., Phase retardation measurement of retinal nerve fiber layer by polarization-sensitive spectral-domain optical coherence tomography and scanning laser polarimetry. *J Biomed Opt*, 2008. **13**(1): 014013.
39. Moon, B.G., K.R. Sung, J.W. Cho, et al., Glaucoma progression detection by retinal nerve fiber layer measurement using scanning laser polarimetry: event and trend analysis. *Korean J Ophthalmol*, 2012. **26**(3): 174–81.
40. Hoffmann, E.M. and A. Schulze, [Glaucoma diagnosis using scanning laser polarimetry]. *Ophthalmologe*, 2009. **106**(8): 696–8, 700–1.
41. Gotzinger, E., M. Pircher, B. Baumann, et al., Retinal nerve fiber layer birefringence evaluated with polarization sensitive spectral domain OCT and scanning laser polarimetry: a comparison. *J Biophotonics*, 2008. **1**(2): 129–39.
42. Fortune, B., L. Wang, G. Cull, et al., Intravitreal colchicine causes decreased RNFL birefringence without altering RNFL thickness. *Invest Ophthalmol Vis Sci*, 2008. **49**(1): 255–61.
43. Zaveri, M.S., A. Conger, A. Salter, et al., Retinal imaging by laser polarimetry and optical coherence tomography evidence of axonal degeneration in multiple sclerosis. *Arch Neurol*, 2008. **65**(7): 924–8.
44. Bagga, H., D.S. Greenfield, W. Feuer, et al., Scanning laser polarimetry with variable corneal compensation and optical coherence tomography in normal and glaucomatous eyes. *Am J Ophthalmol*, 2003. **135**(4): 521–9.
45. Sehi, M., S. Ume, and D.S. Greenfield, Scanning laser polarimetry with enhanced corneal compensation and optical coherence tomography in normal and glaucomatous eyes. *Invest Ophthalmol Vis Sci*, 2007. **48**(5): 2099–104.
46. Michels, S., M. Pircher, W. Geitzenauer, et al., Value of polarisation-sensitive optical coherence tomography in diseases affecting the retinal pigment epithelium. *Br J Ophthalmol*, 2008. **92**(2): 204–9.
47. Merchant, K.Y., D. Su, S.C. Park, et al., Enhanced depth imaging optical coherence tomography of optic nerve head Drusen. *Ophthalmology*, 2013.
48. Hedels, C. and J. Krohn, Enhanced depth imaging optical coherence tomography of optic disc maculopathy without a visible optic pit. *Clin Experiment Ophthalmol*, 2013.
49. Skondra, D., T. Papakostas, and D.G. Vavvas, Enhanced depth imaging optical coherence tomography in age-related macular degeneration. *Semin Ophthalmol*, 2012. **27**(5–6): 209–12.
50. Rahman, W., F.K. Chen, J. Yeoh, et al., Enhanced depth imaging of the choroid in patients with neovascular age-related macular degeneration treated with anti-VEGF therapy versus untreated patients. *Graefes Arch Clin Exp Ophthalmol*, 2013. **251**(6): 1483–8.
51. da Silva, F.T., V.M. Sakata, A. Nakashima, et al., Enhanced depth imaging optical coherence tomography in long-standing Vogt-Koyanagi-Harada disease. *Br J Ophthalmol*, 2013. **97**(1): 70–4.
52. Nakayama, M., H. Keino, A.A. Okada, et al., Enhanced depth imaging optical coherence tomography of the choroid in Vogt-Koyanagi-Harada disease. *Retina*, 2012. **32**(10): 2061–9.
53. Querques, G., R. Lattanzio, L. Querques, et al., Enhanced depth imaging optical coherence tomography in type 2 diabetes. *Invest Ophthalmol Vis Sci*, 2012. **53**(10): 6017–24.
54. Shields, C.L., S. Kaliki, D. Rojanaporn, et al., Enhanced depth imaging optical coherence tomography of small choroidal melanoma: comparison with choroidal nevus. *Arch Ophthalmol*, 2012. **130**(7): 850–6.
55. Shah, S.U., S. Kaliki, C.L. Shields, et al., Enhanced depth imaging optical coherence tomography of

choroidal nevus in 104 cases. *Ophthalmology*, 2012. **119**(5): 1066–72.

56. Park, H.Y., S.H. Jeon, and C.K. Park, Enhanced depth imaging detects lamina cribrosa thickness differences in normal tension glaucoma and primary open-angle glaucoma. *Ophthalmology*, 2012. **119**(1): 10–20.
57. Park, S.C., C.G. De Moraes, C.C. Teng, et al., Enhanced depth imaging optical coherence tomography of deep optic nerve complex structures in glaucoma. *Ophthalmology*, 2012. **119**(1): 3–9.
58. Wong, I.Y., H. Koizumi, and W.W. Lai, Enhanced depth imaging optical coherence tomography. *Ophthalmic Surg Lasers Imaging*, 2011. **42 Suppl**: S75–84.
59. Ikuno, Y., I. Maruko, Y. Yasuno, et al., Reproducibility of retinal and choroidal thickness measurements in enhanced depth imaging and high-penetration optical coherence tomography. *Invest Ophthalmol Vis Sci*, 2011. **52**(8): 5536–40.
60. Imamura, Y., T. Iida, I. Maruko, et al., Enhanced depth imaging optical coherence tomography of the sclera in dome-shaped macula. *Am J Ophthalmol*, 2011. **151**(2): 297–302.
61. Margolis, R. and R.F. Spaide, A pilot study of enhanced depth imaging optical coherence tomography of the choroid in normal eyes. *Am J Ophthalmol*, 2009. **147**(5): 811–5.
62. Spaide, R.F., Enhanced depth imaging optical coherence tomography of retinal pigment epithelial detachment in age-related macular degeneration. *Am J Ophthalmol*, 2009. **147**(4): 644–52.
63. Spaide, R.F., H. Koizumi, and M.C. Pozzoni, Enhanced depth imaging spectral-domain optical coherence tomography. *Am J Ophthalmol*, 2008. **146**(4): 496–500.
64. Hale, G.M. and M.R. Querry, Optical Constants of Water in the 200-nm to 200-microm Wavelength Region. *Appl Opt*, 1973. **12**(3): 555–63.
65. de Bruin, D.M., D.L. Burnes, J. Loewenstein, et al., In vivo three-dimensional imaging of neovascular age-related macular degeneration using optical frequency domain imaging at 1050 nm. *Invest Ophthalmol Vis Sci*, 2008. **49**(10): 4545–52.
66. Lee, E.C., J.F. de Boer, M. Mujat, et al., In vivo optical frequency domain imaging of human retina and choroid. *Opt Express*, 2006. **14**(10): 4403–11.
67. Yasuno, Y., M. Miura, K. Kawana, et al., Visualization of sub-retinal pigment epithelium morphologies of exudative macular diseases by high-penetration optical coherence tomography. *Invest Ophthalmol Vis Sci*, 2009. **50**(1): 405–13.
68. Maruko, I., T. Iida, Y. Sugano, et al., Morphologic analysis in pathologic myopia using high-penetration optical coherence tomography. *Invest Ophthalmol Vis Sci*, 2012. **53**(7): 3834–8.
69. Nagase, S., M. Miura, S. Makita, et al., High-penetration optical coherence tomography with enhanced depth imaging of polypoidal choroidal vasculopathy. *Ophthalmic Surg Lasers Imaging*, 2012. *43 Online*: p. e5–9.
70. Usui, S., Y. Ikuno, A. Miki, et al., Evaluation of the choroidal thickness using high-penetration optical coherence tomography with long wavelength in highly myopic normal-tension glaucoma. *Am J Ophthalmol*, 2012. **153**(1): 10–6 e1.
71. Jaillon, F., S. Makita, E.J. Min, et al., Enhanced imaging of choroidal vasculature by high-penetration and dual-velocity optical coherence angiography. *Biomed Opt Express*, 2011. **2**(5): 1147–58.
72. Nakai, K., F. Gomi, Y. Ikuno, et al., Choroidal observations in Vogt-Koyanagi-Harada disease using high-penetration optical coherence tomography. *Graefes Arch Clin Exp Ophthalmol*, 2012. **250**(7): 1089–95.
73. Chung, S.E., S.W. Kang, J.H. Lee, et al., Choroidal thickness in polypoidal choroidal vasculopathy and exudative age-related macular degeneration. *Ophthalmology*, 2011. **118**(5): p. 840–5.
74. Hong, Y.J., M. Miura, S. Makita, et al., Noninvasive investigation of deep vascular pathologies of exudative macular diseases by high-penetration optical coherence angiography. *Invest Ophthalmol Vis Sci*, 2013. **54**(5): 3621–31.
75. Koizumi, H., T. Yamagishi, T. Yamazaki, et al., Subfoveal choroidal thickness in typical age-related macular degeneration and polypoidal choroidal vasculopathy. *Graefes Arch Clin Exp Ophthalmol*, 2011. **249**(8): 1123–8.
76. Rishi, P., E. Rishi, G. Mathur, et al., Ocular perfusion pressure and choroidal thickness in eyes with polypoidal choroidal vasculopathy, wet-age-related macular degeneration, and normals. *Eye* (Lond), 2013.
77. Klein, T., R. Andre, W. Wieser, et al., Joint aperture detection for speckle reduction and increased collection efficiency in ophthalmic MHz OCT. *Biomed Opt Express*, 2013. **4**(4): 619–34.
78. Wax, A., C. Yang, and J.A. Izatt, *Fourier-domain low-coherence interferometry for light-scattering spectroscopy*. *Opt Lett*, 2003. **28**(14): 1230–2.

Index

Note: locators followed by 'f' and 't' indicate figures and tables.